Current Cancer Research

Series Editor

Wafik El-Deiry

More information about this series at http://www.springer.com/series/7892

Ravi Salgia

Editor

Targeted Therapies for Lung Cancer

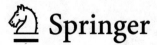 Springer

Editor
Ravi Salgia
Department of Medical Oncology and Therapeutics Research
City of Hope National Medical Center
Duarte, CA, USA

ISSN 2199-2584 ISSN 2199-2592 (electronic)
Current Cancer Research
ISBN 978-3-030-17834-5 ISBN 978-3-030-17832-1 (eBook)
https://doi.org/10.1007/978-3-030-17832-1

This Springer imprint is published by the registered company Springer Nature Switzerland AG
The registered company address is: Gewerbestrasse 11, 6330 Cham, Switzerland

Preface

It is now well established that there is tremendous heterogeneity among cancer cells both at the inter- and intra-tumoral levels. Further, a growing body of work highlights the importance of targeted therapies and personalized medicine in treating cancer patients. In contrast to conventional therapies that are typically administered to the average patient regardless of the patient's genotype, targeted therapies are tailored to patients with specific traits. For example, specific mutations, genetic alterations, and overexpression of actionable targets, or immune markers, contribute to the observed heterogeneity at least in part and may potentially be exploited for delivering personalized medicine. Nonetheless, such genetic changes can be disease-specific (e.g., small-cell lung cancer versus non-small cell lung cancer) and/or target-specific (e.g., KRAS versus EGFR). Furthermore, there are also differences in the frequency with which the genetic variants present in the patient population based on ethnic and age differences. Therefore, discerning this information is key to guiding the right treatment decisions and, hence, enhancing precision medicine.

Targeted Therapies for Lung Cancer addresses these issues manifested in the somatically acquired genetic changes of the targeted gene or immune landscape and provides an up-to-date progress report in several examples against which therapies are currently being targeted in lung cancer. They include small molecules, especially tyrosine kinase inhibitors, immunotherapy, as well as combination therapies such as a receptor tyrosine kinase (RTK) inhibitor together with an immune checkpoint blockade. Each chapter is written by a leading medical oncologist specialized in thoracic oncology and is devoted to a particular target in lung cancer. Experts offer an in-depth review of the literature covering the mechanisms underlying signaling, potential cross talk between the target and downstream signaling, and potential emergence of drug resistance. Some of the unique features of the book are its focus on lung cancer with findings from multiple clinical centers and the most desirable candidates for targeted therapy.

The book is intended to serve as a reference for those interested in familiarizing themselves with the latest information on the subject, especially with regard to current evidence, indications, and clinical trials for the treatment of lung cancer with targeted therapies, immunotherapy, and epigenetic modulators. The book is primarily meant for medical professionals and trainees including students, residents, and fellows interested in treating lung cancer. However, we envisage that the book may also be well suited for scientists as well as advanced graduate students working on lung cancer both in academia and industry.

Duarte, CA, USA   Ravi Salgia
February 2019

Acknowledgments

I would like to thank my wife, Deborah, and children, Sabrina, Meghan, and Nicholas, for who they are and how supportive they have been and the patients and their families for the inspiration. This endeavor would not have been possible without the cooperation and enthusiasm of my esteemed colleagues who graciously agreed to contribute their respective chapters. I would especially like to thank Dr. Prakash Kulkarni for his endless energy, help, and friendship. Finally, I am pleased to acknowledge Ms. Jayashree Dhakshnamoorthy, the Project Coordinator from Springer, for her unstinted support and dedication.

Contents

EGFR Targeted Therapy

Zorawar S. Noor and Jonathan W. Goldman

Abstract The identification of sensitizing mutations in the epidermal growth factor receptor (*EGFR*) gene in patients with non-small cell lung cancer (NSCLC) and the development of EGFR-tyrosine kinase inhibitors (EGFR TKIs) to target these mutations have dramatically improved outcomes for this subset of patients. For patients with *EGFR*-mutated NSCLC, the use of EGFR TKIs is associated with improved efficacy and quality of life compared to chemotherapy. The latest generation EGFR TKI, osimertinib, is highly effective in treating acquired resistance due to the T790M mutation as well as treating central nervous system metastases. As first-line treatment, its use has led to the longest median progression-free survival to date for patients with *EGFR*-mutated NSCLC. Acquired resistance to osimertinib is caused by multiple mechanisms, and numerous trials are currently underway to address this. Future studies should also aim to address the historically refractory *EGFR* exon 20 insertions, and current agents under study are promising.

Keywords Epidermal growth factor receptor (EGFR) mutation · Tyrosine kinase inhibitor (TKI) · Exon 20 insertions · T790M · Osimertinib resistance

Background

Somatic activating mutations in the epidermal growth factor receptor (*EGFR*) gene are the most common targetable molecular alteration in non-small cell lung cancer (NSCLC) [1]. *EGFR* mutations are predominantly found in adenocarcinoma, never smokers, and those of East Asian descent [2, 3]. In the United States and Europe, 10–17% of patients with NSCLC harbor an *EGFR* mutation, and in East Asia the frequency is 35–38% [4–8]. Identifying these mutations is of critical clinical importance given the highly active treatment options available for this subset of patients.

Since the discovery of epidermal growth factor (EGF) in 1962 by Stephen Cohen, and the characterization of its cell surface receptor (now known as EGFR) in 1975,

Z. S. Noor · J. W. Goldman (✉)
David Geffen School of Medicine, University of California Los Angeles, Los Angeles, CA, USA
e-mail: JWGoldman@mednet.ucla.edu

© Springer Nature Switzerland AG 2019   1
R. Salgia (ed.), *Targeted Therapies for Lung Cancer*, Current Cancer Research,
https://doi.org/10.1007/978-3-030-17832-1_1

extensive studies of the receptor and its family have led to revolutionary insights into the fields of growth factor and cancer biology [9–11]. EGFR was one of the first receptor tyrosine kinases (RTK) for which ligand-dependent dimerization was proposed as the mechanism of RTK activity [12]. It was also the first cell surface receptor to be proposed as a target for cancer therapy [13] and the first receptor to have a monoclonal antibody directed against it to inhibit cancer growth [14, 15].

EGFR (HER1, ErbB1) is an RTK expressed on the surface of cells of mesodermal and ectodermal origin, and it mediates cell growth, proliferation, and differentiation in numerous organs [16, 17]. EGFR belongs to the ErbB family of RTKs, which also includes HER2 (ErbB2), HER3 (ErbB3), and HER4 (ErbB4). EGFR binds at least seven highly variable growth factor ligands [18]. Upon stimulation, EGFR undergoes combinatorial homo- or hetero-dimerization with one of the proteins of the HER family, thereby activating an expansive signaling network [16, 19, 20]. The EGFR transmembrane protein has a large extracellular component (with 4 domains, ~620 amino acids) that primarily serves as ligand-binding sites and which is anchored by a short helical transmembrane domain to the intracellular tyrosine kinase domain (TKD) (Fig. 1) [18].

EGFR is believed to play a role in the pathogenesis of lung cancer and is overexpressed in a majority of NSCLCs [21, 22]. However, the clinical importance of EGFR expression in the general NSCLC population is unclear. There was some suggestion that EGFR expression may serve as a predictive biomarker [21], but this has been superseded by mutational analysis after the identification of actionable driver mutations in the *EGFR* gene.

The *EGFR* gene is located on chromosomal region 7p11.2 [23]. *EGFR*-mutated NSCLC is driven by "activating" gain-of-function mutations which cluster around

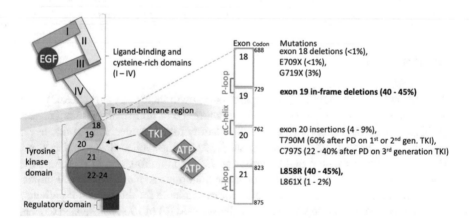

Fig. 1 Schematic representation of the epidermal growth factor receptor (EGFR) and its position on the cellular membrane. The extracellular component consists of four large domains which contain ligand-binding sites for growth factors including epidermal growth factor (EGF). The intracellular component consists of the tyrosine kinase domain followed by the regulatory domain. EGFR tyrosine kinase inhibitors (TKIs) and ATP compete for binding to the phosphate-binding (P) loop. Exon 20 contains two critical features, the alpha-C helix followed by a distal A loop. "ATP" = adenosine triphosphate. "PD" = Progression of disease

the ATP-binding pocket of the TKD and lead to constituent, ligand-independent activation of the EGFR receptor. This in turn promotes prosurvival and antiapoptotic signals such as phosphatidylinositol 3-kinase (PI3K)/protein kinase B (AKT) and extracellular signal-regulated kinase (ERK)/mitogen-activated protein kinase (MAPK) [24]. Approximately 85–90% of activating mutations are either exon 19 in-frame deletions affecting amino acids 747–750 (40–45%) or the point mutation L858R in exon 21 [7, 8, 24, 25]. These mutations are associated with hypersensitivity to small molecule tyrosine kinase inhibitors (TKIs) and are thus termed "sensitizing" *EGFR* mutations, with the exon 19 deletion consistently associated with better survival outcomes with therapy [26–30]. The remaining 10–15% involve exons 18, 20, and 21. Many, but not all, of these mutations have been found to be sensitive to targeted therapy.

First-Generation TKIs and Early Trials in Lung Cancer

EGFR TKIs entered clinical development in late 1990s. First-generation inhibitors, erlotinib, gefitinib, and icotinib [31] bind competitively and reversibly to the ATP-binding site (Fig. 1), preventing autophosphorylation and downstream signaling, thereby preventing EGFR-dependent cell proliferation [32–34]. In 2003, two single-arm phase II trials (IDEAL1 and IDEAL2) demonstrated clinical efficacy of gefitinib in patients with previously treated NSCLC, with response rates of approximately 15% [35, 36]. Of note, more responses were observed in women, patients with adenocarcinoma, never smokers, and those of Asian descent. This compared favorably to chemotherapy, which had an approximately 5% response rate in this population [36]. In 2003, gefitinib became the first US Food and Drug Administration (FDA) approved EGFR TKI for NSCLC.

Soon after, the double-blind placebo-controlled randomized phase III trial (ISEL) failed to find overall survival benefit for gefitinib with best supportive care (BSC) compared to placebo with BSC in unselected NSCLC patients [37]. Considering these results as well as those form IBREESE (gefitinib with BSC vs placebo with BSC), which terminated early and INTEREST (non-inferiority trial of gefitinib vs docetaxel), the FDA withdrew its original approval for gefitinib in 2005 [38, 39]. However, there were already clues to a yet unidentified subset of responders in the trial because the Kaplan-Meier survival curves crossed. There was an early drop off in non-responders, and a clear separation of survival curves at approximately four months. Several follow-up trials evaluated the benefit of adding an EGFR TKI to standard first-line chemotherapy. At least four large randomized controlled trials in unselected, advanced NSCLC patients showed no benefit of the addition of EGFR TKI to standard chemotherapy [40–43]. Once again, these trials were conducted in an unselected group of patients.

The publication of two landmark analyses in 2004 by Lynch et al. and Paez et al. demonstrated that the subset of patients who responded to gefitinib harbored activating *EGFR* mutations (namely, L858R and exon 19 deletions) [7, 8]. This led to a paradigm shift for future trial development, and the history of EGFR TKI clinical trials should be interpreted by differentiating the era of unselected patient enrollment versus the era incorporating EGFR mutation testing. The trial that ushered in this modern era and transformed targeted therapy for NSCLC is the IPASS trial.

EGFR TKIs for Patients with Mutations in *EGFR*

For the first time, the 2009 IPASS trial prospectively demonstrated in a randomized controlled trial that EGFR TKIs were superior to chemotherapy as first-line therapy for patients with EGFR mutations [44]. The biomarker analysis was a preplanned subset analysis of 40% of the 683 randomly assigned patients for whom *EGFR* mutation status could be evaluated, and found an objective response rate (ORR) of 71% and a PFS of 9.5 months for the gefitinib arm compared to 6.3 months for the chemotherapy arm (Table 1) [45]. Over the next half decade, several large trials would be undertaken to look at the efficacy of EGFR TKI vs chemotherapy (Table 1). IFUM fulfilled the European Medicines Agency (EMA) requirement for a single-arm validation trial in Caucasians, confirming the efficacy of gefitinib in Caucasian patients with sensitizing *EGFR* mutations [46]. On July 13, 2015, gefitinib was approved for first-line treatment of patients with metastatic NSCLC with exon 19 deletions or L858R mutations. Erlotinib and gefitinib have both been approved and marketed in numerous countries, whereas icotinib has been approved and widely prescribed only in China [47].

Table 1 Selected trials prospectively comparing first or second generation EGFR TKIs to chemotherapy in EGFR-mutated non-small cell lung cancer

Study	Patients (EGFR mutated)	EGFR TKI	Chemotherapy	Response rate	Median PFS (mo.)	Hazard ratio (*P*)
IPASS (2009)	261	Gefitinib	Carboplatin + paclitaxel	71% vs 47%	9.5 vs 6.3	0.48 (<0.0001)
WJTOG3405 (2009)	172	Gefitinib	Cisplatin + docetaxel	62% vs 32%	9.2 vs 6.3	0.48 (<0.001)
NEJGSG002 (2010)	224	Gefitinib	Carboplatin + paclitaxel	73% vs 31%	10.8 vs 5.4	0.36 (<0.001)
ENSURE (2013)	217	Erlotinib	Cisplatin + gemcitabine	63% vs 34%	11.0 vs 5.5	0.34 (<0.0001)
EURTAC (2012)	173	Erlotinib	Cisplatin + docetaxel	58% vs 15%	9.7 vs 5.2	0.42 (<0.0001)
OPTIMAL (2011)	154	Erlotinib	Carboplatin + gemcitabine	83% vs 36%	13.7 vs 4.6	0.16 (<0.0001)
LUX-Lung 3 (2013)	345	Afatinib	Cisplatin + pemetrexed	56% vs 23%	11.1 vs 6.9	0.47 (<0.0001)
LUX-Lung 6 (2014)	364	Afatinib	Cisplatin + gemcitabine	67% vs 23%	11.0 vs 5.6	0.28 (<0.0001)

Individual trials and meta-analyses have consistently found that EGFR TKIs prolong PFS compared to chemotherapy in patients with *EGFR*-mutated NSCLC; however, until recently, trials have not shown an improvement in OS [48–50]. With good consistency across trials of erlotinib or gefitinib versus chemotherapy, the median PFS is estimated as 11.0 months vs 5.6 months for chemotherapy (HR 0.37, $P < 0.001$) [51]. Randomized phase III trials comparing erlotinib to gefitinib for *EGFR*-mutated NSCLC patients have demonstrated similar efficacy of both [52, 53]. As front-line therapy in patients with *EGFR*-mutated disease, the TKI response rate is 67%, as compared to 30% for chemotherapy (RR 5.68, $P < 0.001$) [50]. The lack of OS benefit has been ascribed to crossover from the chemotherapy arm to an appropriate TKI, within or outside of the clinical trial [51, 54, 55]. Even without the OS benefit, first-line TKI has been the preferred treatment option for *EGFR*-mutated NSCLC due to the ease of an oral therapy, the higher response rate, and an improved quality of life (QOL) [51, 56, 57].

Despite an average of nearly a year of PFS with an EGFR TKI, it was seen that nearly all patients would eventually progress. At the time of progression, continuing gefitinib into subsequent lines of therapy was shown to be detrimental. In the phase III IMPRESS trial, chemotherapy-naïve *EGFR*-mutated patients who progressed on first-line gefitinib were randomized to receive either cisplatin and pemetrexed versus the same chemotherapy plus gefitinib [58]. The study found that continuing gefitinib had a detrimental effect on survival with an OS of 13.4 months compared to 19.5 months for the chemotherapy arm (HR = 1.44, $P = 0.016$) [59]. Data from IMPRESS warns that continuing an EGFR TKI at progression may cause harm, and interestingly, this detriment was associated with a specific secondary mutation, *T790M* (HR 1.49, $P = 0.043$ for T790M+ patients vs HR 1.15, $P = 0.609$ in T790M-patients) [58, 59].

Second-Generation TKIs

The second-generation inhibitors, afatinib and dacomitinib, were introduced as a treatment for those who progressed on a prior generation TKI. Unlike the first-generation inhibitors, the second-generation EGFR TKIs bind covalently and irreversibly [60]. These drugs also tend to have less selective activity, inhibiting other HER family proteins including HER2. Preclinical data of second-generation TKIs was promising, demonstrating potent activity in lung cancer models resistant to first-generation inhibitors [60–63]. The phase IIb/III trial, LUX-Lung 1, randomized patients who had progressive disease after at least three months of treatment on erlotinib or gefitinib to either afatinib or placebo [64]. There was no overall survival benefit (HR 1.08, $P = 0.74$), the ORR on afatinib was 7%, and the PFS was 3.3 months vs 1.1 months (HR 0.38, $P < 0.0001$). The phase II trial of dacomitinib in patients who progressed on chemotherapy and an EGFR TKI was similarly sobering, with an ORR of only 5.2% [65].

Both afatinib and dacomitinib were associated with significant on-target toxicity, primarily rash and diarrhea [64, 65]. Pooled analysis from 21 trials of 1468 patients found statistically higher grade 3 or greater rash with afatinib than with erlotinib or gefitinib (15% vs 8.8% vs 3.5%, respectively) [66]. Grade 3 or higher diarrhea was also more frequent in patients on afatinib than in those on erlotinib or gefitinib (9.6% vs 2.7% vs 1.1%, respectively; odds ratio 3.80 for afatinib vs erlotinib, $P < 0.0001$). More patients discontinued treatment because of an adverse event (AE) on afatinib than erlotinib (7.2% vs 4.1%, $P = 0.040$), but discontinuation rates were similar for afatinib and gefitinib (7.2% vs 7.6%). The treatment interruption rate in trials due to an AE did not vary significantly between afatinib and gefitinib or erlotinib and ranged from 11% to 28% [67]. However, more patients on afatinib required dose reductions. Across trials, discontinuation rates on gefitinib or erlotinib ranged from 6% to 21% (IPASS, OPTIMAL, and EURTAC) [68] as compared to 28.0–53.5% on afatinib (LUX-Lung 3 and LUX-Lung 6) [69]. In the head-to-head phase II trial LUX-Lung 7 randomizing patients to afatinib or gefitinib, 42% of patients required a dose reduction on afatinib, as compared to only 2% with gefitinib [70].

Other trials investigated the possible benefit from a second-generation TKI for front-line therapy. The PFS benefit of afatinib over platinum doublet chemotherapy in the LUX-Lung 3 and LUX-Lung 6 randomized phase III trials (Table 1) is similar to that seen with erlotinib or gefitinib (approximately 11 vs 6 months) [71, 72]. Although there was no OS advantage in the overall population of either trial, pre-planned subgroup analyses in both trials found an OS advantage of the TKI over chemotherapy in patients with an exon 19 deletion [27]. The OS benefit is noteworthy given the lack of OS benefit with TKIs in prior studies.

Two large head-to-head trials have compared second-generation to first-generation TKIs. In LUX-Lung 7, patients with *EGFR*-mutated NSCLC were randomized to afatinib or gefitinib. The trial failed to find an OS improvement, and reported a statistically significant PFS benefit with a difference in the medians of a meager three days (HR 0.74, $P = 0.0178$) [73]. On the other hand, ARCHER 1050, the phase III randomized controlled trial of dacomitinib versus gefitinib as first-line treatment for patients with activating *EGFR* mutations, showed a PFS improvement of 14.7 vs 9.2 months (HR 0.59, $P < 0.0001$) [74]. More strikingly, there was a significant OS advantage for the dacomitinib arm (34.1 vs 26.8 months, HR 0.76, $P = 0.044$) [75]. This is the first head-to-head randomized trial of two TKIs to show an OS advantage. Of note, patients with central nervous system (CNS) metastases and rare *EGFR* mutations were excluded from the trial. In addition, there was significantly higher toxicity, with 51% of subjects experiencing a grade 3 adverse event in the dacomitinib arm (most commonly rash or diarrhea) compared to 30% in the gefitinib arm [74]. Given these factors, the clinical utility of dacomitinib has been questioned, but remains an option. In 2018, dacomitinib was approved by the FDA for the first-line treatment of patients with NSCLC harboring an EGFR exon 19 deletion or L858R mutation [76]. With the recent arrival of the third-generation TKIs, some have said that the second generation has been altogether bypassed, referring to it as the "lost generation" [77, 78].

T790M Mutation

Despite the dramatic responses seen in patients with activating *EGFR* mutations on first- and second-generation EGFR TKIs, unfortunately nearly all patients will eventually develop resistant and progressive cancer. Initial insights into the mechanism of resistance came from analysis of tumor biopsies from a patient who relapsed after two years of complete remission on an EGFR TKI [79]. Tumor DNA sequencing before treatment and at the time of relapse revealed the acquisition of a second mutation, *T790M* in exon 20, which replaces threonine with methionine at position 790. Here, threonine is a "gatekeeper" amino acid because it lies at the entrance to a hydrophobic pocket in the ATP-binding cleft of the EGFR protein, critically determining the specificity of inhibitors.

Initial crystallographic evidence suggested that incorporation of the bulkier methionine side chain sterically hindered the interaction of the first- and second-generation EGFR TKIs [79]. Subsequent analysis showed that the effect was mediated by two factors; not only did methionine block drug binding, it also caused increased ATP affinity at the binding pocket, thereby outcompeting the therapeutic drug [80]. Although second-generation TKIs bind more avidly and irreversibly, and can inhibit T790M-positive clones in vitro, the necessary drug concentrations were not clinically achievable due to skin and gastrointestinal toxicity [81]. In patients treated with first- and second-generation inhibitors, the T790M resistance mutation is detected in approximately 50–60% of patients at the time of progression [82–84]. T790M has generally been associated with a slower rate of growth and an improved prognosis. In a retrospective analysis of 97 patients treated with EGFR TKIs, the PFS was 12.0 months on initial TKI in those who acquired the T790M mutation, as compared to 9.0 months for those who were T790M-negative ($P = 0.021$) [85].

Third-Generation TKIs

Understanding this mechanism of acquired resistance led to the development of third-generation EGFR TKIs. These include rociletinib [86, 87], olmutinib [88], nazartinib [89], avitinib [90], ASP8273 [91], PF-06747775 [92], and osimertinib (AZD9291), the only third-generation EGFR TKI approved for clinical use. Osimertinib is active against exon 19 deletions, exon 21 mutations, and also the exon 20 T790M mutations. It is preferentially selective for mutated *EGFR*, and therefore toxicity at therapeutic doses is lower than for first- and second-generation agents. Notably, osimertinib is able to cross the blood-brain barrier, making it active against disease in the CNS [93].

The safety and tolerability of osimertinib was studied in the phase I trial, AURA. Among 253 patients there were no dose-limiting toxicities observed across all dose levels (20–240 mg) [94]. The most common adverse event was diarrhea (47%), followed by rash, nausea, and decreased appetite. Only 6% of patients discontinued treatment because of a treatment-related adverse event. The phase II AURA extension and AURA2 trial both demonstrated similar tolerability [94]. In the phase III trial (AURA3), grade 3 or higher adverse events occurred in 23% of patients, half of what was experienced in the chemotherapy arm (47%) [95]. Osimertinib toxicity is dose-dependent and is associated with fewer gastrointestinal and dermatologic adverse events than with other approved EGFR TKIs.

The phase III trial of osimertinib (AURA3) randomly assigned 419 patients with advanced T790M-positive NSCLC who had progressed on prior EGFR TKIs to receive either osimertinib or chemotherapy with a platinum agent and pemetrexed [95]. Osimertinib more than doubled PFS when compared to chemotherapy (10.1 vs 4.4 months, HR of 0.30 $P < 0.001$) with an unprecedented response rate of 71% in this resistant population [95]. This led to the FDA granting approval of osimertinib for NSCLC after progression on a prior EGFR TKI with the demonstration of the T790M mutation [96]. Additional data from the United Kingdom confirmed the cost-effectiveness of osimertinib over chemotherapy for this patient population [97].

Even during the initial phase I AURA trial, osimertinib was studied as a potential first-line treatment [98]. In a double-blind randomized controlled trial of untreated *EGFR*-mutated NSCLC patients (FLAURA), the use of osimertinib led to a median PFS of 18.9 months compared to 10.3 months for those treated with first-generation EGFR TKIs, erlotinib or gefitinib. The HR for PD or death was 0.46 ($P < 0.001$), and the benefit of osimertinib over the first-generation EGFR TKI persisted in all subgroup analyses [99]. Patients on osimertinib reported fewer grade 3 or higher adverse events than those on erlotinib or gefitinib (34% vs 45%), and fewer patients experienced rashes (58% vs 78% on erlotinib or gefitinib). On April 18, 2018, the FDA approved osimertinib as first-line therapy for patients with metastatic NSCLC harboring a driver *EGFR* mutation [100]. At the time of publication of the FLAURA dataset, only 18-month OS was available, reported as 83% for the osimertinib arm compared to 71% for first-generation TKIs (HR = 0.63, $P = 0.007$). It remains to be seen if this will result in a significant long-term OS advantage.

Liquid Biopsy to Detect Mutations in *EGFR*

Detection of *EGFR* mutations such as T790M is critical to precision treatment for patients with NSCLC in the era of targeted therapy. "Liquid biopsy" is the method of detecting molecular alterations in circulating tumor DNA (ctDNA) or other nucleic acids from blood or other body fluids. Lack of available tissue for molecular profiling [38, 44, 101–103], risk of biopsy complications [104], significant delay with tissue biopsy [105], and increased cost of biopsy [106], all lead to potential advantages of liquid biopsy. More so, single-site tissue biopsies may not represent the predominant resistance mechanisms in a patient and may miss the emergence of a clinically significant clone [107, 108]. This is due to the marked tumor heterogeneity that has been seen in NSCLC [28, 109–112].

Next-generation sequencing has led to methods which allow ultra-deep sequencing for detection of actionable mutations in *EGFR* [113], de novo resistance mutations [114], and the emergence of acquired resistance during treatment [108, 115, 116]. In January 2015, the EMA approved the use of the therascreen liquid biopsy assay for detection of *EGFR* mutations in patients for whom tissue biopsy is not possible. In June 2016, the Cobas *EGFR* mutation test v2 was approved by the FDA to detect exon 19 deletions and the L858R mutation in plasma, and was extended in September 2016 to cover the T790M resistance mutation as well.

Prospective studies have demonstrated that plasma T790M can predict responders to osimertinib or rociletinib as well as tissue biopsy [113, 117, 118], and even detection of very low allele fractions of T790M in ctDNA may be clinically relevant [113]. Given the advantages over tissue biopsy, liquid biopsy can be considered one of the standard options for detecting acquired resistance mutations [108].

Patients with Brain Metastases

Patients with *EGFR*-mutated NSCLC have a higher risk for developing brain metastasis [119–121]. Historically, whole brain radiation therapy (WBRT) and stereotactic radiosurgery (SRS) have been the standard of care treatment for NSCLC patients with brain metastases. In the era prior to osimertinib use, the median OS after radiotherapy for patients with brain metastases was approximately 14 months [122]. Data regarding the efficacy of EGFR TKI for NSCLC with previously untreated brain metastases is limited since most trials have required prior radiation treatment of brain lesions [123].

A retrospective multi-institutional analysis studied 351 patients with EGFR TKI-naive *EGFR*-mutant NSCLC who developed brain metastases. Patients either received SRS followed by EGFR TKI, WBRT followed by EGFR TKI, or upfront EGFR TKI followed by SRS or WBRT as needed. The OS for the upfront SRS, WBRT, and EGFR TKI cohorts was 46, 30, and 25 months, respectively ($P < 0.001$) [124]. SRS does appear to be a valid option for front-line therapy; however, this approach may vary in the era of osimertinib, which has high efficacy against CNS disease.

In light of cognitive decline and radiation necrosis associated with brain radiation, the use of upfront radiotherapy has been questioned with the availability of osimertinib. In the BLOOM trial, 32 patients who had progressed on prior EGFR TKI therapy and had positive cerebrospinal fluid demonstrating leptomeningeal metastases were treated with 160 mg osimertinib daily [125]. Of 8 patients with neurologic symptoms, 7 had improvement, and one had stable disease. Out of 15 asymptomatic patients, 87% remained asymptomatic. In patients with parenchymal brain metastases, the intracranial ORR was 63% [126].

Although the BLOOM study used a 160 mg dose of osimertinib, both preclinical and clinical data suggest that low-dose osimertinib may have meaningful CNS activity as well [81, 94]. Of 144 patients in AURA3 with CNS metastases, the median PFS was twice as long in the osimertinib cohort vs the chemotherapy cohort (8.5 vs 4.2 months, HR 0.32, CI 0.21–0.49) with an overall response rate of 70% vs 31% ($P = 0.015$) [93, 95]. In the 116 patients with brain metastases in FLAURA, the median PFS was 15.2 with osimertinib compared to 9.6 months with erlotinib or gefitinib (HR 0.47, $P = 0.0009$). Osimertinib's efficacy for brain metastasis and leptomeningeal disease, one of the poorest prognostic groups of NSCLC, further solidifies its role in the treatment of *EGFR*-mutated disease. At this point, there is no clear consensus on whether osimertinib alone should be used upfront for brain metastases or whether WBRT or SRS should be incorporated into the treatment regimen, although many defer WBRT if possible. Further prospective studies are required for these clinically important questions.

Special Populations: Elderly or Poor Performance Status

Since no trials have exclusively enrolled elderly patients, most data is retrospective. One study from 20 centers (OCTOMUT) looked at patients aged 80 or older treated with front-line EGFR TKIs and found that the clinical outcomes and toxicity profile were comparable to those published in the literature [127]. A large retrospective analysis of Japanese patients in the phase IV POLARSTAR study of erlotinib in previously treated NSCLC patients included 7848 patients less than 75 years old, 1911 patients aged 75–84, and 148 patients 85 years or older. It found non-inferior tolerability and efficacy of erlotinib in elderly patients [128]. A meta-analysis actually suggests that EGFR TKIs may have more PFS benefit in elderly patients (HR 0.39, $P = 0.008$) than in younger patients (HR 0.48, $P = 0.04$) [129]. A pooled analysis of NEJ001, NEJ002, and NEJ003 studying first-line gefitinib found that in patients >70 with a good performance status (PS) the median PFS was 14.3 compared to 5.7 months with chemotherapy ($P < 0.001$) [130].

Studies have consistently demonstrated that EGFR TKIs are better tolerated than chemotherapy, although the vast majority of these trials only enrolled patients with an Eastern Cooperative Oncology Group (ECOG) PS of 0 to 2. A single-arm phase II trial of 72 patients with untreated advanced NSCLC and poor PS (2 or 3) found that with gefitinib, 82% reported improvement or no worsening in QOL [131]. The double-blind, placebo-controlled, phase III TOPICAL trial randomized patients with advanced NSCLC deemed unsuitable for chemotherapy because of an ECOG PS >2 or several comorbidities with an estimated life expectancy of at least 8 weeks to erlotinib or placebo. Other than the incidence of rash and diarrhea, adverse events were similar in the two groups, and they concluded that erlotinib could be an option for those for whom chemotherapy is deemed unsuitable [132]. Patients on erlotinib had significantly improved QOL for a cognitive scale ($P = 0.0072$) and physical functioning ($P = 0.0024$) as well as statistically significant improvements in pain, dyspnea, chest pain, hoarseness, and constipation. If only patients with an *EGFR* mutation were enrolled, it would be expected that the benefit would be even more apparent. EGFR TKIs remain a good option for patients with an *EGFR* mutation and poor performance status.

Exon 20 Insertions and Other Rare *EGFR* Mutations

In contrast to sensitizing mutations such as exon 19 deletion and the L858R substitution, in-frame insertions within exon 20 of *EGFR* have been associated with resistance to EGFR TKIs, with response rates <5% to available EGFR TKIs, including the third-generation EGFR TKIs [25, 133–136]. Exon 20 insertions are the third most common type of EGFR mutation and account for 4–9% of EGFR mutations in NSCLC patients [25, 135, 137]. This is a heterogeneous group of about 44 mutations which vary in position and size [137], and three-dimensional structural modeling predicts variable effects on EGFR TKI binding [135]. *EGFR* exon 20 contains an alpha-C helix followed by a loop (Fig. 1). The conformation of the alpha-C helix and the P-loop is altered by exon 20 insertions, leading to steric hindrance and a confined binding pocket [138]. The most deleterious "hot spot" mutations tend to occur distal to the C helix, and represent 80–90% of exon 20 insertions [25, 135].

Few therapies have shown efficacy for patients with *EGFR* exon 20 insertions. The second-generation heat shock protein 90 (HSP90) inhibitors (e.g., ganetespib and luminespib) have had limited success in patients with NSCLC [139–143]. However, luminespib may have clinical activity in patients with exon 20 insertions [144, 145], with a median PFS of 6.1 months in one single arm phase II trial [146], but is associated with ocular toxicity.

Poziotinib is a TKI that covalently and irreversibly inhibits EGFR and HER2, and is unique because of its small terminal group and flexible quinazoline core. Its small size and flexibility allow it to evade the steric hindrance which affects other EGFR TKIs [138]. In a phase II trial of poziotinib, in patients with NSCLC harboring an *EGFR* exon 20 insertion, the ORR at 8 weeks was 58%, and the confirmed ORR at the time of the most recent interim analysis was 38% [147]. The median PFS was 5.6 months. Notably, this was a heavily pretreated group of patients, and the ORR was 62% among those who were previously treated with an EGFR TKI. A multicenter phase II trial of poziotinib is ongoing. Another TKI, AP32788 (TAK-788), was tested in a phase I/II trial of patients with an *EGFR* mutation. Out of 14 evaluable patients, the 9 patients (64%) who achieved a PR or had SD also had an exon 20 insertion [148], demonstrating promising clinical activity for this subset of patients. Poziotinib and AP32788 may represent important future drug options for *EGFR* exon 20 mutation-positive patients.

The incorporation of next-generation sequencing technologies has aided in the characterization of rare mutations in *EGFR*. G719X, deletion 18, and E709X are found in 3.1%, 0.3%, and 0.3% of patients with lung cancer (X connotes one of several possible amino acids). The G719X mutations can be found in combination with S768I and L861Q mutations which account for 1.1% and 0.9% of cases, respectively [137]. In an analysis of 32 patients with metastatic NSCLC with the uncommon *EGFR* mutations S68I, L861Q, and/or G719X (originally enrolled in LUX-Lung 2, LUX-Lung 3, and LUX-Lung 6), the ORR by independent radiology review was 66%. Among the 21 responders, 52% responded for a year or longer [149, 150]. This led to the FDA expanding its approval of afatinib to cover these uncommon non-resistant *EGFR* mutations in January 2018. There is some preclinical data suggesting osimertinib activity for some of these mutations, as well [137]. There are a range of EGFR mutations with varying sensitivity to EGFR TKIs, and the precise detection of these mutations will help to further refine EGFR targeted therapy.

Anti-EGFR Monoclonal Antibodies

In comparison to EGFR TKIs, anti-EGFR monoclonal antibodies have had little role in the treatment of NSCLC. The humanized IgG1 anti-EGFR monoclonal antibody, cetuximab, has been tested in several combinations and has generally demonstrated meager clinical success for an unselected NSCLC population. In patients with stage III NSCLC, the addition of cetuximab to concurrent chemoradiation and consolidation carboplatin plus paclitaxel provided no OS benefit and was associated with more grade 3 or greater toxic effects (86% vs 70%, $P < 0.0001$) [151]. The addition of cetuximab to platinum-based chemotherapy for advanced NSCLC was examined in two large randomized phase III trials: FLEX in patients with "EGFR-expressing" tumors by histology or cytology and BMS099 in unselected patients. There was no change in PFS, and the OS advantage was 1.3 months ($P = 0.04$ for FLEX, and $P = 0.169$ for BMS099) [152, 153]. More recently, in the randomized phase III SWOG S0819 trial of 1313 treatment-naive patients with advanced NSCLC, the addition of cetuximab to carboplatin plus paclitaxel (and if appropriate, bevacizumab) failed to add an improvement in OS [154]. Subset analysis of patients with tumors with EGFR high copy number or amplification by fluorescence in situ hybridization (FISH) also failed to find any OS benefit. Weekly administration, additional cost, minimal or no survival advantage, and side effects (primarily grade 3 rash) led to cetuximab not being approved by either the EMA or FDA [155].

Despite their lack of success in unselected NSCLC patients, anti-EGFR monoclonal antibodies have shown some efficacy in squamous NSCLC. Although squamous NSCLC harbor a low frequency of EGFR mutations, they tend to have higher rates of EGFR overexpression compared to lung adenocarcinoma [156]. In fact, the EGFR TKIs, erlotinib and afatinib, have also demonstrated efficacy in squamous NSCLC, and afatinib has an FDA approval for pretreated squamous cell carcinoma of the lung [157, 158]. In a prespecified subset analysis of 111 patients in SWOG S0819 with squamous histology, the median overall survival was 11.8 months in the cetuximab arm vs 6.1 months for carboplatin and paclitaxel arm (HR = 0.58, $P = 0.007$) [154].

The second-generation fully humanized IgG1 anti-EGFR monoclonal antibody, necitumumab, was added to gemcitabine/cisplatin for patients with advanced squamous NSCLC in the randomized phase III trial, SQUIRE. There was a slight OS advantage (11.5 vs 9.9 months for the gemcitabine/cisplatin, HR 0.84, $P = 0.01$), at the expense of more grade 3 adverse events reported in patients receiving necitumumab (72% vs 62%) [159]. In 2015, the FDA approved necitumumab in combination with gemcitabine and cisplatin for squamous NSCLC [160]. In light of other therapies such as combination chemoimmunotherapy or docetaxel plus ramucirumab [161, 162], the role of anti-EGFR therapy for squamous NSCLC has been debated [163, 164]. Recently, the National Comprehensive Cancer Network Panel unanimously voted to delete necitumumab plus gemcitabine and cisplatin from its list of recommended therapies, citing "toxicity, cost, and limited improvement in efficacy when compared to cisplatin/gemcitabine" [165].

The most significant area of clinical success of EGFR monoclonal antibodies for NSCLC is in combination with EGFR TKIs. In a phase Ib study of 126 heavily pretreated patients who had acquired resistance to erlotinib or gefitinib, the combination of afatinib with cetuximab led to an ORR of 29% and median PFS 4.7 months (regardless of T790M mutation status) [166, 167]. This suggests that at the time of acquired resistance a certain proportion of patients retain dependence on EGFR-mediated signaling that may be overcome with dual EGFR blockade. Given the improved efficacy and toxicity profile of osimertinib compared to afatinib across trials, there are at least three ongoing phase I trials of osimertinib in combination with necitumumab [168].

Addition of Chemotherapy to First-Line EGFR TKI

It has been hypothesized that the addition of chemotherapy to EGFR TKI could postpone the emergence of acquired resistance. The first trial to assess an EGFR TKI plus chemotherapy compared to an EGFR TKI alone in an exclusively *EGFR* mutation-positive population was a randomized phase II trial conducted in Asia of 191 patients with advanced NSCLC with activating *EGFR* mutations who received pemetrexed with gefitinib or gefitinib alone [169]. The combination prolonged PFS to 15.8 months vs 10.9 months, which was intriguing but did not reach statistical significance (HR = 0.68, $P = 0.18$). There is an ongoing confirmatory phase III study, AGAIN (JCOG1404/WJOG8214L), in which patients are randomized to gefitinib or gefitinib with cisplatin and pemetrexed as first-line treatment. Currently, it is unclear whether the addition of chemotherapy to an EGFR TKI offers benefit, and single-agent EGFR TKI remains the standard of care first-line treatment [165].

Bevacizumab Added to EGFR TKI

Bevacizumab is a humanized monoclonal antibody against the vascular endothelial growth factor receptor (VEGFR). The addition of bevacizumab to chemotherapy has been shown to improve OS and PFS in patients with NSCLC [170, 171]. In unselected patients with advanced, pretreated NSCLC, the double-blind phase III trial (BeTa) randomized patients to bevacizumab and erlotinib or erlotinib alone. Addition of bevacizumab to erlotinib resulted in a minimal PFS advantage of 3.4 months as compared to 1.7 months with erlotinib alone (HR 0.62, 95% CI 0.52–0.75), without any OS advantage [172]. Post hoc subset analysis failed to demonstrate any PFS or OS benefit among patients harboring EGFR mutations in this population [172].

More recent trials prospectively examining the use of bevacizumab with an EGFR TKI in patients selected for *EGFR* mutations have shown more promising results. In the randomized phase II study (JO25567) of upfront bevacizumab with erlotinib in patients with activating EGFR mutations, the PFS was 16.0 months in the erlotinib plus bevacizumab group compared to 9.7 months in the erlotinib group (HR 0.54, $P = 0.0015$) [30]. The most common grade 3 adverse reactions included hypertension (60% vs 10%), rash (25% vs 19%), and proteinuria (8% vs 0). In another randomized phase III trial (NEJ026) of patients with treatment-naive *EGFR*-mutated NSCLC, the study met its primary endpoint for PFS at the interim analysis with a PFS of 16.9 months in the bevacizumab and erlotinib arm compared to 13.3 months in the erlotinib arm (HR = 0.605, $P = 0.0157$) [173]. Both randomized trials provide evidence for combining an EGFR TKI with bevacizumab as first-line therapy, and in 2016 the European Medicines Agency (EMA) approved the combination, although no OS benefit has been found at this time.

Current combination studies are evaluating similar strategies, including some with osimertinib as the TKI and others with ramucirumab as a VEGFR monoclonal antibody. Randomized phase II trials of osimertinib and bevacizumab versus osimertinib are ongoing (BOOSTER; NCT03133546) as is the phase III CAURAL trial with an arm of osimertinib with bevacizumab (NCT02454933). The RELAY study (NCT02411448) is a randomized phase Ib/III study to investigate the safety and efficacy of ramucirumab and erlotinib, and it has a substudy arm looking at combination treatment with osimertinib. These trials may help define a potential role for VEGF pathway inhibitors in the first-line treatment for *EGFR*-mutated patients.

Immune Checkpoint Inhibition

Immune checkpoint inhibitors (ICIs) have dramatically changed the treatment landscape and prognosis of advanced NSCLC [174, 175], yet response rates to monotherapy in unselected patients are generally less than 20%. Therefore, there is a critical need to define those patients who are most likely to benefit. Blocking the programmed-death ligand 1 (PD-L1) or its receptor (PD-1) has demonstrated less success in patients with *EGFR* mutations compared to those with wild-type *EGFR*. A recent analysis of 1588 patients with NSCLC who had progressed on at least one prior therapy and were treated with nivolumab showed a lower ORR in the those with *EGFR*-mutated disease of 8.8%, compared to 19.6% for those with wild-type *EGFR* ($P = 0.007$) [176]. A meta-analysis of ICIs in metastatic NSCLC disease showed no benefit of an ICI compared to docetaxel for *EGFR*-mutated patients [177], further dampening the excitement for using ICIs in this population.

The combination of PD-L1 blockade and EGFR TKI has also been explored. However, this appears to be associated with significant toxicity. In the phase Ib TATTON trial, the combination of osimertinib and durvalumab was associated with interstitial lung disease in 38% of patients [178]. The study arm was closed prematurely as was the phase III CAURAL trial (NCT02454933) of osimertinib plus durvalumab [179].

In general, immune checkpoint inhibition for *EGFR*-mutated NSCLC has been disappointing, reflecting the different pathogenesis of this oncogene-driven subset of NSCLC. In part, this may be due to low tobacco exposure and the low resultant mutation burden and neo-antigen expression seen in EGFR-positive disease. One exception is the IMpower 150 trial of carboplatin, paclitaxel, and bevacizumab (BCP) compared to the same regimen with the PDL1 inhibitor, atezolizumab (ABCP) for patients with non-squamous NSCLC [180]. In patients without an *EGFR* or *ALK* mutation, there was a 4.5 month OS benefit (median OS 19.2 months vs 14.7 months, HR = 0.78, *P* = 0.016) in the ABCP arm. The combination is FDA approved for patients with non-squamous NSCLC without *EGFR* or *ALK* mutations [181]. This trial included 80 patients with an *EGFR* mutation and 34 with *EML4-ALK* fusion, another actionable NSCLC mutation; among these patients taken as a group, PFS was longer with ABCP than with BCP (median, 9.7 months vs 6.1 months; unstratified hazard ratio, 0.59; 95% CI, 0.37–0.94). Although this dataset contains relatively few patients, ABCP does offer a treatment option for *EGFR*-mutated NSCLC, particularly at the point that EGFR-targeted therapy options have been exhausted.

Resistance to Osimertinib and Future Directions

There are multiple causes of resistance to third-generation inhibitors, including *EGFR* or mesenchymal–epithelial transition factor (*MET*) amplification [182]; acquisition of resistance mutations such as C797S, L718X, and L792X [183]; and small cell transformation [168, 184, 185]. At the time of progression on osimertinib, approximately 22–40% of patients can be found to have the C797S point mutation in exon 20, a tertiary mutation that removes an important cysteine residue [114, 186]. Unlike the reversible EGFR TKIs, a defining feature of second- and third-generation inhibitors is covalent bonding to the cysteine at the 797 position, a residue at the edge of the EGFR ATP-binding cleft [80]. Due to a mutation changing the cysteine to a serine, covalent inhibitors can no longer bind to the protein. The T790M and C797S can exist in a cis position, in which a single allele has both the T790M and the C797S mutations, or in a trans position, with T790M and C797S on different alleles. Preclinical data and some clinical data suggest that the cis relationship is predominant and would be resistant to all known EGFR TKIs [187–189]. In contrast, if C797S and T790M are in the trans position, combined or alternating first-generation and third-generation inhibitors may be beneficial [190, 191].

The C797S mutation prevents binding of covalent inhibitors to EGFR at the ATP-binding pocket, but this may theoretically be circumvented by binding to a different site than the catalytic active site. EAI045 is one such selective allosteric inhibitor that was identified in high-throughput screens. It binds tightly to an allosteric site created by displacement of the C helix in the inactive confirmation of EGFR [192, 193]. EAI045 demonstrates selectivity and efficacy in mouse models harboring the EGFR C797S mutation (L858R/T790M/C797S) in combination with cetuximab [193]. The synergy with cetuximab seems critical to EAI045's activity against C797S-mutated NSCLC. It remains to be seen whether other ongoing high-throughput screens will identify other potent allosteric inhibitors of EGFR and whether they will rely on the use of combination EGFR blockade as well [194].

Brigatinib is a small molecule inhibitor of both ALK and EGFR [195]. In preclinical models, "triple-mutant EGFR"-positive cells (activating *EGFR* mutation/ T790M/C797S) responded to the combination of brigatinib with an anti-EGFR monoclonal antibody, cetuximab or panitumumab [196]. Single-agent activity of brigatinib in a phase I/II trial was only 5% [197], possibly compounded by low plasma concentrations [196], but the addition of an anti-EGFR monoclonal antibody remains to be clinically tested. The preclinical data with brigatinib and EAI045 in laboratory models with a C797S mutation demonstrate that combination therapies with an anti-EGFR monoclonal antibody may lead to overcoming resistance to osimertinib.

HER2 and MET amplification have been recognized as EGFR-independent mechanisms of acquired resistance to osimertinib, and result in continued activation of ERK and AKT [168, 198]. In patients with MET activation, the MET inhibitor, crizotinib, shows activity in preclinical models and case reports [182, 199, 200]. In the phase Ib/II TATTON trial, the combination of osimertinib with the MET inhibitor savolitinib was studied in patients with T790M EGFR-mutated NSCLC and MET amplification. In those who had not previously received a third-generation EGFR TKI, 43% of patients achieved a PR. In those previously treated with a third-generation EGFR TKI the PR rate was 20% [201]. To target both MET and EGFR, the bispecific antibody, LY3164530, was tested in a phase I trial in patients with advanced and metastatic cancer [202]. The authors concluded that the significant toxicities along with a lack of potential predictive biomarkers limited future development, but other dual-targeted agents are under development, including JNJ-61186372.

In HER2 amplified cells with acquired resistance to osimertinib, trastuzumab emtansine has shown preclinical activity [203]. In an animal tumor model that initially responds to osimertinib but eventually relapses, the addition of cetuximab and trastuzumab to osimertinib resulted in rapid and durable inhibition of tumor recurrence [204]. The authors also demonstrated benefit with the addition of an anti-HER3 antibody. There is an ongoing phase I trial of the HER3-targeting antibody drug conjugate, U3-1402, in patients with NSCLC and an activating EGFR mutation who either progressed on osimertinib or are T790M negative at the time of disease progression [205].

Conclusion

The discovery of *EGFR* mutations in NSCLC and the development of EGFR TKIs to target them have helped define the modern era of precision medicine. Our understanding of the molecular mechanisms of disease and resistance has allowed us to deliver innovative ways of targeting this disease, and expanded our ability to treat patients. The latest generation of EGFR TKI, osimertinib, has shown dramatic benefits, first in overcoming T790M-mediated resistance, and more recently as the first-line therapy with the longest PFS. Given its efficacy in treating CNS metastases, we are likely to redefine the optimal sequence of treatment for this special population of patients while optimizing quality of life. We have already embarked upon the next challenge of treating acquired resistance to third-generation inhibitors with several new compounds in clinical trials. Multiple mechanisms occur in acquired resistance, and future directions to overcome this might involve combination therapy targeted to the specific resistance genotype. Whereas no effective options have been available for patients with the exon 20 insertion, early clinical data show promising results for poziotinib and AP32788. We await further reports on these agents as well as others to target rare mutations in *EGFR*. The story of the discovery of targeted treatment for *EGFR*-mutated NSCLC has taught us that a deep understanding of the molecular mechanisms of disease can lead to powerful personalized treatment.

References

1. Rotow J, Bivona TG. Understanding and targeting resistance mechanisms in NSCLC. Nat Rev Cancer. 2017;17(11):637–58. https://doi.org/10.1038/nrc.2017.84.
2. Shigematsu H, Lin L, Takahashi T, Nomura M, Suzuki M, Wistuba II, et al. Clinical and biological features associated with epidermal growth factor receptor gene mutations in lung cancers. J Natl Cancer Inst. 2005;97(5):339–46. https://doi.org/10.1093/jnci/dji055.
3. Tsao AS, Tang XM, Sabloff B, Xiao L, Shigematsu H, Roth J, et al. Clinicopathologic characteristics of the EGFR gene mutation in non-small cell lung cancer. J Thorac Oncol. 2006;1(3):231–9.
4. Rosell R, Moran T, Queralt C, Porta R, Cardenal F, Camps C, et al. Screening for epidermal growth factor receptor mutations in lung cancer. N Engl J Med. 2009;361(10):958–67. https://doi.org/10.1056/NEJMoa0904554.
5. Zhang YL, Yuan JQ, Wang KF, Fu XH, Han XR, Threapleton D, et al. The prevalence of EGFR mutation in patients with non-small cell lung cancer: a systematic review and meta-analysis. Oncotarget. 2016;7(48):78985–93. https://doi.org/10.18632/oncotarget.12587.
6. Pao W, Miller V, Zakowski M, Doherty J, Politi K, Sarkaria I, et al. EGF receptor gene mutations are common in lung cancers from "never smokers" and are associated with sensitivity of tumors to gefitinib and erlotinib. Proc Natl Acad Sci U S A. 2004;101(36):13306–11. https://doi.org/10.1073/pnas.0405220101.
7. Lynch TJ, Bell DW, Sordella R, Gurubhagavatula S, Okimoto RA, Brannigan BW, et al. Activating mutations in the epidermal growth factor receptor underlying responsiveness of non-small-cell lung cancer to gefitinib. N Engl J Med. 2004;350(21):2129–39. https://doi.org/10.1056/NEJMoa040938.
8. Paez JG, Janne PA, Lee JC, Tracy S, Greulich H, Gabriel S, et al. EGFR mutations in lung cancer: correlation with clinical response to gefitinib therapy. Science. 2004;304(5676):1497–500. https://doi.org/10.1126/science.1099314.
9. Cohen S. Isolation of a mouse submaxillary gland protein accelerating incisor eruption and eyelid opening in the new-born animal. J Biol Chem. 1962;237:1555–62.
10. Burgess AW, Cho H-S, Eigenbrot C, Ferguson KM, Garrett TPJ, Leahy DJ, et al. An open-and-shut case? Recent insights into the activation of EGF/ErbB receptors. Mol Cell. 2003;12(3):541–52. https://doi.org/10.1016/S1097-2765(03)00350-2.

11. Carpenter G, Lembach KJ, Morrison MM, Cohen S. Characterization of the binding of 125-I-labeled epidermal growth factor to human fibroblasts. J Biol Chem. 1975;250(11):4297–304.
12. Yarden Y, Schlessinger J. Epidermal growth factor induces rapid, reversible aggregation of the purified epidermal growth factor receptor. Biochemistry. 1987;26(5):1443–51.
13. de Larco JE, Todaro GJ. Epithelioid and fibroblastic rat kidney cell clones: epidermal growth factor (EGF) receptors and the effect of mouse sarcoma virus transformation. J Cell Physiol. 1978;94(3):335–42. https://doi.org/10.1002/jcp.1040940311.
14. Mendelsohn J, Masui H, Goldenberg A. Anti-epidermal growth factor receptor monoclonal antibodies may inhibit A431 tumor cell proliferation by blocking an autocrine pathway. Trans Assoc Am Phys. 1987;100:173–8.
15. Dokala A, Thakur SS. Extracellular region of epidermal growth factor receptor: a potential target for anti-EGFR drug discovery. Oncogene. 2017;36(17):2337–44. https://doi.org/10.1038/onc.2016.393.
16. Yarden Y, Sliwkowski MX. Untangling the ErbB signalling network. Nat Rev Mol Cell Biol. 2001;2(2):127–37. https://doi.org/10.1038/35052073.
17. Ullrich A, Coussens L, Hayflick JS, Dull TJ, Gray A, Tam AW, et al. Human epidermal growth factor receptor cDNA sequence and aberrant expression of the amplified gene in A431 epidermoid carcinoma cells. Nature. 1984;309:418. https://doi.org/10.1038/309418a0.
18. Lemmon MA, Schlessinger J, Ferguson KM. The EGFR family: not so prototypical receptor tyrosine kinases. Cold Spring Harb Perspect Biol. 2014;6(4):a020768. https://doi.org/10.1101/cshperspect.a020768.
19. Garrett TPJ, McKern NM, Lou M, Elleman TC, Adams TE, Lovrecz GO, et al. Crystal structure of a truncated epidermal growth factor receptor extracellular domain bound to transforming growth factor α. Cell. 2002;110(6):763–73. https://doi.org/10.1016/S0092-8674(02)00940-6.
20. Schlessinger J. Cell signaling by receptor tyrosine kinases. Cell. 2000;103(2):211–25.
21. Hirsch FR, Varella-Garcia M, Cappuzzo F. Predictive value of EGFR and HER2 overexpression in advanced non-small-cell lung cancer. Oncogene. 2009;28:S32. https://doi.org/10.1038/onc.2009.199.
22. Prabhakar CN. Epidermal growth factor receptor in non-small cell lung cancer. Transl Lung Cancer Res. 2015;4(2):110–8. https://doi.org/10.3978/j.issn.2218-6751.2015.01.01.
23. Testa JR, Siegfried JM. Chromosome abnormalities in human non-small cell lung cancer. Cancer Res. 1992;52(9 Suppl):2702s–6s.
24. Sharma SV, Bell DW, Settleman J, Haber DA. Epidermal growth factor receptor mutations in lung cancer. Nat Rev Cancer. 2007;7(3):169–81. https://doi.org/10.1038/nrc2088.
25. Yasuda H, Park E, Yun CH, Sng NJ, Lucena-Araujo AR, Yeo WL, et al. Structural, biochemical, and clinical characterization of epidermal growth factor receptor (EGFR) exon 20 insertion mutations in lung cancer. Sci Transl Med. 2013;5(216):216ra177. https://doi.org/10.1126/scitranslmed.3007205.
26. Wang Y, Li RQ, Ai YQ, Zhang J, Zhao PZ, Li YF, et al. Exon 19 deletion was associated with better survival outcomes in advanced lung adenocarcinoma with mutant EGFR treated with EGFR-TKIs as second-line therapy after first-line chemotherapy: a retrospective analysis of 128 patients. Clin Transl Oncol. 2015;17(9):727–36. https://doi.org/10.1007/s12094-015-1300-4.
27. Yang JC-H, Wu Y-L, Schuler M, Sebastian M, Popat S, Yamamoto N, et al. Afatinib versus cisplatin-based chemotherapy for *EGFR* mutation-positive lung adenocarcinoma (LUX-Lung 3 and LUX-Lung 6): analysis of overall survival data from two randomised, phase 3 trials. Lancet Oncol. 2015;16(2):141–51. https://doi.org/10.1016/S1470-2045(14)71173-8.
28. Zhang Y, Sheng J, Kang S, Fang W, Yan Y, Hu Z, et al. Patients with exon 19 deletion were associated with longer progression-free survival compared to those with L858R mutation after first-line EGFR-TKIs for advanced non-small cell lung cancer: a meta-analysis. PLoS One. 2014;9(9):e107161. https://doi.org/10.1371/journal.pone.0107161.

29. Ichihara E, Hotta K, Nogami N, Kuyama S, Kishino D, Fujii M, et al. Phase II trial of gefitinib in combination with bevacizumab as first-line therapy for advanced non-small cell lung cancer with activating EGFR gene mutations: the Okayama Lung Cancer Study Group Trial 1001. J Thorac Oncol. 2015;10(3):486–91. https://doi.org/10.1097/jto.0000000000000434.

30. Seto T, Kato T, Nishio M, Goto K, Atagi S, Hosomi Y, et al. Erlotinib alone or with bevacizumab as first-line therapy in patients with advanced non-squamous non-small-cell lung cancer harbouring EGFR mutations (JO25567): an open-label, randomised, multicentre, phase 2 study. Lancet Oncol. 2014;15(11):1236–44. https://doi.org/10.1016/s1470-2045(14)70381-x.

31. Qu J, Wang YN, Xu P, Xiang DX, Yang R, Wei W, et al. Clinical efficacy of icotinib in lung cancer patients with different EGFR mutation status: a meta-analysis. Oncotarget. 2017;8(20):33961–71. https://doi.org/10.18632/oncotarget.15475.

32. Moyer JD, Barbacci EG, Iwata KK, Arnold L, Boman B, Cunningham A, et al. Induction of apoptosis and cell cycle arrest by CP-358,774, an inhibitor of epidermal growth factor receptor Tyrosine Kinase. Cancer Res. 1997;57(21):4838–48.

33. Barker AJ, Gibson KH, Grundy W, Godfrey AA, Barlow JJ, Healy MP, et al. Studies leading to the identification of ZD1839 (IRESSA): an orally active, selective epidermal growth factor receptor tyrosine kinase inhibitor targeted to the treatment of cancer. Bioorg Med Chem Lett. 2001;11(14):1911–4.

34. Ward WH, Cook PN, Slater AM, Davies DH, Holdgate GA, Green LR. Epidermal growth factor receptor tyrosine kinase. Investigation of catalytic mechanism, structure-based searching and discovery of a potent inhibitor. Biochem Pharmacol. 1994;48(4):659–66.

35. Fukuoka M, Yano S, Giaccone G, Tamura T, Nakagawa K, Douillard JY, et al. Multi-institutional randomized phase II trial of gefitinib for previously treated patients with advanced non-small-cell lung cancer (the IDEAL 1 trial) [corrected]. J Clin Oncol. 2003;21(12):2237–46. https://doi.org/10.1200/jco.2003.10.038.

36. Kris MG, Natale RB, Herbst RS, et al. Efficacy of gefitinib, an inhibitor of the epidermal growth factor receptor tyrosine kinase, in symptomatic patients with non–small cell lung cancer: a randomized trial. JAMA. 2003;290(16):2149–58. https://doi.org/10.1001/jama.290.16.2149.

37. Thatcher N, Chang A, Parikh P, Rodrigues Pereira J, Ciuleanu T, von Pawel J, et al. Gefitinib plus best supportive care in previously treated patients with refractory advanced non-small-cell lung cancer: results from a randomised, placebo-controlled, multicentre study (Iressa survival evaluation in lung cancer). Lancet. 2005;366(9496):1527–37. https://doi.org/10.1016/s0140-6736(05)67625-8.

38. Kim ES, Hirsh V, Mok T, Socinski MA, Gervais R, Wu YL, et al. Gefitinib versus docetaxel in previously treated non-small-cell lung cancer (INTEREST): a randomised phase III trial. Lancet. 2008;372(9652):1809–18. https://doi.org/10.1016/s0140-6736(08)61758-4.

39. Kazandjian D, Blumenthal GM, Yuan W, He K, Keegan P, Pazdur R. FDA approval of Gefitinib for the treatment of patients with metastatic EGFR mutation-positive non-small cell lung cancer. Clin Cancer Res. 2016;22(6):1307–12. https://doi.org/10.1158/1078-0432.Ccr-15-2266.

40. Herbst RS, Giaccone G, Schiller JH, Natale RB, Miller V, Manegold C, et al. Gefitinib in combination with paclitaxel and carboplatin in advanced non-small-cell lung cancer: a phase III trial–INTACT 2. J Clin Oncol. 2004;22(5):785–94. https://doi.org/10.1200/jco.2004.07.215.

41. Giaccone G, Herbst RS, Manegold C, Scagliotti G, Rosell R, Miller V, et al. Gefitinib in combination with gemcitabine and cisplatin in advanced non-small-cell lung cancer: a phase III trial–INTACT 1. J Clin Oncol. 2004;22(5):777–84. https://doi.org/10.1200/jco.2004.08.001.

42. Gatzemeier U, Pluzanska A, Szczesna A, Kaukel E, Roubec J, De Rosa F, et al. Phase III study of erlotinib in combination with cisplatin and gemcitabine in advanced non-small-cell lung cancer: the Tarceva lung cancer investigation trial. J Clin Oncol. 2007;25(12):1545–52. https://doi.org/10.1200/jco.2005.05.1474.

43. Herbst RS, Prager D, Hermann R, Fehrenbacher L, Johnson BE, Sandler A, et al. TRIBUTE: a phase III trial of erlotinib hydrochloride (OSI-774) combined with carboplatin and paclitaxel

chemotherapy in advanced non-small-cell lung cancer. J Clin Oncol. 2005;23(25):5892–9. https://doi.org/10.1200/jco.2005.02.840.

44. Mok TS, Wu Y-L, Thongprasert S, Yang C-H, Chu D-T, Saijo N, et al. Gefitinib or carboplatin–paclitaxel in pulmonary adenocarcinoma. N Engl J Med. 2009;361(10):947–57. https://doi.org/10.1056/NEJMoa0810699.

45. Fukuoka M, Wu YL, Thongprasert S, Sunpaweravong P, Leong SS, Sriuranpong V, et al. Biomarker analyses and final overall survival results from a phase III, randomized, open-label, first-line study of gefitinib versus carboplatin/paclitaxel in clinically selected patients with advanced non-small-cell lung cancer in Asia (IPASS). J Clin Oncol. 2011;29(21):2866–74. https://doi.org/10.1200/jco.2010.33.4235.

46. Douillard JY, Ostoros G, Cobo M, Ciuleanu T, McCormack R, Webster A, et al. First-line gefitinib in Caucasian EGFR mutation-positive NSCLC patients: a phase-IV, open-label, single-arm study. Br J Cancer. 2014;110(1):55–62. https://doi.org/10.1038/bjc.2013.721.

47. Shen YW, Zhang XM, Li ST, Lv M, Yang J, Wang F, et al. Efficacy and safety of icotinib as first-line therapy in patients with advanced non-small-cell lung cancer. Onco Targets Ther. 2016;9:929–35. https://doi.org/10.2147/ott.S98363.

48. Bria E, Milella M, Cuppone F, Novello S, Ceribelli A, Vaccaro V, et al. Outcome of advanced NSCLC patients harboring sensitizing EGFR mutations randomized to EGFR tyrosine kinase inhibitors or chemotherapy as first-line treatment: a meta-analysis. Ann Oncol. 2011;22(10):2277–85. https://doi.org/10.1093/annonc/mdq742.

49. Petrelli F, Borgonovo K, Cabiddu M, Barni S. Efficacy of EGFR tyrosine kinase inhibitors in patients with EGFR-mutated non-small-cell lung cancer: a meta-analysis of 13 randomized trials. Clin Lung Cancer. 2012;13(2):107–14. https://doi.org/10.1016/j.cllc.2011.08.005.

50. Gao G, Ren S, Li A, Xu J, Xu Q, Su C, et al. Epidermal growth factor receptor-tyrosine kinase inhibitor therapy is effective as first-line treatment of advanced non-small-cell lung cancer with mutated EGFR: a meta-analysis from six phase III randomized controlled trials. Int J Cancer. 2012;131(5):E822–9. https://doi.org/10.1002/ijc.27396.

51. Lee CK, Davies L, Wu YL, Mitsudomi T, Inoue A, Rosell R, et al. Gefitinib or Erlotinib vs chemotherapy for EGFR mutation-positive lung cancer: individual patient data meta-analysis of overall survival. J Natl Cancer Inst. 2017;109(6) https://doi.org/10.1093/jnci/djw279.

52. Yang JJ, Zhou Q, Yan HH, Zhang XC, Chen HJ, Tu HY, et al. A phase III randomised controlled trial of erlotinib vs gefitinib in advanced non-small cell lung cancer with EGFR mutations. Br J Cancer. 2017;116(5):568–74. https://doi.org/10.1038/bjc.2016.456.

53. Urata Y, Katakami N, Morita S, Kaji R, Yoshioka H, Seto T, et al. Randomized phase III study comparing Gefitinib with Erlotinib in patients with previously treated advanced lung adenocarcinoma: WJOG 5108L. J Clin Oncol. 2016;34(27):3248–57. https://doi.org/10.1200/jco.2015.63.4154.

54. Lee CK, Brown C, Gralla RJ, Hirsh V, Thongprasert S, Tsai CM, et al. Impact of EGFR inhibitor in non-small cell lung cancer on progression-free and overall survival: a meta-analysis. J Natl Cancer Inst. 2013;105(9):595–605. https://doi.org/10.1093/jnci/djt072.

55. Paz-Ares L, Soulieres D, Moecks J, Bara I, Mok T, Klughammer B. Pooled analysis of clinical outcome for EGFR TKI-treated patients with EGFR mutation-positive NSCLC. J Cell Mol Med. 2014;18(8):1519–39. https://doi.org/10.1111/jcmm.12278.

56. Thongprasert S, Duffield E, Saijo N, Wu YL, Yang JC, Chu DT, et al. Health-related quality-of-life in a randomized phase III first-line study of gefitinib versus carboplatin/paclitaxel in clinically selected patients from Asia with advanced NSCLC (IPASS). J Thorac Oncol. 2011;6(11):1872–80. https://doi.org/10.1097/JTO.0b013e31822adaf7.

57. Chen G, Feng J, Zhou C, Wu YL, Liu XQ, Wang C, et al. Quality of life (QoL) analyses from OPTIMAL (CTONG-0802), a phase III, randomised, open-label study of first-line erlotinib versus chemotherapy in patients with advanced EGFR mutation-positive non-small-cell lung cancer (NSCLC). Ann Oncol. 2013;24(6):1615–22. https://doi.org/10.1093/annonc/mdt012.

58. Soria JC, Wu YL, Nakagawa K, Kim SW, Yang JJ, Ahn MJ, et al. Gefitinib plus chemotherapy versus placebo plus chemotherapy in EGFR-mutation-positive non-small-cell lung cancer after progression on first-line gefitinib (IMPRESS): a phase 3 randomised trial. Lancet Oncol. 2015;16(8):990–8. https://doi.org/10.1016/s1470-2045(15)00121-7.

59. Mok TSK, Kim SW, Wu YL, Nakagawa K, Yang JJ, Ahn MJ, et al. Gefitinib plus chemotherapy versus chemotherapy in epidermal growth factor receptor mutation-positive non-small-cell lung cancer resistant to first-line Gefitinib (IMPRESS): overall survival and biomarker analyses. J Clin Oncol. 2017;35(36):4027–34. https://doi.org/10.1200/jco.2017.73.9250.

60. Li D, Ambrogio L, Shimamura T, Kubo S, Takahashi M, Chirieac LR, et al. BIBW2992, an irreversible EGFR/HER2 inhibitor highly effective in preclinical lung cancer models. Oncogene. 2008;27:4702. https://doi.org/10.1038/onc.2008.109. https://www.nature.com/articles/onc2008109#supplementary-information.

61. Engelman JA, Zejnullahu K, Gale CM, Lifshits E, Gonzales AJ, Shimamura T, et al. PF00299804, an irreversible pan-ERBB inhibitor, is effective in lung cancer models with EGFR and ERBB2 mutations that are resistant to gefitinib. Cancer Res. 2007;67(24):11924–32. https://doi.org/10.1158/0008-5472.Can-07-1885.

62. Gonzales AJ, Hook KE, Althaus IW, Ellis PA, Trachet E, Delaney AM, et al. Antitumor activity and pharmacokinetic properties of PF-00299804, a second-generation irreversible pan-erbB receptor tyrosine kinase inhibitor. Mol Cancer Ther. 2008;7(7):1880–9. https://doi.org/10.1158/1535-7163.Mct-07-2232.

63. Yonesaka K, Kudo K, Nishida S, Takahama T, Iwasa T, Yoshida T, et al. The pan-HER family tyrosine kinase inhibitor afatinib overcomes HER3 ligand heregulin-mediated resistance to EGFR inhibitors in non-small cell lung cancer. Oncotarget. 2015;6(32):33602–11. https://doi.org/10.18632/oncotarget.5286.

64. Miller VA, Hirsh V, Cadranel J, Chen YM, Park K, Kim SW, et al. Afatinib versus placebo for patients with advanced, metastatic non-small-cell lung cancer after failure of erlotinib, gefitinib, or both, and one or two lines of chemotherapy (LUX-Lung 1): a phase 2b/3 randomised trial. Lancet Oncol. 2012;13(5):528–38. https://doi.org/10.1016/s1470-2045(12)70087-6.

65. Reckamp KL, Giaccone G, Camidge DR, Gadgeel SM, Khuri FR, Engelman JA, et al. A phase 2 trial of dacomitinib (PF-00299804), an oral, irreversible pan-HER (human epidermal growth factor receptor) inhibitor, in patients with advanced non-small cell lung cancer after failure of prior chemotherapy and erlotinib. Cancer. 2014;120(8):1145–54. https://doi.org/10.1002/cncr.28561.

66. Takeda M, Okamoto I, Nakagawa K. Pooled safety analysis of EGFR-TKI treatment for EGFR mutation-positive non-small cell lung cancer. Lung Cancer. 2015;88(1):74–9. https://doi.org/10.1016/j.lungcan.2015.01.026.

67. Wang LY, Cui JJ, Guo AX, Yin JY. Clinical efficacy and safety of afatinib in the treatment of non-small-cell lung cancer in Chinese patients. Onco Targets Ther. 2018;11:529–38. https://doi.org/10.2147/ott.S136579.

68. Califano R, Tariq N, Compton S, Fitzgerald DA, Harwood CA, Lal R, et al. Expert consensus on the management of adverse events from EGFR Tyrosine Kinase inhibitors in the UK. Drugs. 2015;75(12):1335–48. https://doi.org/10.1007/s40265-015-0434-6.

69. Yang CJ, Tsai MJ, Hung JY, Lee MH, Tsai YM, Tsai YC, et al. The clinical efficacy of Afatinib 30 mg daily as starting dose may not be inferior to Afatinib 40 mg daily in patients with stage IV lung adenocarcinoma harboring exon 19 or exon 21 mutations. BMC Pharmacol Toxicol. 2017;18(1):82. https://doi.org/10.1186/s40360-017-0190-1.

70. Park K, Tan E-H, O'Byrne K, Zhang L, Boyer M, Mok T, et al. Afatinib versus gefitinib as first-line treatment of patients with EGFR mutation-positive non-small-cell lung cancer (LUX-Lung 7): a phase 2B, open-label, randomised controlled trial. Lancet Oncol. 2016;17(5):577–89. https://doi.org/10.1016/S1470-2045(16)30033-X.

71. Sequist LV, Yang JC, Yamamoto N, O'Byrne K, Hirsh V, Mok T, et al. Phase III study of afatinib or cisplatin plus pemetrexed in patients with metastatic lung adenocarcinoma with EGFR mutations. J Clin Oncol. 2013;31(27):3327–34. https://doi.org/10.1200/jco.2012.44.2806.

72. Wu YL, Zhou C, Hu CP, Feng J, Lu S, Huang Y, et al. Afatinib versus cisplatin plus gemcitabine for first-line treatment of Asian patients with advanced non-small-cell lung cancer harbouring EGFR mutations (LUX-Lung 6): an open-label, randomised phase 3 trial. Lancet Oncol. 2014;15(2):213–22. https://doi.org/10.1016/s1470-2045(13)70604-1.

73. Paz-Ares L, Tan EH, O'Byrne K, Zhang L, Hirsh V, Boyer M, et al. Afatinib versus gefitinib in patients with EGFR mutation-positive advanced non-small-cell lung cancer: overall survival data from the phase IIb LUX-Lung 7 trial. Ann Oncol. 2017;28(2):270–7. https://doi.org/10.1093/annonc/mdw611.
74. Wu YL, Cheng Y, Zhou X, Lee KH, Nakagawa K, Niho S, et al. Dacomitinib versus gefitinib as first-line treatment for patients with EGFR-mutation-positive non-small-cell lung cancer (ARCHER 1050): a randomised, open-label, phase 3 trial. Lancet Oncol. 2017;18(11):1454–66. https://doi.org/10.1016/s1470-2045(17)30608-3.
75. Mok TS, Cheng Y, Zhou X, Lee KH, Nakagawa K, Niho S, et al. Improvement in overall survival in a randomized study that compared Dacomitinib with Gefitinib in patients with advanced non–small-cell lung cancer and EGFR-activating mutations. J Clin Oncol. 2018;36(22):2244–50. https://doi.org/10.1200/JCO.2018.78.7994.
76. FDA. VIZIMPRO (dacomitinib) tablets, for oral use. https://www.accessdata.fda.gov/drugsatfda_docs/label/2018/211288s000lbl.pdf.
77. Addeo A. Dacomitinib in NSCLC: a positive trial with little clinical impact. Lancet Oncol. 2018;19(1):e4. https://doi.org/10.1016/S1470-2045(17)30923-3.
78. Ou SHI, Soo RA. Dacomitinib in lung cancer: a "lost generation" EGFR tyrosine-kinase inhibitor from a bygone era? Drug Des Devel Ther. 2015;9:5641–53. https://doi.org/10.2147/dddt.S52787.
79. Kobayashi S, Boggon TJ, Dayaram T, Jänne PA, Kocher O, Meyerson M, et al. EGFR mutation and resistance of non–small-cell lung cancer to Gefitinib. N Engl J Med. 2005;352(8):786–92. https://doi.org/10.1056/NEJMoa044238.
80. Yun C-H, Mengwasser KE, Toms AV, Woo MS, Greulich H, Wong K-K, et al. The T790M mutation in EGFR kinase causes drug resistance by increasing the affinity for ATP. Proc Natl Acad Sci. 2008;105(6):2070–5. https://doi.org/10.1073/pnas.0709662105.
81. Cross DAE, Ashton SE, Ghiorghiu S, Eberlein C, Nebhan CA, Spitzler PJ, et al. AZD9291, an irreversible EGFR TKI, overcomes T790M-mediated resistance to EGFR inhibitors in lung cancer. Cancer Discov. 2014;4(9):1046–61. https://doi.org/10.1158/2159-8290.Cd-14-0337.
82. Oxnard GR, Arcila ME, Sima CS, Riely GJ, Chmielecki J, Kris MG, et al. Acquired resistance to EGFR Tyrosine Kinase inhibitors in EGFR-mutant lung cancer: distinct natural history of patients with tumors harboring the T790M mutation. Clin Cancer Res. 2011;17(6):1616–22. https://doi.org/10.1158/1078-0432.Ccr-10-2692.
83. Yu HA, Arcila ME, Rekhtman N, Sima CS, Zakowski MF, Pao W, et al. Analysis of tumor specimens at the time of acquired resistance to EGFR-TKI therapy in 155 patients with EGFR-mutant lung cancers. Clin Cancer Res. 2013;19(8):2240–7. https://doi.org/10.1158/1078-0432.Ccr-12-2246.
84. Sequist LV, Waltman BA, Dias-Santagata D, Digumarthy S, Turke AB, Fidias P, et al. Genotypic and histological evolution of lung cancers acquiring resistance to EGFR inhibitors. Sci Transl Med. 2011;3(75):75ra26. https://doi.org/10.1126/scitranslmed.3002003.
85. Gaut D, Sim MS, Yue Y, Wolf BR, Abarca PA, Carroll JM, et al. Clinical implications of the T790M mutation in disease characteristics and treatment response in patients with epidermal growth factor receptor (EGFR)-mutated non-small-cell lung cancer (NSCLC). Clin Lung Cancer. 2018;19(1):e19–28. https://doi.org/10.1016/j.cllc.2017.06.004.
86. Sequist LV, Soria JC, Goldman JW, Wakelee HA, Gadgeel SM, Varga A, et al. Rociletinib in EGFR-mutated non-small-cell lung cancer. N Engl J Med. 2015;372(18):1700–9. https://doi.org/10.1056/NEJMoa1413654.
87. Sequist LV, Soria J-C, Camidge DR. Update to Rociletinib data with the RECIST confirmed response rate. N Engl J Med. 2016;374(23):2296–7. https://doi.org/10.1056/NEJMc1602688.
88. Park K, Jänne PA, Yu CJ, Bazhenova L, Paz-Ares L, Baek E, et al. 412OA global phase II study of olmutinib (HM61713) in patients with T790M-positive NSCLC after failure of first-line EGFR-TKI. Ann Oncol. 2017;28(suppl_10):mdx671.001. https://doi.org/10.1093/annonc/mdx671.001.

89. Kim D-W, Tan DS-W, Ponce Aix S, Sequist LV, Smit EF, Hida T, et al. Preliminary phase II results of a multicenter, open-label study of nazartinib (EGF816) in adult patients with treatment-naïve EGFR-mutant non-small cell lung cancer (NSCLC). J Clin Oncol. 2018;36(15_suppl):9094. https://doi.org/10.1200/JCO.2018.36.15_suppl.9094.

90. Wang H, Zhang L, Zheng X, Zhang X, Si X, Wang M. The ability of avitinib to penetrate the blood brain barrier and its control of intra−/extra- cranial disease in patients of non-small cell lung cancer (NSCLC) harboring EGFR T790M mutation. J Clin Oncol. 2017;35(15_suppl):e20613. https://doi.org/10.1200/JCO.2017.35.15_suppl.e20613.

91. Murakami H, Nokihara H, Hayashi H, Seto T, Park K, Azuma K, et al. Clinical activity of ASP8273 in Asian patients with non-small-cell lung cancer with EGFR activating and T790M mutations. Cancer Sci. 2018;109(9):2852–62. https://doi.org/10.1111/cas.13724.

92. Husain H, Martins RG, Goldberg SB, Senico P, Ma W, Masters J, et al. 1358PFirst-in-human phase I study of PF-06747775, a third-generation mutant selective EGFR tyrosine kinase inhibitor (TKI) in metastatic EGFR mutant NSCLC after progression on a first-line EGFR TKI. Ann Oncol. 2017;28(suppl_5):mdx380.060. https://doi.org/10.1093/annonc/mdx380.060.

93. Wu YL, Ahn MJ, Garassino MC, Han JY, Katakami N, Kim HR, et al. CNS efficacy of Osimertinib in patients with T790M-positive advanced non-small-cell lung cancer: data from a randomized phase III trial (AURA3). J Clin Oncol. 2018:Jco2018779363. https://doi.org/10.1200/jco.2018.77.9363.

94. Gao X, Le X, Costa DB. The safety and efficacy of osimertinib for the treatment of EGFR T790M mutation positive non-small-cell lung cancer. Expert Rev Anticancer Ther. 2016;16(4):383–90. https://doi.org/10.1586/14737140.2016.1162103.

95. Mok TS, Wu YL, Ahn MJ, Garassino MC, Kim HR, Ramalingam SS, et al. Osimertinib or Platinum-Pemetrexed in EGFR T790M-positive lung cancer. N Engl J Med. 2017;376(7):629–40. https://doi.org/10.1056/NEJMoa1612674.

96. Osimertinib (TAGRISSO). U.S. Food and Drug Administration (FDA). https://www.fda.gov/drugs/informationondrugs/approveddrugs/ucm549683.htm. Accessed 12 Oct 2018.

97. Bertranou E, Bodnar C, Dansk V, Greystoke A, Large S, Dyer M. Cost-effectiveness of osimertinib in the UK for advanced EGFR-T790M non-small cell lung cancer. J Med Econ. 2018;21(2):113–21. https://doi.org/10.1080/13696998.2017.1377718.

98. Ramalingam SS, Yang JC, Lee CK, Kurata T, Kim DW, John T, et al. Osimertinib as first-line treatment of EGFR mutation-positive advanced non-small-cell lung cancer. J Clin Oncol. 2018;36(9):841–9. https://doi.org/10.1200/jco.2017.74.7576.

99. Soria JC, Ohe Y, Vansteenkiste J, Reungwetwattana T, Chewaskulyong B, Lee KH, et al. Osimertinib in untreated EGFR-mutated advanced non-small-cell lung cancer. N Engl J Med. 2018;378(2):113–25. https://doi.org/10.1056/NEJMoa1713137.

100. FDA approves osimertinib for first-line treatment of metastatic NSCLC with most common EGFR mutations. U.S. Food & Drug Administation (FDA). https://www.fda.gov/drugs/informationondrugs/approveddrugs/ucm605113.htm. Accessed 13 Oct 2018.

101. Sundaresan TK, Sequist LV, Heymach JV, Riely GJ, Janne PA, Koch WH, et al. Detection of T790M, the acquired resistance EGFR mutation, by Tumor Biopsy versus noninvasive blood-based analyses. Clin Cancer Res. 2016;22(5):1103–10. https://doi.org/10.1158/1078-0432.ccr-15-1031.

102. Vanderlaan PA, Yamaguchi N, Folch E, Boucher DH, Kent MS, Gangadharan SP, et al. Success and failure rates of tumor genotyping techniques in routine pathological samples with non-small-cell lung cancer. Lung Cancer. 2014;84(1):39–44. https://doi.org/10.1016/j.lungcan.2014.01.013.

103. Folch E, Yamaguchi N, VanderLaan PA, Kocher ON, Boucher DH, Goldstein MA, et al. Adequacy of lymph node transbronchial needle aspirates using convex probe endobronchial ultrasound for multiple tumor genotyping techniques in non-small-cell lung cancer. J Thorac Oncol. 2013;8(11):1438–44. https://doi.org/10.1097/JTO.0b013e3182a471a9.

104. Overman MJ, Modak J, Kopetz S, Murthy R, Yao JC, Hicks ME, et al. Use of research biopsies in clinical trials: are risks and benefits adequately discussed? J Clin Oncol. 2013;31(1):17–22. https://doi.org/10.1200/jco.2012.43.1718.

105. Sacher AG, Paweletz C, Dahlberg SE, Alden RS, O'Connell A, Feeney N, et al. Prospective validation of rapid plasma genotyping for the detection of EGFR and KRAS mutations in advanced lung cancer. JAMA Oncol. 2016;2(8):1014–22. https://doi.org/10.1001/jamaoncol.2016.0173.

106. Lokhandwala T, Bittoni MA, Dann RA, D'Souza AO, Johnson M, Nagy RJ, et al. Costs of diagnostic assessment for lung cancer: a medicare claims analysis. Clin Lung Cancer. 2017;18(1):e27–34. https://doi.org/10.1016/j.cllc.2016.07.006.

107. Piotrowska Z, Niederst MJ, Mino-Kenudson M, Morales-Oyarvide V, Fulton L, Lockerman E, et al. Variation in mechanisms of acquired resistance among EGFR-mutant NSCLC patients with more than 1 Postresistant Biopsy. Int J Radiat Oncol Biol Phys. 90(5):S6–7. https://doi.org/10.1016/j.ijrobp.2014.08.032.

108. Goldman JW, Noor ZS, Remon J, Besse B, Rosenfeld N. Are liquid biopsies a surrogate for tissue EGFR testing? Ann Oncol. 2018;29(suppl_1):i38–46. https://doi.org/10.1093/annonc/mdx706.

109. Zhang J, Fujimoto J, Zhang J, Wedge DC, Song X, Zhang J, et al. Intratumor heterogeneity in localized lung adenocarcinomas delineated by multiregion sequencing. Science. 2014;346(6206):256–9. https://doi.org/10.1126/science.1256930.

110. de Bruin EC, McGranahan N, Mitter R, Salm M, Wedge DC, Yates L, et al. Spatial and temporal diversity in genomic instability processes defines lung cancer evolution. Science (New York, NY). 2014;346(6206):251–6. https://doi.org/10.1126/science.1253462.

111. Lawrence MS, Stojanov P, Polak P, Kryukov GV, Cibulskis K, Sivachenko A, et al. Mutational heterogeneity in cancer and the search for new cancer-associated genes. Nature. 2013;499(7457):214–8. https://doi.org/10.1038/nature12213.

112. Jamal-Hanjani M, Wilson GA, McGranahan N, Birkbak NJ, Watkins TBK, Veeriah S, et al. Tracking the evolution of non-small-cell lung cancer. N Engl J Med. 2017;376(22):2109–21. https://doi.org/10.1056/NEJMoa1616288.

113. Remon J, Caramella C, Jovelet C, Lacroix L, Lawson A, Smalley S, et al. Osimertinib benefit in EGFR-mutant NSCLC patients with T790M-mutation detected by circulating tumour DNA. Ann Oncol. 2017;28(4):784–90. https://doi.org/10.1093/annonc/mdx017.

114. Thress KS, Paweletz CP, Felip E, Cho BC, Stetson D, Dougherty B, et al. Acquired EGFR C797S mutation mediates resistance to AZD9291 in non-small cell lung cancer harboring EGFR T790M. Nat Med. 2015;21(6):560–2. https://doi.org/10.1038/nm.3854.

115. de Bruin EC, McGranahan N, Mitter R, Salm M, Wedge DC, Yates L, et al. Spatial and temporal diversity in genomic instability processes defines lung cancer evolution. Science. 2014;346(6206):251–6. https://doi.org/10.1126/science.1253462.

116. Guibert NM, Paweletz C, Hu Y, Feeney NB, Plagnol V, Poole V, et al. Early detection of competing resistance mutations using plasma next-generation sequencing (NGS) in patients (pts) with EGFR-mutant NSCLC treated with osimertinib. J Clin Oncol. 2017;35(15_suppl):11529. https://doi.org/10.1200/JCO.2017.35.15_suppl.11529.

117. Oxnard GR, Thress KS, Alden RS, Lawrance R, Paweletz CP, Cantarini M, et al. Association between plasma genotyping and outcomes of treatment with Osimertinib (AZD9291) in advanced non-small-cell lung cancer. J Clin Oncol. 2016;34(28):3375–82. https://doi.org/10.1200/jco.2016.66.7162.

118. Goldman JW, Karlovich C, Sequist LV, Melnikova V, Franovic A, Gadgeel SM, et al. EGFR genotyping of matched urine, plasma, and tumor tissue in patients with non–small-cell lung cancer treated with Rociletinib, an EGFR Tyrosine Kinase inhibitor. JCO Precis Oncol. 2018;(2):1–13. https://doi.org/10.1200/po.17.00116.

119. Ge M, Zhuang Y, Zhou X, Huang R, Liang X, Zhan Q. High probability and frequency of EGFR mutations in non-small cell lung cancer with brain metastases. J Neuro-Oncol. 2017;135(2):413–8. https://doi.org/10.1007/s11060-017-2590-x.

120. Shin DY, Na II, Kim CH, Park S, Baek H, Yang SH. EGFR mutation and brain metastasis in pulmonary adenocarcinomas. J Thorac Oncol. 2014;9(2):195–9. https://doi.org/10.1097/jto.0000000000000069.

121. Hsiao SH, Chou YT, Lin SE, Hsu RC, Chung CL, Kao YR, et al. Brain metastases in patients with non-small cell lung cancer: the role of mutated-EGFRs with an exon 19 deletion or L858R point mutation in cancer cell dissemination. Oncotarget. 2017;8(32):53405–18. https://doi.org/10.18632/oncotarget.18509.

122. Mak KS, Gainor JF, Niemierko A, Oh KS, Willers H, Choi NC, et al. Significance of targeted therapy and genetic alterations in EGFR, ALK, or KRAS on survival in patients with non–small cell lung cancer treated with radiotherapy for brain metastases. Neuro-Oncology. 2015;17(2):296–302. https://doi.org/10.1093/neuonc/nou146.

123. Martínez P, Mak RH, Oxnard GR. Targeted therapy as an alternative to whole-brain radiotherapy in egfr-mutant or alk-positive non–small-cell lung cancer with brain metastases. JAMA Oncol. 2017;3(9):1274–5. https://doi.org/10.1001/jamaoncol.2017.1047.

124. Magnuson WJ, Lester-Coll NH, Wu AJ, Yang TJ, Lockney NA, Gerber NK, et al. Management of brain metastases in Tyrosine Kinase inhibitor–Naïve epidermal growth factor receptor–mutant non–small-cell lung cancer: a retrospective multi-institutional analysis. J Clin Oncol. 2017;35(10):1070–7. https://doi.org/10.1200/JCO.2016.69.7144.

125. Yang JC, Cho BC, Kim CH, Kim S, Lee J, Su W, et al. Osimertinib for patients (pts) with leptomeningeal metastases (LM) from EGFR-mutant non-small cell lung cancer (NSCLC): updated results from the BLOOM study. J Clin Oncol. 2017;35(15_suppl):2020. https://doi.org/10.1200/JCO.2017.35.15_suppl.2020.

126. Ahn M-J, Kim D-W, Cho BC, Kim S-W, Lee J-S, Ahn JS, et al. Phase I study (BLOOM) of AXD3759, a BBB penetrable EGFR inhibitor, in TKI naïve EGFRm NSCLC patients in CNS metastases. J Clin Oncol. 2017;35(suppl 18):abst 2006.

127. Corre R, Gervais R, Guisier F, Tassy L, Vinas F, Lamy R, et al. Octogenarians with EGFR-mutated non-small cell lung cancer treated by tyrosine-kinase inhibitor: a multicentric real-world study assessing tolerance and efficacy (OCTOMUT study). Oncotarget. 2018;9(9):8253–62. https://doi.org/10.18632/oncotarget.23836.

128. Yoshioka H, Komuta K, Imamura F, Kudoh S, Seki A, Fukuoka M. Efficacy and safety of erlotinib in elderly patients in the phase IV POLARSTAR surveillance study of Japanese patients with non-small-cell lung cancer. Lung Cancer. 2014;86(2):201–6. https://doi.org/10.1016/j.lungcan.2014.09.015.

129. Roviello G, Zanotti L, Cappelletti MR, Gobbi A, Dester M, Paganini G, et al. Are EGFR tyrosine kinase inhibitors effective in elderly patients with EGFR-mutated non-small cell lung cancer? Clin Exp Med. 2018;18(1):15–20. https://doi.org/10.1007/s10238-017-0460-7.

130. Morikawa N, Minegishi Y, Inoue A, Maemondo M, Kobayashi K, Sugawara S, et al. First-line gefitinib for elderly patients with advanced NSCLC harboring EGFR mutations. A combined analysis of North-East Japan Study Group studies. Expert Opin Pharmacother. 2015;16(4):465–72. https://doi.org/10.1517/14656566.2015.1002396.

131. Spigel DR, Hainsworth JD, Burkett ER, Burris HA, Yardley DA, Thomas M, et al. Single-agent gefitinib in patients with untreated advanced non-small-cell lung cancer and poor performance status: a Minnie pearl cancer research network phase II trial. Clin Lung Cancer. 2005;7(2):127–32. https://doi.org/10.3816/CLC.2005.n.028.

132. Lee SM, Khan I, Upadhyay S, Lewanski C, Falk S, Skailes G, et al. First-line erlotinib in patients with advanced non-small-cell lung cancer unsuitable for chemotherapy (TOPICAL): a double-blind, placebo-controlled, phase 3 trial. Lancet Oncol. 2012;13(11):1161–70. https://doi.org/10.1016/s1470-2045(12)70412-6.

133. Oxnard GR, Lo PC, Nishino M, Dahlberg SE, Lindeman NI, Butaney M, et al. Natural history and molecular characteristics of lung cancers harboring EGFR exon 20 insertions. J Thorac Oncol. 2013;8(2):179–84. https://doi.org/10.1097/JTO.0b013e3182779d18.

134. Yasuda H, Kobayashi S, Costa DB. EGFR exon 20 insertion mutations in non-small-cell lung cancer: preclinical data and clinical implications. Lancet Oncol. 2012;13(1):e23–31. https://doi.org/10.1016/s1470-2045(11)70129-2.

135. Arcila ME, Nafa K, Chaft JE, Rekhtman N, Lau C, Reva BA, et al. *EGFR* Exon 20 insertion mutations in lung adenocarcinomas: prevalence, molecular heterogeneity, and clinicopathologic characteristics. Mol Cancer Ther. 2013;12(2):220–9. https://doi.org/10.1158/1535-7163. Mct-12-0620.

136. Yang M, Xu X, Cai J, Ning J, Wery JP, Li QX. NSCLC harboring EGFR exon-20 insertions after the regulatory C-helix of kinase domain responds poorly to known EGFR inhibitors. Int J Cancer. 2016;139(1):171–6. https://doi.org/10.1002/ijc.30047.

137. Kobayashi Y, Mitsudomi T. Not all epidermal growth factor receptor mutations in lung cancer are created equal: perspectives for individualized treatment strategy. Cancer Sci. 2016;107(9):1179–86. https://doi.org/10.1111/cas.12996.

138. Robichaux JP, Elamin YY, Tan Z, Carter BW, Zhang S, Liu S, et al. Mechanisms and clinical activity of an EGFR and HER2 exon 20–selective kinase inhibitor in non–small cell lung cancer. Nat Med. 2018;24(5):638–46. https://doi.org/10.1038/s41591-018-0007-9.

139. Socinski MA, Goldman J, El-Hariry I, Koczywas M, Vukovic V, Horn L, et al. A multicenter phase II study of ganetespib monotherapy in patients with genotypically defined advanced non-small cell lung cancer. Clin Cancer Res. 2013;19(11):3068–77. https://doi.org/10.1158/1078-0432.Ccr-12-3381.

140. Ramalingam S, Goss G, Rosell R, Schmid-Bindert G, Zaric B, Andric Z, et al. A randomized phase II study of ganetespib, a heat shock protein 90 inhibitor, in combination with docetaxel in second-line therapy of advanced non-small cell lung cancer (GALAXY-1). Ann Oncol. 2015;26(8):1741–8. https://doi.org/10.1093/annonc/mdv220.

141. Pillai R, Fennell D, Kovcin V, Ciuleanu T, Ramlau R, Kowalski D, et al. PL03.09: phase 3 study of Ganetespib, a heat shock protein 90 inhibitor, with Docetaxel versus Docetaxel in advanced non-small cell lung cancer (GALAXY-2). J Thorac Oncol. 2017;12(1):S7–8. https://doi.org/10.1016/j.jtho.2016.11.009.

142. Johnson ML, Yu HA, Hart EM, Weitner BB, Rademaker AW, Patel JD, et al. Phase I/II study of HSP90 inhibitor AUY922 and Erlotinib for EGFR-mutant lung cancer with acquired resistance to epidermal growth factor receptor Tyrosine Kinase inhibitors. J Clin Oncol. 2015;33(15):1666–73. https://doi.org/10.1200/jco.2014.59.7328.

143. Pillai RN, Ramalingam SS. Throwing more cold water on heat shock protein 90 inhibitors in NSCLC. J Thorac Oncol. 2018;13(4):473–4. https://doi.org/10.1016/j.jtho.2018.02.010.

144. Felip E, Barlesi F, Besse B, Chu Q, Gandhi L, Kim SW, et al. Phase 2 study of the HSP-90 inhibitor AUY922 in previously treated and molecularly defined patients with advanced non-small cell lung cancer. J Thorac Oncol. 2018;13(4):576–84. https://doi.org/10.1016/j.jtho.2017.11.131.

145. Noor Z, Goldman JW, Lawler W, Melancon D, Telivala B, Braiteh F, et al. P2.13-39 a phase Ib trial of the HSP90 inhibitor AUY922 in combination with Pemetrexed in metastatic non-squamous, non-small cell lung cancer patients. J Thorac Oncol. 2018;13(10, Supplement):S813–S4. https://doi.org/10.1016/j.jtho.2018.08.1434.

146. Piotrowska Z, Costa DB, Huberman M, Oxnard GR, Gainor JF, Heist RS, et al. Activity of AUY922 in NSCLC patients with EGFR exon 20 insertions. J Clin Oncol. 2015;33(15_suppl):8015. https://doi.org/10.1200/jco.2015.33.15_suppl.8015.

147. Heymach J, Negrao M, Robichaux J, et al. OA02.06 a phase II trial of Poziotinib in EGFR and HER2 Exon 20 mutant non-small cell lung cancer (NSCLC). J Thorac Oncol. 2018;13:S323–S4.

148. Doebele RC, Riely GJ, Spira AI, Horn L, Piotrowska Z, Costa DB, et al. First report of safety, PK, and preliminary antitumor activity of the oral EGFR/HER2 exon 20 inhibitor TAK-788 (AP32788) in non–small cell lung cancer (NSCLC). J Clin Oncol. 2018;36(15_suppl):9015. https://doi.org/10.1200/JCO.2018.36.15_suppl.9015.

149. FDA. GILOTRIF (afatinib). FDA. 2018. https://www.accessdata.fda.gov/drugsatfda_docs/label/2018/201292s014lbl.pdf. Accessed 1 Nov 2018.
150. Yang JC, Sequist LV, Geater SL, Tsai CM, Mok TS, Schuler M, et al. Clinical activity of afatinib in patients with advanced non-small-cell lung cancer harbouring uncommon EGFR mutations: a combined post-hoc analysis of LUX-Lung 2, LUX-Lung 3, and LUX-Lung 6. Lancet Oncol. 2015;16(7):830–8. https://doi.org/10.1016/s1470-2045(15)00026-1.
151. Bradley JD, Paulus R, Komaki R, Masters G, Blumenschein G, Schild S, et al. Standard-dose versus high-dose conformal radiotherapy with concurrent and consolidation carboplatin plus paclitaxel with or without cetuximab for patients with stage IIIA or IIIB non-small-cell lung cancer (RTOG 0617): a randomised, two-by-two factorial phase 3 study. Lancet Oncol. 2015;16(2):187–99. https://doi.org/10.1016/s1470-2045(14)71207-0.
152. Pirker R, Pereira JR, Szczesna A, von Pawel J, Krzakowski M, Ramlau R, et al. Cetuximab plus chemotherapy in patients with advanced non-small-cell lung cancer (FLEX): an open-label randomised phase III trial. Lancet. 2009;373(9674):1525–31. https://doi.org/10.1016/s0140-6736(09)60569-9.
153. Lynch TJ, Patel T, Dreisbach L, McCleod M, Heim WJ, Hermann RC, et al. Cetuximab and first-line taxane/carboplatin chemotherapy in advanced non-small-cell lung cancer: results of the randomized multicenter phase III trial BMS099. J Clin Oncol. 2010;28(6):911–7. https://doi.org/10.1200/jco.2009.21.9618.
154. Herbst RS, Redman MW, Kim ES, Semrad TJ, Bazhenova L, Masters G, et al. Cetuximab plus carboplatin and paclitaxel with or without bevacizumab versus carboplatin and paclitaxel with or without bevacizumab in advanced NSCLC (SWOG S0819): a randomised, phase 3 study. Lancet Oncol. 2018;19(1):101–14. https://doi.org/10.1016/s1470-2045(17)30694-0.
155. Sgambato A, Casaluce F, Maione P, Rossi A, Ciardiello F, Gridelli C. Cetuximab in advanced non-small cell lung cancer (NSCLC): the showdown? J Thorac Dis. 2014;6(6):578–80. https://doi.org/10.3978/j.issn.2072-1439.2014.06.14.
156. Nakamura H, Kawasaki N, Taguchi M, Kabasawa K. Survival impact of epidermal growth factor receptor overexpression in patients with non-small cell lung cancer: a meta-analysis. Thorax. 2006;61(2):140.
157. Shepherd FA, Rodrigues Pereira J, Ciuleanu T, Tan EH, Hirsh V, Thongprasert S, et al. Erlotinib in previously treated non–small-cell lung cancer. N Engl J Med. 2005;353(2):123–32. https://doi.org/10.1056/NEJMoa050753.
158. Soria J-C, Felip E, Cobo M, Lu S, Syrigos K, Lee KH, et al. Afatinib versus erlotinib as second-line treatment of patients with advanced squamous cell carcinoma of the lung (LUX-Lung 8): an open-label randomised controlled phase 3 trial. Lancet Oncol. 2015;16(8):897–907. https://doi.org/10.1016/S1470-2045(15)00006-6.
159. Thatcher N, Hirsch FR, Luft AV, Szczesna A, Ciuleanu TE, Dediu M, et al. Necitumumab plus gemcitabine and cisplatin versus gemcitabine and cisplatin alone as first-line therapy in patients with stage IV squamous non-small-cell lung cancer (SQUIRE): an open-label, randomised, controlled phase 3 trial. Lancet Oncol. 2015;16(7):763–74. https://doi.org/10.1016/s1470-2045(15)00021-2.
160. FDA. PORTRAZZA (necitumumab) injection, for intravenous use – FDA. FDA. 2015. https://www.accessdata.fda.gov/drugsatfda_docs/label/2015/125547s000lbl.pdf. Accessed 30 Oct 2018.
161. Paz-Ares L, Luft A, Vicente D, Tafreshi A, Gümüş M, Mazières J, et al. Pembrolizumab plus chemotherapy for squamous non–small-cell lung cancer. N Engl J Med. 2018; https://doi.org/10.1056/NEJMoa1810865.
162. Garon EB, Ciuleanu TE, Arrieta O, Prabhash K, Syrigos KN, Goksel T, et al. Ramucirumab plus docetaxel versus placebo plus docetaxel for second-line treatment of stage IV non-small-cell lung cancer after disease progression on platinum-based therapy (REVEL): a multicentre, double-blind, randomised phase 3 trial. Lancet. 2014;384(9944):665–73. https://doi.org/10.1016/s0140-6736(14)60845-x.

163. Hirsch FR, Herbst RS, Gandara DR. EGFR tyrosine kinase inhibitors in squamous cell lung cancer. Lancet Oncol. 2015;16(8):872–3. https://doi.org/10.1016/S1470-2045(15)00126-6.

164. di Noia V, D'Argento E, Pilotto S, Grizzi G, Caccese M, Iacovelli R, et al. Necitumumab in the treatment of non-small-cell lung cancer: clinical controversies. Expert Opin Biol Ther. 2018;18(9):937–45. https://doi.org/10.1080/14712598.2018.1508445.

165. NCCN. NCCN Clinical practice guidelines in oncology – non-small cell lung cancer. NCCN. org. 2018. https://www.nccn.org/professionals/physician_gls/pdf/nscl.pdf. Accessed 30 Oct 2018.

166. Janjigian YY, Smit EF, Groen HJ, Horn L, Gettinger S, Camidge DR, et al. Dual inhibition of EGFR with afatinib and cetuximab in kinase inhibitor-resistant EGFR-mutant lung cancer with and without T790M mutations. Cancer Discov. 2014;4(9):1036–45. https://doi.org/10.1158/2159-8290.Cd-14-0326.

167. Smit E, Soria JC, Janjigian YY, Groen HJM, Pao W, Calvo E, et al. 86OAfatinib (A) plus cetuximab (C) in the treatment of patients (pts) with NSCLC: the story so far. Ann Oncol. 2017;28(suppl_2):mdx091.06-mdx.06. https://doi.org/10.1093/annonc/mdx091.006.

168. Tang Z-H, Lu J-J. Osimertinib resistance in non-small cell lung cancer: mechanisms and therapeutic strategies. Cancer Lett. 2018;420:242–6. https://doi.org/10.1016/j.canlet.2018.02.004.

169. Cheng Y, Murakami H, Yang PC, He J, Nakagawa K, Kang JH, et al. Randomized phase II trial of Gefitinib with and without Pemetrexed as first-line therapy in patients with advanced nonsquamous non small cell lung cancer with activating epidermal growth factor receptor mutations. J Clin Oncol. 2016;34(27):3258–66. https://doi.org/10.1200/jco.2016.66.9218.

170. Sandler A, Gray R, Perry MC, Brahmer J, Schiller JH, Dowlati A, et al. Paclitaxel–carboplatin alone or with bevacizumab for non–small-cell lung cancer. N Engl J Med. 2006;355(24):2542–50. https://doi.org/10.1056/NEJMoa061884.

171. Sandler A, Yi J, Dahlberg S, Kolb MM, Wang L, Hambleton J, et al. Treatment outcomes by tumor histology in Eastern Cooperative Group Study E4599 of bevacizumab with paclitaxel/carboplatin for advanced non-small cell lung cancer. J Thorac Oncol. 2010;5(9):1416–23. https://doi.org/10.1097/JTO.0b013e3181da36f4.

172. Herbst RS, Ansari R, Bustin F, Flynn P, Hart L, Otterson GA, et al. Efficacy of bevacizumab plus erlotinib versus erlotinib alone in advanced non-small-cell lung cancer after failure of standard first-line chemotherapy (BeTa): a double-blind, placebo-controlled, phase 3 trial. Lancet. 2011;377(9780):1846–54. https://doi.org/10.1016/s0140-6736(11)60545-x.

173. Furuya N, Fukuhara T, Saito H, Watanabe K, Sugawara S, Iwasawa S, et al. Phase III study comparing bevacizumab plus erlotinib to erlotinib in patients with untreated NSCLC harboring activating EGFR mutations: NEJ026. J Clin Oncol. 2018;36(15_suppl):9006. https://doi.org/10.1200/JCO.2018.36.15_suppl.9006.

174. Garon EB, Rizvi NA, Hui R, Leighl N, Balmanoukian AS, Eder JP, et al. Pembrolizumab for the treatment of non–small-cell lung cancer. N Engl J Med. 2015;372(21):2018–28. https://doi.org/10.1056/NEJMoa1501824.

175. Gandhi L, Rodríguez-Abreu D, Gadgeel S, Esteban E, Felip E, De Angelis F, et al. Pembrolizumab plus chemotherapy in metastatic non–small-cell lung cancer. N Engl J Med. 2018;378(22):2078–92. https://doi.org/10.1056/NEJMoa1801005.

176. Garassino MC, Gelibter AJ, Grossi F, Chiari R, Soto Parra H, Cascinu S, et al. Italian Nivolumab expanded access program in nonsquamous non-small cell lung cancer patients: results in never-smokers and EGFR-mutant patients. J Thorac Oncol. 2018;13(8):1146–55. https://doi.org/10.1016/j.jtho.2018.04.025.

177. Lee CK, Man J, Lord S, Links M, Gebski V, Mok T, et al. Checkpoint inhibitors in metastatic EGFR-Mutated non-small cell lung cancer-a meta-analysis. J Thorac Oncol. 2017;12(2):403–7. https://doi.org/10.1016/j.jtho.2016.10.007.

178. Ahn MJ, Yang J, Yu H, Saka H, Ramalingam S, Goto K, et al. 136O: Osimertinib combined with durvalumab in EGFR-mutant non-small cell lung cancer: results from the TATTON phase Ib trial. J Thorac Oncol. 2016;11(4):S115. https://doi.org/10.1016/S1556-0864(16)30246-5.

179. Mezquita L, Planchard D. Durvalumab for the treatment of non-small cell lung cancer. Expert Rev Respir Med. 2018;12(8):627–39. https://doi.org/10.1080/17476348.2018.1494575.
180. Socinski MA, Jotte RM, Cappuzzo F, Orlandi F, Stroyakovskiy D, Nogami N, et al. Atezolizumab for first-line treatment of metastatic nonsquamous NSCLC. N Engl J Med. 2018;378(24):2288–301. https://doi.org/10.1056/NEJMoa1716948.
181. FDA. TECENTRIQ (atezolizumab) injection, for intravenous use. https://www.accessdata.fda.gov/drugsatfda_docs/label/2018/761034s009lbl.pdf. Accessed 14 Jan 2019.
182. Ortiz-Cuaran S, Scheffler M, Plenker D, Dahmen L, Scheel AH, Fernandez-Cuesta L, et al. Heterogeneous mechanisms of primary and acquired resistance to third-generation EGFR inhibitors. Clin Cancer Res. 2016;22(19):4837.
183. Yang Z, Yang N, Ou Q, Xiang Y, Jiang T, Wu X, et al. Investigating novel resistance mechanisms to third-generation EGFR Tyrosine Kinase inhibitor Osimertinib in non–small cell lung cancer patients. Clin Cancer Res. 2018;24(13):3097.
184. Yu HA, Tian SK, Drilon AE, Borsu L, Riely GJ, Arcila ME, et al. Acquired resistance of EGFR-mutant lung cancer to a T790M-specific EGFR inhibitor: emergence of a third mutation (C797S) in the EGFR Tyrosine Kinase domain. JAMA Oncol. 2015;1(7):982–4. https://doi.org/10.1001/jamaoncol.2015.1066.
185. Kim TM, Song A, Kim D-W, Kim S, Ahn Y-O, Keam B, et al. Mechanisms of acquired resistance to AZD9291: a mutation-selective, irreversible EGFR inhibitor. J Thorac Oncol. 2015;10(12):1736–44. https://doi.org/10.1097/JTO.0000000000000688.
186. Oxnard GR, Hu Y, Mileham KF, Husain H, Costa DB, Tracy P, et al. Assessment of resistance mechanisms and clinical implications in patients with EGFR T790M-positive lung cancer and acquired resistance to Osimertinib. JAMA Oncol. 2018; https://doi.org/10.1001/jamaoncol.2018.2969.
187. Ou SI, Cui J, Schrock AB, Goldberg ME, Zhu VW, Albacker L, et al. Emergence of novel and dominant acquired EGFR solvent-front mutations at Gly796 (G796S/R) together with C797S/R and L792F/H mutations in one EGFR (L858R/T790M) NSCLC patient who progressed on osimertinib. Lung Cancer. 2017;108:228–31. https://doi.org/10.1016/j.lungcan.2017.04.003.
188. Hidaka N, Iwama E, Kubo N, Harada T, Miyawaki K, Tanaka K, et al. Most T790M mutations are present on the same EGFR allele as activating mutations in patients with non-small cell lung cancer. Lung Cancer. 2017;108:75–82. https://doi.org/10.1016/j.lungcan.2017.02.019.
189. Niederst MJ, Hu H, Mulvey HE, Lockerman EL, Garcia AR, Piotrowska Z, et al. The Allelic context of the C797S mutation acquired upon treatment with third-generation EGFR inhibitors impacts sensitivity to subsequent treatment strategies. Clin Cancer Res. 2015;21(17):3924–33. https://doi.org/10.1158/1078-0432.Ccr-15-0560.
190. Wang Z, Yang JJ, Huang J, Ye JY, Zhang XC, Tu HY, et al. Lung adenocarcinoma harboring EGFR T790M and in trans C797S responds to combination therapy of first- and third-generation EGFR TKIs and shifts allelic configuration at resistance. J Thorac Oncol. 2017;12(11):1723–7. https://doi.org/10.1016/j.jtho.2017.06.017.
191. Arulananda S, Do H, Musafer A, Mitchell P, Dobrovic A, John T. Combination Osimertinib and Gefitinib in C797S and T790M EGFR-mutated non-small cell lung cancer. J Thorac Oncol. 2017;12(11):1728–32. https://doi.org/10.1016/j.jtho.2017.08.006.
192. Zhao P, Yao M-Y, Zhu S-J, Chen J-Y, Yun C-H. Crystal structure of EGFR T790M/C797S/V948R in complex with EAI045. Biochem Biophys Res Commun. 2018;502(3):332–7. https://doi.org/10.1016/j.bbrc.2018.05.154.
193. Jia Y, Yun C-H, Park E, Ercan D, Manuia M, Juarez J, et al. Overcoming EGFR(T790M) and EGFR(C797S) resistance with mutant-selective allosteric inhibitors. Nature. 2016;534:129. https://doi.org/10.1038/nature17960.
194. Westover D, Qiao H, Ichihara E, Meador CB, Lovly CM. Mechanisms of Osimertinib resistance in EGFR mutant lung cancer. J Thorac Oncol. 2017;12(8):S1546. https://doi.org/10.1016/j.jtho.2017.06.063.

195. Huang W-S, Liu S, Zou D, Thomas M, Wang Y, Zhou T, et al. Discovery of Brigatinib (AP26113), a phosphine oxide-containing, potent, orally active inhibitor of anaplastic lymphoma kinase. J Med Chem. 2016;59(10):4948–64. https://doi.org/10.1021/acs.jmedchem.6b00306.
196. Uchibori K, Inase N, Araki M, Kamada M, Sato S, Okuno Y, et al. Brigatinib combined with anti-EGFR antibody overcomes osimertinib resistance in EGFR-mutated non-small-cell lung cancer. Nat Commun. 2017;8:14768. https://www.nature.com/articles/ncomms14768#supplementary-information. https://doi.org/10.1038/ncomms14768.
197. Gettinger SN, Bazhenova LA, Langer CJ, Salgia R, Gold KA, Rosell R, et al. Activity and safety of brigatinib in ALK-rearranged non-small-cell lung cancer and other malignancies: a single-arm, open-label, phase 1/2 trial. Lancet Oncol. 2016;17(12):1683–96. https://doi.org/10.1016/s1470-2045(16)30392-8.
198. Planchard D, Loriot Y, André F, Gobert A, Auger N, Lacroix L, et al. EGFR-independent mechanisms of acquired resistance to AZD9291 in EGFR T790M-positive NSCLC patients. Ann Oncol. 2015;26(10):2073–8. https://doi.org/10.1093/annonc/mdv319.
199. Ou S-HI, Agarwal N, Ali SM. High MET amplification level as a resistance mechanism to osimertinib (AZD9291) in a patient that symptomatically responded to crizotinib treatment post-osimertinib progression. Lung Cancer. 2016;98:59–61. https://doi.org/10.1016/j.lungcan.2016.05.015.
200. York ER, Varella-Garcia M, Bang TJ, Aisner DL, Camidge DR. Tolerable and effective combination of full-dose crizotinib and osimertinib targeting MET amplification sequentially emerging after T790M positivity in EGFR-mutant non–small cell lung cancer. J Thorac Oncol. 2017;12(7):e85–8. https://doi.org/10.1016/j.jtho.2017.02.020.
201. Ahn M, Han J, Sequist L, Cho BC, Lee JS, Kim S, et al. OA 09.03 TATTON Ph Ib expansion Cohort: Osimertinib plus Savolitinib for Pts with EGFR-Mutant MET-Amplified NSCLC after progression on prior EGFR-TKI. J Thorac Oncol. 2017;12(11):S1768. https://doi.org/10.1016/j.jtho.2017.09.377.
202. Patnaik A, Gordon M, Tsai F, Papadopoulous K, Rasco D, Beeram SM, et al. A phase I study of LY3164530, a bispecific antibody targeting MET and EGFR, in patients with advanced or metastatic cancer. Cancer Chemother Pharmacol. 2018;82(3):407–18. https://doi.org/10.1007/s00280-018-3623-7.
203. La Monica S, Cretella D, Bonelli M, Fumarola C, Cavazzoni A, Digiacomo G, et al. Trastuzumab emtansine delays and overcomes resistance to the third-generation EGFR-TKI osimertinib in NSCLC EGFR mutated cell lines. J Exp Clin Cancer Res. 2017;36(1):174. https://doi.org/10.1186/s13046-017-0653-7.
204. Romaniello D, Mazzeo L, Mancini M, Marrocco I, Noronha A, Kreitman MS, et al. A combination of approved antibodies overcomes resistance of lung cancer to Osimertinib by blocking bypass pathways. Clin Cancer Res. 2018; https://doi.org/10.1158/1078-0432.Ccr-18-0450.
205. Janne PA, Yu HA, Johnson ML, Vigliotti M, Shipitofsky N, Guevara FM, et al. Phase 1 study of the anti-HER3 antibody drug conjugate U3-1402 in metastatic or unresectable EGFR-mutant NSCLC. J Clin Oncol. 2018;36(15_suppl):TPS9110–TPS. https://doi.org/10.1200/JCO.2018.36.15_suppl.TPS9110.

Anaplastic Lymphoma Kinase

Nicolas A. Villanueva, Nicholas P. Giustini, and Lyudmila A. Bazhenova

Abstract Anaplastic lymphoma kinase (ALK) is a transmembrane receptor tyrosine kinase, which is a member of the insulin receptor superfamily. Fusions in ALK result in constitutively activated signaling which is susceptible to inhibition by ALK tyrosine kinase inhibitors (TKIs). In this chapter we are describing management of patients with ALK-fused lung cancer. We will discuss molecular basis of ALK fusion including different fusion partners and variants, testing for ALK, targeting ALK with TKI, and managing resistance. Targeting ALK oncogenic driver has been an example of rapid drug development with the first ALK inhibitor approved in 2011 just 4 years after the first publication of ALK discovery by Soda et al. In the following years, we have discovered second- and third-generation ALK inhibitors which are able to circumvent ALK resistance and distinguished by better CNS penetration.

Keywords Anaplastic lymphoma kinase · Insulin receptor superfamily · Lung cancer · Echinoderm microtubule-associated protein-like 4 · EML4-ALK fusion gene

Anaplastic Lymphoma Kinase

Anaplastic lymphoma kinase (ALK) fusion in non-small cell lung cancer (NSCLC) was first described by Soda and colleagues in 2007. Using a retrovirus-mediated complementary DNA expression system, they discovered that a small inversion in the chromosome 2p results in a product consisting of portions of the echinoderm microtubule-associated protein-like 4 (EML4) gene and the ALK gene. The fusion had transforming properties in mouse 3T3 fibroblast model and was targetable by ALK inhibitor WHI-P154 [1].

N. A. Villanueva · N. P. Giustini · L. A. Bazhenova (✉)
UC San Diego Health Moores Cancer Center, San Diego, CA, USA
e-mail: Lbazhenova@ucsd.edu

© Springer Nature Switzerland AG 2019　　　　　　　　　　　　　　　　　31
R. Salgia (ed.), *Targeted Therapies for Lung Cancer*, Current Cancer Research,
https://doi.org/10.1007/978-3-030-17832-1_2

The Structure of ALK Gene and Gene Fusions

The human ALK gene is located at chromosome region 2p23.2–p23.1. As one of the members of the receptor tyrosine kinase (RTK) family, ALK contains an extracellular domain (ECD), a transmembrane domain, and an intracellular domain (ICD) [2]. In mice, *alk* is expressed in the nervous system [3, 4]. Therefore, it has been postulated that the biological functions of mammalian ALK are related to the development and function of the nervous system. The precise activation mechanism of wild-type ALK is not known with the canonical RTK activation mechanism though ligand binding thought to be the most likely.

The oncogenic EML4-ALK fusion gene results from chromosomal translocation within the short arm of chromosome 2, where EML4 and ALK genes are located 12 Mb apart with opposite orientation. Other reported fusion partners include KIF5B and KLC1-ALK [5, 6]. ALK fusion partner may cause dimerization (or oligomerization) of the ALK fusion protein independent of ligand binding, causing oncogenic ALK activation.

The break points for the translocations of ALK genes are typically located at exons 19–20 or exons 20–21. ALK fusion proteins usually contain the complete ALK kinase domain which is placed under promoter control of another gene as a result of a fusion. The break point in a partner gene is variable generating several ALK fusion variants [7]. The break point of ALK is constantly located before the 5′-end of exon 20 at the start of the kinase domain. The most commonly reported variant is variant 1 which is detected in a third of ALK-fused NSCLC patients. Overall, the three major variants (v1: E13;A20, v2: E20;A20, and v3: E6;A20) account for more than 90% of lung cancers associated with EML4-ALK.The significance of different variants is not clear. Preclinical data points to differential sensitivity of ALK variants to ALK inhibitors which may be explained by differences in protein stability in EML4-ALK-expressing cells [8, 9].

In a single institution retrospective analysis of 35 patients treated with crizotinib, longer progression-free survival (PFS) has been reported in variant 1 patients compared to non-variant 1 (11 vs. 4.2 months, respectively; $P < 0.05$). Response rates were similar (74% and 63%, respectively; $P < 0.0318$) [10]. In another retrospective study of 92 patients, a differential in PFS between variant 1 and non-variant 1 was not confirmed (12.3 vs. 15.8 months, respectively, $P = 0.482$). However, variant 2 showed improved PFS compared to non-variant 2 (34.53 vs 12.30 months, respectively, $P = 0.021$) [11]. Yet, a third retrospective study of 51 patients separated patients into variant 3 vs. other groups and showed improved 2-year PFS at 2 year in non-variant 3 patients (76% vs. 26.4% respectively, P 0.034) [12]. This is corroborated by a dataset by Lin who showed that ALK variant 3 patients were more likely to develop resistance mutations especially G1202R (57% vs. 30%; $P = 0.023$ for all resistant mutations and 32% vs. 0%; $P = 0.001$ for G1202R) [13]. The main weakness of all those studies is its retrospective nature which is probably responsible for contradicting results. In this light, results of the ALEX trial provide a tie breaker. ALEX trial was a randomized trial comparing alectinib to crizotinib in treatment-naïve ALK-positive NSCLC patients [14]. There was no significant PFS difference across variant types for patients treated with crizotinib or alectinib using either plasma or tissue [15].

Frequency of ALK Fusions in NSCLC

ALK fusion oncogene happens in about 3–13% of patients with NSCLC [1, 16–18]. In the lung cancer mutational consortium dataset, the frequency of ALK alteration was reported to be 8% [19]. ALK fusions commonly occur in nonsmokers and with rare exceptions are mutually exclusive with other driver mutations [20]. ALK fusions have been described in other cancers such as colorectal, breast, renal cell, esophageal, and ovarian, anaplastic thyroid carcinoma, and diffuse large B-cell lymphoma at low frequencies [21].

Diagnosis of EML4-ALK Fusion

Fluorescent In Situ Hybridization

Fluorescent in situ hybridization (FISH) assay using a break-apart probe (Abbott Molecular Diagnostics) was the first assay used to select patients for ALK therapy. ALK positivity was defined as 15 or more cells showing a split signal.

Immunohistochemistry

Immunohistochemistry (IHC) is an easier and more economical testing alternative. Potentially IHC can be interpreted with a smaller biopsy size and variety of samples such as fluid or cytology cell blocks in addition to tissue blocks. The ALK (D5F3) CDx Assay (Ventana) has been approved by the US FDA as a stand-alone test.

RT-PCR and Non-multiplexed Platforms

RT-PCR is a very sensitive method which provides information about fusion partners. However, the high sensitivity of the test is achieved only when the fusion pattern is within a detectable range of primer pairs, requiring a comprehensive primer dataset. The main downside of RT-PCR is not being able to detect irregular variants with deletions in the annealing site of the primers or non-EML4 fusions unless primers for non-EML4 fusions are specifically designed. Comparative quantitative RT-PCR which is based on differential expression of 3′ and 5′ transcript in ALK fusions is immune to problems arising from not knowing an exact fusion partner.

Next-Generation Sequencing

Next-generation sequencing (NGS) and massively parallel or deep sequencing are related terms that describe a DNA sequencing technology which has revolutionized genomic research. NGS platforms perform sequencing of millions of small fragments of DNA in parallel. Bioinformatics analyses are used to piece together these fragments by mapping the individual reads to the human reference genome. Hybrid capture-based NGS gene panels have been shown to have utility in detecting ALK fusions including complex fusions that can be missed by FISH or IHC [22, 23].

Clinical Efficacy of ALK Inhibitors

There has been a rapid expansion of ALK inhibitors since crizotinib was designated for breakthrough approval by the FDA in 2011. Currently, there are three generations of ALK inhibitors, with each class possessing a higher affinity against the ALK gene, improved central nervous system (CNS) activity, and the capability of overcoming select acquired mutations. These ALK inhibitors are small molecule ATP-competitive inhibitors of the ALK tyrosine kinase domain [24]. Below we describe their clinical efficacy, current indications, and associated toxicities.

First-Generation ALK Inhibitor

Crizotinib was initially discovered as a potent selective inhibitor of MET proto-oncogene, receptor tyrosine kinase (c-MET), but was also found to have activity against ALK [24]. Preclinical trials demonstrated that crizotinib interrupted tyrosine phosphorylation in cells containing the ALK fusion protein, resulting in downstream cell cycle arrest and apoptosis. The subsequent phase I study of crizotinib in ALK-positive solid tumors refractory to standard treatments revealed activity in two patients with NSCLC during the dose-escalation phase, prompting an expanded cohort of these patients [25]. Eighty-two patients with ALK-rearranged NSCLC were treated with crizotinib 250 mg twice daily and produced an overall response rate (ORR) of 57% (95% CI, 46–68%). Treatment was well-tolerated with the most common toxicities being nausea, diarrhea, lower extremity edema, elevated transaminases, and visual disturbances; these effects were reversible with dose interruption. It should be noted that interstitial lung disease (ILD) was a rare adverse event (AE) associated with crizotinib occurring in 1.0% of patients. Subsequent studies evaluated crizotinib in ALK-positive NSCLC and are summarized in Table 1 [26–31].

Two subsequent phase III studies were conducted in previously treated (PROFILE 1007) and treatment-naïve (PROFILE 1014) NSCLC that compared crizotinib to chemotherapy [28, 29]. Both studies met their primary endpoints of PFS, but an overall survival (OS) advantage was not seen due to the allowance of crossover of

Table 1 Crizotinib trials for ALK-positive NSCLC

	Crizotinib			
Trial name (phase, line of therapy)	PROFILE 1001 [26] (phase I, 2L)	PROFILE 1005 [27] (phase II, 2L)	PROFILE 1007 [28] (phase III, 2L)	PROFILE 1014 [29] (phase III, 1L)
Comparator arm	N/A	N/A	Pemetrexed or docetaxel (1:1)	Platinum doublet (1:1)
N	149	1066	347	343
ORR (%)	60.8 (95% CI 52.3–68.9)	54 (95% CI, 51–57)[a], 41 (95% CI, 33–49)[b]	65 vs. 20	74 vs. 45
Median DOR	49.1 weeks (95% CI 39.3–75.4)	11.8 months (95% CI, 10.4–12.8)[a], 9.5 months (95% CI 6.9–15.2)[b]	32.1 weeks vs. 24.4 weeks	11.3 months vs. 5.3 months
Median PFS (months)	9.7 (95% CI 7.7–12.8)	8.4 (95% CI, 7.1–9.7)[a], 6.9 (95% CI, 5.6–9.4)	7.7 vs. 3.0 (HR 0.49, 95% CI, 0.37–0.64, $p < 0.001$)	10.9 vs. 7.0 (HR 0.45, 95% CI, 0.35–0.60, $p < 0.001$)
N baseline BM	N/A	275/888 (31%) pooled patients [30]		79 (23%) [31]
IC-ORR (%) ITT population	N/A	18 (95% CI, 5–40) = untreated BM 33 (95% 13–59) = previously treated BM		77 vs. 28 (treated BM)

BM Brain metastases, *DOR* duration of response, *IC-ORR* intracranial objective response rate, *ITT* intention-to-treat, *N/A* non-applicable, *ORR* objective response rate, *PFS* progression-free survival, *1L* first line, *2L* second line
[a]Central ALK tested
[b]Local ALK tested

the chemotherapy arms to receive crizotinib upon disease progression. The phase III PROFILE 1014 study randomized 343 treatment-naïve ALK-positive NSCLC patients to crizotinib or platinum doublet chemotherapy [29]. The median PFS was longer with crizotinib at 10.9 months vs. 7.0 months (HR 0.45, 95% CI, 0.35–0.60, $p < 0.001$). Additionally, crizotinib was associated with a higher ORR (74% vs. 45%), duration of response (DOR) (11.3 months vs. 5.3 months), improved quality of life (QoL), and cancer-related symptoms. Recently, long-term follow-up reported an OS benefit when adjusted for crossover with a median OS of 59.8 months vs. 19.2 months (HR 0.345, 95% bootstrap CI, 0.081–0.718) [32]. This trial established crizotinib as the standard frontline treatment for ALK-positive NSCLC.

Second-Generation ALK Inhibitors

Ceritinib, alectinib, and brigatinib are second-generation ALK inhibitors with increased affinity against the ALK fusion gene and have improved CNS efficacy as compared to crizotinib. All three agents are currently FDA-approved for patients intolerant to or who experience disease progression with crizotinib. Ceritinib is 20-fold more potent as compared to crizotinib and also overcomes select resistance mutations associated with prior crizotinib treatment [33]. It was the first in its class to be FDA-approved for crizotinib-resistance ALK-positive NSCLC based upon the phase III ASCEND-5 study. The study randomized 231 previously treated patients with advanced ALK-positive NSCLC and gave certinib 750 mg once daily or single-agent chemotherapy [34]. Crossover was allowed following disease progression. Certinib resulted in a significantly longer PFS (5.4 months vs. 1.6 months, HR 0.49, 95% CI, 0.36–0.67, $p < 0.0001$), higher ORR (39.1% vs. 6.9%) with a median DOR of 6.9 months (95% CI, 5.4–8.9 months), and improved cancer-related symptoms. The most common AE of any grade were diarrhea, nausea, vomiting, decreased appetite, and elevations in alanine aminotransferase (ALT) and aspartate amino-transferase (AST). Dose adjustments or interruptions occurred in 80% of patients in the ceritinib group. Similar to crizotinib, ILD was rarely seen; there were 15 deaths (13%) in the certinib arm but none were treatment-related. Ceritinib was then tested in the frontline space with the phase III ASCEND-4 study comparing certinib to platinum doublet chemotherapy in treatment-naïve ALK-positive NSCLC [35]. As with crizotinib in the PROFILE 1014 study, certinib was associated with a longer median PFS (16.6 months vs. 8.1 months, HR 0.55, 95% CI 0.42–0.73, $p < 0.00001$), ORR (72.5% vs. 26.7%), DOR (23.9 months vs. 11.1 months), and cancer-related symptoms over upfront chemotherapy. Gastrointestinal toxicities remained a promi-nent AE with ceritinib, prompting evaluation with a lower dose. The ongoing phase I ASCEND-8 study is comparing lower doses of 450 mg and 600 mg once daily with a low-fat meal compared to the standard 750 mg once daily fasted dose [36]. Currently reported results are encouraging, showing that the 450 mg once daily dose produces similar systemic concentrations, comparable ORR, and improved tolerability compared with the standard 750 mg once daily fasted dose [36, 37].

Alectinib is another selective ALK inhibitor that is able to overcome resistance mutations from prior crizotinib exposure [38]. The phase II, single-arm study in North America enrolled 87 patients with advanced ALK-positive NSCLC who pro-gressed on crizotinib [39]. Alectinib 600 mg twice daily resulted in an ORR of 52% (95% CI, 40–61%), median DOR of 13.5 months (95% CI, 6.7–NR months), and median PFS of 8.1 months (95% CI, 6.2–12.6 months). The most common AE of any grade were constipation, fatigue, myalgia, and peripheral edema. Grade 3–4 elevations in ALT, AST, and creatinine phosphokinase (CPK) were most common but occurred in <10% of patients. There was one alectinib-related death due to hem-orrhage in a patient taking anticoagulation. Overall, alectinib was very well-tolerated with dose interruptions, reductions, and discontinuations occurring in 36%, 16%, and 2% of patients, respectively. Alectinib was further evaluated in the frontline set-ting compared to the standard of care crizotinib in the phase III J-ALEX and ALEX studies [14, 40]. Both trials randomized treatment-naïve ALK-positive NSCLC patients 1:1 to alectinib or crizotinib. The J-ALEX study only recruited patients from Japan and used a lower alectinib dose of 300 mg twice daily, based upon their phase I AF-001JP Japanese study [41]. The ALEX study recruited 303 patients from 98 centers internationally and used the standard alectinib dose of 600 mg twice daily. The inclusion criteria were similar between studies; the ALEX study additionally stratified patients based upon ECOG performance status (0 or 1 vs. 2), race (Asian vs. non-Asian), and the presence or absence of baseline brain metastases. The primary endpoint of PFS for both studies was significantly higher with alectinib. The investigator-assessed PFS was significantly longer in the alectinib arm (not reached vs. 11.1 months, HR 0.47, 95% CI, 0.34–0.65, $p < 0.001$). All subgroups benefited from alectinib. The ORR were similar between arms (82.9% vs. 75.5%, $p = 0.09$) and responses were durable; the 12-month event-free rate was 72.5% and 44.1%, respectively. The median OS was not estimable at the time of initial data analysis; the 12-month OS rate was 84.3% and 82.5% (HR 0.76, 95% CI, 0.48–1.20), respectively. Consistent with the phase I study, alectinib was well-tolerated; as compared to crizotinib, alectinib was associated with more anemia (20% vs. 5%), myalgia (16% vs. 2%), weight gain (10% vs. 0%), and photosensitivity reaction (5% vs. 0%). Crizotinib was associated with more gastrointestinal toxicities. There were similar grade 5 toxicities between crizotinib and alectinib (3% vs. 5%), and two were related to crizotinib but none were related to alectinib. Treatment reduction, interruption, and discontinuation were similar between arms, occurring with alectinib in 16%, 19%, and 11%, respectively. Following the results of the ALEX study, alectinib was granted regular approval by the FDA in November 2017 and became another frontline option for treatment-naïve ALK-positive NSCLC.

Brigatinib is the last second-generation ALK inhibitor, similarly more potent as compared to crizotinib and, like the other drugs in its class, can overcome select resistance mutations [42]. It was granted accelerated FDA approval in April 2017 for patients who progress or are intolerant to crizotinib, joining ceritinib and alectinib in this indication. Approval was based upon the results of the phase II ALTA study which included 222 patients who developed disease progression on crizotinib, randomized 1:1 to brigatinib 90 mg once daily (arm A) or 180 mg once daily with a 7-day lead-in at 90 mg once daily (arm B) [43]. Patients in arm A were allowed to receive the 180 mg once daily dose upon disease progression. Both arms produced similar investigator-assessed ORR (45% vs. 54%), and responses were durable (median DOR 13.8 months vs. 11.1 months). The median PFS was numerically longer in arm B at 12.9 months versus 9.2 months in arm A. The most common AE of any grade were nausea, vomiting, headache, and fatigue. Notable grade ≥ 3 AE (arms A/B) were hypertension (6%/6%), elevated CPK (3%/9%), elevated lipase (4%/3%), and pneumonia (3%/5%). Unique to brigatinib is the occurrence of pulmonary symptoms (dyspnea, cough, pneumonia, pneumonitis) occurring within 24–48 hours of treatment initiation [44]. These symptoms were believed to be due to a higher brigatinib starting dose that was mediated with the introduction of a 7-day lead-in at 90 mg once daily. There were 14 patients (6%) who experienced pulmonary AE, with a median time to onset of 2 days (range, 1–9 days). Six patients required dose interruption with successful reintroduction and one death that was not attributable to brigatinib. The improved median PFS in arm B led to its use in the phase III frontline study which randomized 275 treatment-naïve patients 1:1 to brigatinib or crizotinib (ALTA-1 L). The estimated 12-month PFS was 67% (95% CI, 56–75%) versus 43% (95% CI, 32–53%); HR 0.49 (95% CI 0.33–0.74, $p < 0.001$). Confirmed ORR were achieved in 71% vs. 60%, and responses were durable at the time of data analysis; the 12-month DOR was 78% vs. 48%. The survival data is not yet mature. The AE profile was similar to the phase II study; there were higher rates of elevated CPK (39% vs. 15%), cough (25% vs. 16%), hypertension (23% vs. 7%), and elevated lipase levels (19% vs. 12%) without any cases of pancreatitis. Grade 3–5 toxicities were similar between arms; there were 14 fatal events (7 in the brigatinib arm, 7 in the crizotinib arm) but none were treatment-related. The ALTA-1 L study established brigatinib as another potential treatment option with alectinib in the frontline space; it is currently pending FDA approval for this indication.

Third-Generation ALK Inhibitor

Lorlatinib is the sole third-generation ALK inhibitor at this time; it is approved for ALK-positive NSCLC patients who progressed on at least two ALK inhibitors with one being crizotinib or who progressed on alectinib or ceritinib if either is used in the frontline setting. Preclinical studies demonstrate that lorlatinib is a potent ALK and ROS1 inhibitor that can successfully penetrate the blood-brain barrier and overcome common resistance mutations seen with second-generation ALK TKIs, including G1202R [45]. The first-in-human phase I study in ALK or ROS1-positive NSCLC included 54 patients; 41 (76%) were ALK-positive, 28 (52%) had at ≥ 2 prior TKIs, and 39 (72%) had baseline brain metastases [46]. The most common AE were hypercholesterolemia, hypertriglyceridemia, peripheral edema, peripheral neuropathy, and transient cognitive effects. Gastrointestinal toxicities were uncommon. There were no dose-limiting toxicities or treatment-related deaths. The recommended phase II dose was 100 mg once daily. The single-arm, multicenter, phase II study enrolled 276 patients into one of six expansion cohorts (EXP1–6) based upon the patient's ALK or ROS1 status and prior treatment history [47]. Treatment-naïve patients were placed in EXP1 ($N = 30$), while different groups of prior ALK TKI failure were placed in EXP2–5 ($N = 198$). Patients with ROS1-positive NSCLC were placed in EXP6. In EXP1, ORR were seen in 27 patients (90%, 95% CI, 73.5–97.9%) with 85% of responses ongoing at the median follow-up of 6.9 months. In EXP2–5, responses were seen in 93 patients (47%, 95% CI, 39.9–54.2%) with 68% of responses ongoing. In patients who previously received crizotinib ($N = 59$), the ORR was 69.5% with 78% of responses ongoing. Responses were also seen in patients who received a second-generation ALK TKI as their last therapy; ORR were 37.1%, 40.4%, and 37.5% for alectinib ($N = 62$), ceritinib ($N = 47$), and brigatinib ($N = 8$), respectively. Furthermore, in patients who received two to three prior ALK TKIs ($N = 111$), the ORR was 38.7% with 60% ongoing responses at median follow-up of 7.2 months. The safety profile was overall similar to the phase I without any additional concerns. Tables 2 and 3 summarize the clinical trials evaluating the second- and third-generation ALK inhibitors for crizotinib-refractory and crizotinib-naïve ALK-positive NSCLC, respectively.

Table 2 Trials of second- and third-generation ALK inhibitors for crizotinib-refractory ALK-positive NSCLC

	Ceritinib			Alectinib				Brigatinib		Lorlatinib	
Trial name (phase)	ASCEND-1 [91] (phase I)	ASCEND-2 [92] (phase II)	ASCEND-5 [34] (phase III)	AF-002JG [53] (phase I/II)	NP28673 [93] (Global phase II)	NP28761 [39] (North American phase II)	ALUR [94] (phase III)	Phase I/II [44] muticohort	ALTA [43] (phase II)	Phase I [46]	Phase II [47] multicohort
Comparator arm	N/A	N/A	Pemetrexed or docetaxel (1:1)	N/A	N/A	N/A	Pemetrexed or docetaxel (2:1)	N/A	Brigatinib 90 mg, 90 mg → 180 mg (1:1)[a]	N/A	N/A; EXP2–5 w/ prior ALK TKI
N	163	140	231	47	138	87	107	137 (71 ALK-mutated)	222	54 (41 ALK-mutated)	276 (EXP2–5, 198)
ORR (%)	57 (95% CI, 49–64%)	38.6 (95% CI, 30.5–47.2)	39.1 vs. 6.9	55	50.8 (95% CI, 41.6–60.0)	52 (95% CI, 40–65)	37.5 vs. 2.9[b] (HR 2.9, 95% CI 0.346, 95% CI, 0.15–0.53)	72[b] (95% CI, 60–82)	45 vs. 54[b]	46[b] (95% CI, 31–63)	47 (95% CI, 39.9–54.2)
Median DOR (months)	8.3 (95% CI, 6.8–9.7)	9.7 (95% CI 7.1–11.1)	6.9 vs. 8.3	Not provided	15.2 (95% CI, 11.2–24.9)	13.5 (95% CI, 6.7–NE)	9.3 vs. 2.7[b]	11.2[b] (95% CI, 7.6–29.7)	13.8 vs. 11.1[b]	12.4[b] (95% CI, 6.5–NE)	NE (11.1–NE)
Median PFS (months)	6.9 (95% CI, 19.6–NE)	5.7 (95% CI, 5.4–7.6)	5.4 vs. 1.6 (HR 0.49, 95% CI, 0.36–0.67, p < 0.0001)	Not provided	8.9 (95% CI, 5.6–12.8)	8.1 (95% CI, 6.2–12.6)	9.6 vs. 1.4[b] (HR 0.15, 95% CI, 0.08–0.29, p < 0.001)	14.5[b] (95% CI, 9.2–NE) in crizotinib-refractory (N = 42)	9.2 vs. 12.9[b] (no PFS statistical comparison)	9.6[b] (95% CI 3.4–16.6)	7.3 (95% CI, 5.6–11.0)

(continued)

Table 2 (continued)

	Ceritinib			Alectinib				Brigatinib		Lorlatinib	
N BM	98 (60%)	100 (71.4%)	133 (58%)	21 (45%)	84 (61%)	52 (60%)	76 (71%)	50 (63%)	154 (69%)	32 (78%)	133 (67%)
IC-ORR (%) ITT population	18	33	35 vs. 5[c]	5/9 (56%)[c]	46.4 (95% CI, 35.5–57.7)	40 (95% CI, 27–55)	36 vs. C[b] (p < 0.C01)	39[b]	42 vs. 67[c]	31[b]	63[c] (95% CI, 51.5–73.4)

BM Brain metastases, *DOR* duration of response, *IC-ORR* intracranial objective response rate, *ITT* intention-to-treat, *N/A* non-applicable, *NE* not-estimable, *ORR* objective response rate, *PFS* progression-free survival

[a]The phase II ALTA study evaluated brigatinib 90 mg once daily with 90 mg lead-in for 7 days followed by 180 mg once daily

[b]Investigator-review. Remaining are based upon independent review

[c]Measurable BM

Table 3 Trials of second-generation ALK inhibitors for crizotinib-naïve ALK-positive NSCLC

	Ceritinib				Alectinib			Brigatinib
Trial name (indication)	ASCEND-1 [91] (phase I)	ASCEND-3 [95] (phase II)	ASCEND-4 [35] (phase III)	ASCEND-8 [37] (phase I)	AF001JP[a] [41] (Japan) (phase I/II)	J-ALEX [40] (Japan, phase III)	ALEX [14] (International, phase III)	ALTA-1 L [55] (phase III)
Comparator arm	N/A	N/A	Platinum doublet	Certinib 450 mg fed, 600 mg fed, 750 mg fasted (1:1:1)	N/A	Crizotinib (1:1)	Crizotinib (1:1)	Crizotinib (1:1)
N	83	124	376	198 (73, 51, 74)	Phase I = 24 phase II = 46	207	303	275
ORR (%)	72 (95% CI, 61–82)	63.7 (95% CI, 54.6–72.2)[b]	72.5 vs. 26.7	78.1, 72.5, 75.7	93.5 (95% CI, 82.1–98.6) in phase II	92 vs. 79	82.9 vs. 75.5[b] (p = 0.09)	71 vs. 60
Median DOR (months)	17 (95% CI, 11.3–NE)	9.3 (95% CI, 9.1–NE)[b]	23.9 vs. 11.1	NE, 20.7, 15.4	7.1 (range, 1–11)	NE vs. 11.1	NE vs. 11.1[b]	NE vs. 11.1
Median PFS (months)	18.4 (95% CI, 11.1–NE)	11.1 (95% CI, 9.3–NE)[b]	16.6 vs. 8.1 (HR 0.55, 95% CI 0.42–0.73, p < 0.00001)	NE, 17.0, 12.2	NE	NE vs. 10.2 (HR 0.34, 95% CI, 0.17–0.71, p < 0.0001)	NE vs. 11.1[b] (HR 0.47, 95% CI, 0.34–0.65, p < 0.001)	NE vs. 9.8 (HR 0.49, 95% CI, 0.33–0.74, p < 0.001)
N (brain mets)	26 (31%)	50 (40%)	121 (32%)	Not provided	15 (33%) in phase II	43 (21%)	122 (40%)	81 (29%)
IC-ORR (%) ITT-population	42	10/17 (58.8%)[c]	46.3 vs. 21.2	Not provided	Not provided	Not provided	59 vs. 26[a]	67 vs. 17

BM Brain metastases, *DOR* duration of response, *IC-ORR* intracranial objective response rate, *ITT* intention-to-treat, *N/A* non-applicable, *NE* not-estimable, *ORR* objective response rate, *PFS* progression-free survival

[a]The phase II recommended dose in AF001JP was alectinib 300 mg twice daily which was studied in the Japanese phase III J-ALEX study. The international phase III ALEX study used the FDA-approved dose of alectinib 600 mg twice daily

[b]Investigator-review. Remaining are based upon independent review

[c]Measurable BM

CNS Efficacy

Approximately 25% of patients with ALK-rearranged NSCLC will develop brain metastases [48]. Although crizotinib has improved outcomes for patients with advanced ALK-positive NSCLC, the CNS remains a common site of treatment failure [30]. In the PROFILE 1014 study, the intracranial disease control rate (IC-DCR), defined as the percent of patients achieving at least stable disease intracranially, was significantly longer at up to 24 weeks (56% vs. 25%, $p = 0.006$) with crizotinib vs. chemotherapy [31]. Despite providing initial control of intracranial disease, the intracranial time to progression (IC-TTP), defined as the time from randomization to intracranial progressive disease (IC-PD), was not significantly different from patients who received chemotherapy (HR 0.60, 95% CI 0.34–1.05, $p = 0.069$ in the intention to treat population (ITT)). Intracranial-only PD was more common with crizotinib than chemotherapy (24% vs. 10%). It is believed that the mechanism of IC-PD with crizotinib is attributed to its poor CNS penetration due to P-glycoprotein (PGP) efflux transporters that decrease the concentration of crizotinib in this space [49, 50].

The second-generation ALK TKIs demonstrate improved CNS efficacy due to their increased potency and improved CNS penetration. In the post-crizotinib studies, approximately 60–70% of patients have baseline brain metastases [34, 39, 43, 47]. These studies included asymptomatic untreated or treated brain metastases completed at least 14 days before enrollment. In the ASCEND-5 study comparing certinib to single-agent chemotherapy, the median PFS continued to favor ceritinib regardless of baseline brain metastases (4.4 months vs. 1.4 months, HR 0.50, 95% CI, 0.33–0.76) [34]. Intracranial and extracranial responses were similar, but ceritinib failure in the CNS alone occurred in 51% vs. 67%, respectively. Certinib, like crizotinib, is a PGP substrate and may explain the eventual CNS failure despite being a more potent drug [51]. In contrast to ceritinib, alectinib is not a substrate of the PGP efflux system supporting its improved CNS activity [52]. This finding was further validated in the phase I/II study of alectinib in crizotinib-resistant ALK-positive NSCLC, where there was a linear relationship between alectinib cerebrospinal fluid (CSF) and systemic concentrations [53]. In pooled analysis of this cohort, patients with untreated brain metastases ($N = 41$) demonstrated an intracranial ORR (IC-ORR) of 58.5% (95% CI, 42.1–73.7%) of which 48.8% achieved an intracranial complete response (IC-CR) [54]. Intracranial responses were durable, lasting a median of 11.1 months (95% CI, 10.3–NR months) among patients with measurable or nonmeasurable baseline brain metastases ($N = 136$). In the ALEX study, alectinib also reported similar IC-ORR of 81% (38% with IC-CR) and 59% (45% with IC-CR) in patients with measurable disease ($N = 21$) and measurable or nonmeasurable disease ($N = 64$), respectively. The responses were more durable and delayed the incidence of CNS progression with alectinib as compared to crizotinib. The IC-DOR in patients with measurable CNS disease was 17.3 months (95% CI, 14.8–NR months) vs. 5.5 months (95% CI 2.1–17.3 months), respectively. In the ITT population, the 12-month cumulative incidence of CNS progression was 9.4% (95% CI, 5.4%–14.7%) versus 41.4% (95% CI, 33.2–49.4), respectively [14].

Brigatinib was similarly efficacious in both phase I/II crizotinib-failure cohorts and ALK-inhibitor-naïve cohorts in the phase III ALTA-1 L study. The ALTA-1 L study reported an independent review committee (IRC)-assessed IC-ORR of 67% (95% CI, 51–81%) with 37% achieving IC-CR among alectinib-treated patients with measurable or nonmeasurable baseline brain metastases ($N = 43$). Responses were durable and delayed the incidence of CNS progression as compared to crizotinib. The cumulative incidence of CNS progression was 9% vs. 19% (HR 0.30, 95% CI 0.15–0.60). The improved CNS efficacy of alectinib and brigatinib as compared to crizotinib in the phase III studies should be a taken into account when deciding upfront ALK TKI therapy.

Finally, lorlatinib has been associated with improved CNS efficacy and its ability to overcome common resistance mutations associated with second-generation ALK inhibitors, making it an exciting drug. In the patients with prior ALK TKI failure ($N = 81$), the IRC-assessed IC-ORR was 63% (95% CI, 51.5–73.4%) with 20% achieving an IC-CR. The intracranial responses were durable, with a median DOR of 14.5 months (95% CI, 8.4–14.5 months). In patients who received ≥2 prior ALK TKIs ($N = 49$), the IRC-assessed IC-ORR was comparable at 53.1% (95% CI, 38.3–67.5%) and a similar median DOR of 14.5 months (95% CI 6.9–14.5 months) [47]. Lorlatinib produces a high intracranial response that is durable, even in the most heavily pretreated ALK-positive NSCLC. Tables 2 and 3 summarize the intracranial activity of second- and third-generation ALK inhibitors for crizotinib-refractory and crizotinib-naïve ALK-positive NSCLC, respectively.

Sequencing ALK Inhibitors

Currently, there are five ALK TKIs for the treatment of advanced ALK-mutated NSCLC, of which crizotinib, ceritinib, and alectinib are FDA-approved in the front-line setting (brigatinib is likely to be also approved for this indication). Prior to the seminal publication of the J-ALEX and ALEX studies, crizotinib and certinib were first-line options followed by ceritinib (if not previously exposed), alectinib, or brigatinib upon disease progression. In the post-ALEX era, alectinib joined crizotinib and ceritinib as the potential first-line option, with many selecting alectinib given its PFS advantage and improved AE profile over crizotinib. Questions remain on whether upfront alectinib improves OS as compared to serial ALK TKI use with crizotinib followed by ceritinib or alectinib upon disease progression. There is no data to currently answer this clinical question as the survival data from the ALEX trials are not yet mature. Keeping in mind the limitations with combining data from different studies, we can estimate the PFS between alectinib and serial ALK TKI treatment with crizotinib followed by alectinib. The median PFS of crizotinib in the phase III ALEX trial was 10.4 months (95% CI, 7.7–14.6 months) and of alectinib in the phase II trial following crizotinib failure was 8.1 months (95% CI, 6.2–12.6 months), which estimates a total median PFS of crizotinib followed by alectinib upon progression of 18.5 months (range, 13.9–27.2 months) [14, 39]. For comparison, in the ALEX trial, alectinib was associated with a median PFS of 25.7 months (95% CI, 19.9–NR). Given the current available data, alectinib is a reasonable first-line treatment option for advanced ALK-positive NSCLC given its prolonged PFS and favorable AE profile as compared to crizotinib. Following the publication of the ALTA-1 L study, brigatinib will likely be added as an option for treatment-naïve patients. There are no planned head-to-head trials comparing alectinib to brigatinib, both of which demonstrated a significantly longer PFS compared to crizotinib. Understanding the limitations of cross-trial comparisons, the HR for PFS are similar between alectinib (HR 0.50, 95% CI, 0.36–0.70) and brigatinib (HR 0.49, 95% CI, 0.33–0.74) [14, 55]. Additionally, the systemic and intracranial responses are comparable with longer delays in CNS progression versus upfront crizotinib. Both drugs are well-tolerated with slightly different side effect profiles. Brigatinib is administered once daily with a 7-day lead-in, while alectinib is administered twice daily. When brigatinib is approved in the frontline setting, patients will need to make an individualized decision based upon these factors as both agents are equally efficacious in the upfront setting.

Patients with advanced ALK-positive NSCLC now have a plethora of treatment options before resorting to systemic chemotherapy. Newer generation ALK TKIs are more potent, durable, and with an improved side effect profile as compared to crizotinib. These agents also possess improved CNS activity to overcome the failure of crizotinib in this space. The current dilemma now is figuring out how best to sequence the currently available ALK TKIs and the next generation of drugs. Ensartinib (X-396) and entrectinib are two novel TKIs with activity against ALK that show promise in early phase studies [56, 57]. Additionally, lorlatinib (NCT03052608) and ensartinib (NCT02767804) are also being compared to crizotinib in the frontline setting for treatment-naïve ALK-positive NSCLC.

Mechanisms of Resistance

Types of Resistance

ALK-mediated NSCLC is classified as an oncogene addicted cancer, which depends upon the ALK pathway for proliferation and will either undergo apoptosis or transition to a quiescent cell state in the presence of an ALK inhibitor. Eventually, both in vivo and in vitro, tumors will develop resistance through multiple mechanisms, which will be discussed here. While pharmacologic resistance can develop through issues with compliance, absorption through the GI tract, differences in enzymatic metabolism including drug interactions, and differences in penetration of the blood-brain barrier, these mechanisms are issues of inadequate drug exposure [58]. Mechanisms to be further explored here entail acquired biological resistance or resistance that occurs in the setting of adequate drug exposure after initial response to ALK TKI therapy.

ALK-Dependent Mechanisms of Resistance

Secondary Mutations

ALK-dependent mechanisms of overcoming these TKIs include methods of increasing the ALK signal to downstream cellular pathways. Secondary mutations in the ALK tyrosine kinase domain alter the activity of the kinase often by weakening or blocking binding of the aforementioned TKIs. Largely these are point mutations that alter a single amino acid, changing the binding domain. These mutations will be discussed by generation of ALK TKI as they have been discovered with the use of these drugs.

As sole first-generation ALK TKI, crizotinib drove early trials and aided in the discovery of secondary mutations. L1196 is considered the ALK gatekeeper residue—the critical amino acid that lies deep within the ATP-binding pocket and affects drug binding—with the L1196M mutation affecting drug binding via steric hindrance as well as stabilization of the active protein conformation. This residue is considered analogous to the EGFR gatekeeper T790M, which is implicated in 50–65% of EGFR-resistant cases. However, as opposed to the EGFR T790M, L1196M is not implicated in a majority of resistant cases, much like with the gatekeeper of CML with T315I [59–61].

C1156Y is on the edge of the kinase-binding pocket and may somewhat inhibit binding; however, more likely the mechanism of resistance is allosteric interference [60]. Similarly, L1152R does not affect the binding pocket but decreases downstream ALK effects [62]. Other mutations discovered include G1202R and S1206Y, which are located at the solvent front of the kinase domain and likely interfere with ALK activity through steric hindrance and possibly through conformational changes [63]. 1151Tins is thought to cause a change in affinity of ALK for ATP, decreasing activity [63]. G1269A also interferes with ALK activity through steric hindrance [61]. Finally, D1203N induces resistance through an unknown mechanism [64].

With regard to second-generation ALK TKIs, ceritinib selects for resistance most commonly through G1202R, F1174C, and F1174 L; the latter two are thought to stabilize the active conformation of the kinase domain leading to increased ATP binding. In addition, a novel mutation G1202del was identified, which is thought to shift the 1203 aspartate leading to steric interference [65]. In addition, case reports noted G1123S sterically inhibits binding and/or interferes with the glycine-rich loop important in TKI binding [66]. Lastly, L1152R was shown to confer resistance to ceritinib [67]. A study of patients who progressed on ceritinib did show C1156Y as possibly contributing to resistance; however, both biopsy samples in this study showed compound mutations, one with I1171N and the other with V1180L [65].

Alectinib selects for resistance through G1202R, 1151Tins, I1171T, I1171S, I1171N, and V1180 L with I1171 and V1180 L mutations destabilizing the alectinib and ALK complex through steric interference; I1171 is also thought to stabilize the activated ALK conformation [63, 65, 66, 68–71]. Brigatinib also selects for G1202R with some partial resistance contributed from the G1202del mutation [65]. The newest generation ALK TKI, lorlatinib, has been shown to be effective against all known mutations, except L1198F through steric interference. However, while this mutation provided resistance to lorlatinib, it re-induced sensitivity to crizotinib [72].

Amplification

Amplification of the ALK gene, or copy number gain (CNG) defined as an ALK to centromere 2 ratio of ≥2.0, can lead to increased expression of ALK. This method of increasing ALK has been noted in a small percentage of patients who progress on crizotinib therapy, without other identifiable mutations [61, 63]. Amplification has also been posited as an intermediate step between sensitivity and resistance via other mechanisms, as a cellular line of ALK+ cells developed CNG and partial resistance to crizotinib and then later developed secondary mutations and resistance to higher doses of crizotinib [73]. When occurring after first-generation therapy and without other mutations, this mechanism can often be overcome with second-generation or later therapy, as these are more potent ALK TKIs.

ALK-Independent Mechanisms of Resistance

Bypass Signaling Pathways

ALK-independent resistance occurs when oncogenically addicted cells exposed to an ALK TKI subvert the ALK pathway as the driving force for proliferation and instead upregulate alternate signaling pathways to activate the downstream drivers PI3K/AKT, JAK3-STAT3, and RAS/ERK.

An alternative pathway ripe for adjunct targeting is via EGFR. In vitro studies of a patient who progressed on crizotinib therapy identified both a secondary mutation and strongly increased EGFR and MET phosphorylation without an EGFR mutation or amplification via upregulation of the EGFR ligand amphiregulin. Partial inhibition of growth was achieved with an ALK TKI; however, a pan-ERBB inhibitor was significantly more effective in restricting growth [62]. Another in vitro study created ceritinib-resistant cells without secondary or amplification mutations from a parental EML4-ALK rearranged NSCLC cell line. The resistant cell line exhibited decreased ALK phosphorylation and concomitantly exhibited increased EGFR phosphorylation not via EGFR mutation or amplification, but via upregulated TGFα, an EGFR ligand. This was confirmed by knockout of TGFα in these cells resulting in increased sensitivity to ceritinib [74].

In crizotinib-resistant EML4-ALK cells without secondary mutations, increased phosphorylation of EGFR and related HER2 and HER3 proteins was detected, mediated by increased EGF, a ligand for this family of proteins. This finding was confirmed by exposing the cells to an irreversible EGFR TKI, which induced apoptosis. Finally, incubation of the parental cell line—prior to exposure with crizotinib—to exogenous EGF induced resistance to crizotinib [75]. Similarly, two separate cell lines without secondary mutations were generated with resistance to alectinib and ceritinib, respectively. Phosphorylated EGFR, IGF-1R, and HER3 levels were increased with a downstream increase in phosphorylated AKT and ERK mediated by NRG1, another EGFR ligand. As in the previous example, exogenous NRG1 incubation induced ALK resistance in the parental cells (prior to ALK TKI exposure) [76].

As opposed to EGFR-driven alternative signaling, KIT has also been implicated. In a crizotinib resistance tumor sample, KIT gene amplification with increased KIT protein levels was driven by SCF, the KIT ligand. In an in vitro sample, treatment with imatinib, a KIT inhibitor, reversed the resistant phenotype [63]. Indeed, EGFR mutations, KRAS mutations, ErbB phosphorylation, KIT amplification, IFG-1R pathway activation, and increased EGFR ligands have all been implicated as resistance mechanisms in ALK+ NSCLC [77].

Transformation

Change in morphology has also been shown as an ALK-independent mechanism of inducing resistance. Epithelial to mesenchymal transition (EMT) occurs when epithelial cells transition to mesenchymal cell in order to become more motile and invasive through the loss of junctions, apical-basal polarity, and reorganization of their cytoskeletons primarily via TGF-β [78]. This transition was noted as a resistance mechanism in a crizotinib-resistant cell line which phenotypically changed to spindle-shaped cells as well as exhibiting a decrease in E-cadherin and increase in vimentin and AXL driven by TGF-β1 [79]. Alternatively, rarely transformation into small cell lung cancer has been noted in case reports, with preservation of ALK positivity in the small cell sample [80–85]. While the exact mechanism is unknown, loss of the retinoblastoma gene is implicated in transformation of EGFR-positive NSCLC to small cell lung cancer and may occur via a similar mechanism in ALK-positive NSCLC [86].

Overcoming Resistance

When progression on ALK TKI therapy occurs, identification of oligoprogressive disease—stability of disease overall with limited areas of progression—should be elucidated. As crizotinib does not effectively penetrate the blood-brain barrier, CNS-only progression may be managed by CNS radiation alone with continuation of crizotinib assuming the extracranial disease is stable, or switching to a second generation ALK TKI with better brain penetrance. Alternatively, oligoprogression outside the CNS (in four or fewer sites) amenable to local ablative therapy via either surgery or radiation should be treated to remove or suppress clones that have locally developed resistance mechanisms. In a study of patients who continued on crizotinib after oligoprogression treated with local ablative therapy, treatment led to extended disease control by greater than 6 months [87].

Patients with diffuse systemic progression on ALK TKI could be considered for a post-progression biopsy. As discussed earlier, secondary resistance mutations to ALK TKIs can occur and vary based upon the type of ALK TKI used. Patients who develop resistance to crizotinib will often respond to second-generation TKIs as these are more potent, and can overcome CNG and secondary resistance mutations. Furthermore, the second-generation TKIs are FDA-approved following crizotinib regardless of post-progression testing and in this setting, ALK resistance mutations only occur in 20% of patients [65]. For patients progressing on second-generation TKIs, ALK resistance mutations are seen at a higher rate in 56% of patients, so post-progression biopsies can be considered. These mutations are heterogenous and can impact TKI selection. Patients with F1174 mutations after ceritinib therapy are still sensitive to alectinib and brigatinib, while patients with I1171 mutations after alectinib are still sensitive to ceritinib. Patients with G1202R mutations are pan-resistant to second-generation ALK TKIs but are sensitive to lorlatinib and brigatinib. Resistance generated to lorlatinib through L1198F can be overcome with the use of the first-generation ALK TKI crizotinib [43, 65, 70, 72]. There is emerging evidence that ALK resistance mutations may serve as a biomarker for response to lorlatinib in select patients. Patients enrolled in the lorlatinib phase II multicohort study [47] were evaluated in the setting of the presence or absence of ALK resistance mutations detected on tissue or plasma molecular profiling [96]. Patients who only received crizotinib derived similar outcomes regardless of the presence or absence of ALK resistance mutations. However, patients who previously received one or more second generation ALK TKIs had a higher ORR if an ALK resistance mutation was found in either the tissue (69% vs. 27%, respectively) or plasma (62% vs. 32%, respectively). Moreover, in patients with ALK resistance mutations detected in the tissue, PFS was significantly longer (11.0 months vs. 5.4 months, HR 0.47; 95% CI, 0.27–0.83) with a median DOR of 24.4 months compared to 4.3 months, respectively. This data suggests that in patients previously treated with a second-generation ALK TKI, the persistence of an ALK-dependent mechanism of resistance may predict a better response to lorlatinib. It should be noted that in this heavily pretreated population, even in the absence of ALK resistance mutations, response rates are still ~30%. Further confirmatory studies are needed.

Once treatment with TKIs has been exhausted, chemotherapy and clinical trial options should be considered. In this context, ALK TKI continuation can be considered as removal of ALK suppression may cause flare up of a population of cells that were previously in a quiescent state as noted in EGFR NSCLC patients [88]. With regard to the choice of chemotherapy, pemetrexed use in ALK+ versus wild-type patients has been associated with ORR of 46.7% and PFS of 9.2 months compared to 16.2% and 2.9 months, respectively. The proposed mechanism of this sensitivity is twofold. Lower levels of thymidylate synthase in ALK+ NSCLC are targeted by pemetrexed. In addition, ATIC, an enzyme that catalyzes a portion of purine biosynthesis, is posited to be a substrate for ALK-mediated phosphorylation and is also targeted by pemetrexed [89, 90]. Finally, multiple clinical trials with the use of ALK TKI in combination with PD-1/PD-L1 inhibitors are underway [59].

Conclusion

ALK-rearranged NSCLC is uncommon but a very treatable population of advanced NSCLC. Testing all newly diagnosed advanced NSCLC patients for ALK gene rearrangements with any of the approved diagnostic tests (FISH, IHC, RT-PCR, NGS) should be standard of care with a high index of suspicion in nonsmokers. We now have three generations of ALK TKIs that are increasingly more effective, durable, and actively penetrate into the CNS. Clinicians have options when deciding frontline therapy and should consider not only the TKI efficacy but also the side effect profile, drug administration, and presence of baseline brain metastases. Unfortunately, resistance will inevitably develop via ALK-dependent and ALK-independent mechanisms. The more potent newer-generation ALK TKIs can overcome common ALK-dependent mechanisms such as point mutations and ALK gene amplifications. Post-progression biopsies can be considered to evaluate for mechanisms of resistance but remain an active area of research. The landscape for ALK-positive NSCLC continues to evolve in our understanding and management of this disease.

References

1. Soda M, Choi YL, Enomoto M, et al. Identification of the transforming EML4-ALK fusion gene in non-small-cell lung cancer. Nature. 2007;448:561–6.
2. Morris SW, Naeve C, Mathew P, et al. ALK, the chromosome 2 gene locus altered by the t(2;5) in non-Hodgkin's lymphoma, encodes a novel neural receptor tyrosine kinase that is highly related to leukocyte tyrosine kinase (LTK). Oncogene. 1997;14:2175–88.
3. Iwahara T, Fujimoto J, Wen D, et al. Molecular characterization of ALK, a receptor tyrosine kinase expressed specifically in the nervous system. Oncogene. 1997;14:439–49.
4. Vernersson E, Khoo NK, Henriksson ML, et al. Characterization of the expression of the ALK receptor tyrosine kinase in mice. Gene Expr Patterns. 2006;6:448–61.
5. Takeuchi K, Choi YL, Togashi Y, et al. KIF5B-ALK, a novel fusion oncokinase identified by an immunohistochemistry-based diagnostic system for ALK-positive lung cancer. Clin Cancer Res. 2009;15:3143–9.
6. Togashi Y, Soda M, Sakata S, et al. KLC1-ALK: a novel fusion in lung cancer identified using a formalin-fixed paraffin-embedded tissue only. PLoS One. 2012;7:e31323.
7. Sasaki T, Rodig SJ, Chirieac LR, et al. The biology and treatment of EML4-ALK non-small cell lung cancer. Eur J Cancer. 2010;46:1773–80.
8. Heuckmann JM, Balke-Want H, Malchers F, et al. Differential protein stability and ALK inhibitor sensitivity of EML4-ALK fusion variants. Clin Cancer Res. 2012;18:4682–90.
9. Koivunen JP, Mermel C, Zejnullahu K, et al. EML4-ALK fusion gene and efficacy of an ALK kinase inhibitor in lung cancer. Clin Cancer Res. 2008;14:4275–83.
10. Yoshida T, Oya Y, Tanaka K, et al. Differential crizotinib response duration among ALK fusion variants in ALK-positive non-small-cell lung cancer. J Clin Oncol. 2016;34:3383–9.
11. Li Y, Zhang T, Zhang J, et al. Response to crizotinib in advanced ALK-rearranged non-small cell lung cancers with different ALK-fusion variants. Lung Cancer. 2018;118:128–33.
12. Woo CG, Seo S, Kim SW, et al. Differential protein stability and clinical responses of EML4-ALK fusion variants to various ALK inhibitors in advanced ALK-rearranged non-small cell lung cancer. Ann Oncol. 2017;28:791–7.

13. Lin JJ, Zhu VW, Yoda S, et al. Impact of EML4-ALK variant on resistance mechanisms and clinical outcomes in ALK-positive lung cancer. J Clin Oncol. 2018;36:1199–206.
14. Peters S, Camidge DR, Shaw AT, et al. Alectinib versus crizotinib in untreated ALK-positive non-small-cell lung cancer. N Engl J Med. 2017;377:829–38.
15. Dziadziuszko RTSM, Camidge DR, Shaw AT, Noe J, Nowicka M, Liu T, Mitry E, Peters S. Impact of the EML4-ALK variant on the efficacy of alectinib (ALC) in untreated ALK+ advanced NSCLC (aNSCLC) in the global phase III ALEX study. Ann Oncol. 2018;29. https://academic.oup.com/annonc/article/29/suppl_8/mdy292.002/5141572
16. Inamura K, Takeuchi K, Togashi Y, et al. EML4-ALK fusion is linked to histological characteristics in a subset of lung cancers. J Thorac Oncol. 2008;3:13–7.
17. Inamura K, Takeuchi K, Togashi Y, et al. EML4-ALK lung cancers are characterized by rare other mutations, a TTF-1 cell lineage, an acinar histology, and young onset. Mod Pathol. 2009;22:508–15.
18. Martelli MP, Sozzi G, Hernandez L, et al. EML4-ALK rearrangement in non-small cell lung cancer and non-tumor lung tissues. Am J Pathol. 2009;174:661–70.
19. Kris MG, Johnson BE, Berry LD, et al. Using multiplexed assays of oncogenic drivers in lung cancers to select targeted drugs. JAMA. 2014;311:1998–2006.
20. Shaw AT, Yeap BY, Mino-Kenudson M, et al. Clinical features and outcome of patients with non-small-cell lung cancer who harbor EML4-ALK. J Clin Oncol. 2009,27.4247–53.
21. Hallberg B, Palmer RH. Mechanistic insight into ALK receptor tyrosine kinase in human cancer biology. Nat Rev Cancer. 2013;13:685–700.
22. Drilon A, Wang L, Arcila ME, et al. Broad, hybrid capture-based next-generation sequencing identifies actionable genomic alterations in lung adenocarcinomas otherwise negative for such alterations by other genomic testing approaches. Clin Cancer Res. 2015;21:3631–9.
23. Peled N, Palmer G, Hirsch FR, et al. Next-generation sequencing identifies and immunohistochemistry confirms a novel crizotinib-sensitive ALK rearrangement in a patient with metastatic non-small-cell lung cancer. J Thorac Oncol. 2012;7:e14–6.
24. Christensen JG, Zou HY, Arango ME, et al. Cytoreductive antitumor activity of PF-2341066, a novel inhibitor of anaplastic lymphoma kinase and c-Met, in experimental models of anaplastic large-cell lymphoma. Mol Cancer Ther. 2007;6:3314–22.
25. Kwak EL, Bang YJ, Camidge DR, et al. Anaplastic lymphoma kinase inhibition in non-small-cell lung cancer. N Engl J Med. 2010;363:1693–703.
26. Camidge DR, Bang YJ, Kwak EL, et al. Activity and safety of crizotinib in patients with ALK-positive non-small-cell lung cancer: updated results from a phase 1 study. Lancet Oncol. 2012;13:1011–9.
27. Blackhall F, Ross Camidge D, Shaw AT, et al. Final results of the large-scale multinational trial PROFILE 1005: efficacy and safety of crizotinib in previously treated patients with advanced/metastatic ALK-positive non-small-cell lung cancer. ESMO Open. 2017;2:e000219.
28. Shaw AT, Kim DW, Nakagawa K, et al. Crizotinib versus chemotherapy in advanced ALK-positive lung cancer. N Engl J Med. 2013;368:2385–94.
29. Solomon BJ, Mok T, Kim DW, et al. First-line crizotinib versus chemotherapy in ALK-positive lung cancer. N Engl J Med. 2014;371:2167–77.
30. Costa DB, Shaw AT, Ou SH, et al. Clinical experience with crizotinib in patients with advanced ALK-rearranged non-small-cell lung Cancer and brain metastases. J Clin Oncol. 2015;33:1881–8.
31. Solomon BJ, Cappuzzo F, Felip E, et al. Intracranial efficacy of crizotinib versus chemotherapy in patients with advanced ALK-positive non-small-cell lung cancer: results from PROFILE 1014. J Clin Oncol. 2016;34:2858–65.
32. Solomon BJ, Kim DW, Wu YL, et al. Final overall survival analysis from a study comparing first-line crizotinib versus chemotherapy in ALK-mutation-positive non-small-cell lung cancer. J Clin Oncol. 2018;36:2251–8.
33. Friboulet L, Li N, Katayama R, et al. The ALK inhibitor ceritinib overcomes crizotinib resistance in non-small cell lung cancer. Cancer Discov. 2014;4:662–73.

34. Shaw AT, Kim TM, Crinò L, et al. Ceritinib versus chemotherapy in patients with ALK-rearranged non-small-cell lung cancer previously given chemotherapy and crizotinib (ASCEND-5): a randomised, controlled, open-label, phase 3 trial. Lancet Oncol. 2017;18:874–86.
35. Soria JC, Tan DSW, Chiari R, et al. First-line ceritinib versus platinum-based chemotherapy in advanced ALK-rearranged non-small-cell lung cancer (ASCEND-4): a randomised, open-label, phase 3 study. Lancet. 2017;389:917–29.
36. Cho BC, Kim DW, Bearz A, et al. ASCEND-8: a randomized phase 1 study of ceritinib, 450 mg or 600 mg, taken with a low-fat meal versus 750 mg in fasted state in patients with anaplastic lymphoma kinase (ALK)-rearranged metastatic non-small cell lung cancer (NSCLC). J Thorac Oncol. 2017;12:1357–67.
37. Cho BC, Obermannova R, Orlov SV, et al. LBA59Primary efficacy and updated safety of ceritinib (450 mg or 600 mg) with food vs 750 mg fasted in ALK+ metastatic NSCLC (ASCEND-8). Ann Oncol. 2018;29:mdy424.071.
38. Kodama T, Tsukaguchi T, Yoshida M, et al. Selective ALK inhibitor alectinib with potent antitumor activity in models of crizotinib resistance. Cancer Lett. 2014;351:215–21.
39. Shaw AT, Gandhi L, Gadgeel S, et al. Alectinib in ALK-positive, crizotinib-resistant, non-small-cell lung cancer: a single-group, multicentre, phase 2 trial. Lancet Oncol. 2016;17:234–42.
40. Hida T, Nokihara H, Kondo M, et al. Alectinib versus crizotinib in patients with ALK-positive non-small-cell lung cancer (J-ALEX): an open-label, randomised phase 3 trial. Lancet. 2017;390:29–39.
41. Seto T, Kiura K, Nishio M, et al. CH5424802 (RO5424802) for patients with ALK-rearranged advanced non-small-cell lung cancer (AF-001JP study): a single-arm, open-label, phase 1-2 study. Lancet Oncol. 2013;14:590–8.
42. Zhang S, Anjum R, Squillace R, et al. The potent ALK inhibitor brigatinib (AP26113) overcomes mechanisms of resistance to first- and second-generation ALK inhibitors in preclinical models. Clin Cancer Res. 2016;22:5527–38.
43. Kim DW, Tiseo M, Ahn MJ, et al. Brigatinib in patients with crizotinib-refractory anaplastic lymphoma kinase-positive non-small-cell lung Cancer: a randomized, multicenter phase II trial. J Clin Oncol. 2017;35:2490–8.
44. Gettinger SN, Bazhenova LA, Langer CJ, et al. Activity and safety of brigatinib in ALK-rearranged non-small-cell lung cancer and other malignancies: a single-arm, open-label, phase 1/2 trial. Lancet Oncol. 2016;17:1683–96.
45. Zou HY, Friboulet L, Kodack DP, et al. PF-06463922, an ALK/ROS1 inhibitor, overcomes resistance to first and second generation ALK inhibitors in preclinical models. Cancer Cell. 2015;28:70–81.
46. Shaw AT, Felip E, Bauer TM, et al. Lorlatinib in non-small-cell lung cancer with ALK or ROS1 rearrangement: an international, multicentre, open-label, single-arm first-in-man phase 1 trial. Lancet Oncol. 2017;18:1590–9.
47. Solomon BJ, Besse B, Bauer TM, et al. Lorlatinib in patients with ALK-positive non-small-cell lung cancer: results from a global phase 2 study. Lancet Oncol. 2018;19:1654–67.
48. Rangachari D, Yamaguchi N, VanderLaan PA, et al. Brain metastases in patients with EGFR-mutated or ALK-rearranged non-small-cell lung cancers. Lung Cancer. 2015;88:108–11.
49. Costa DB, Kobayashi S, Pandya SS, et al. CSF concentration of the anaplastic lymphoma kinase inhibitor crizotinib. J Clin Oncol. 2011;29:e443–5.
50. Johnson TW, Richardson PF, Bailey S, et al. Discovery of (10R)-7-amino-12-fluoro-2,10,16-trimethyl-15-oxo-10,15,16,17-tetrahydro-2H-8,4-(m etheno)pyrazolo[4,3-h][2,5,11]-benzoxadiazacyclotetradecine-3-carbonitrile (PF-06463922), a macrocyclic inhibitor of anaplastic lymphoma kinase (ALK) and c-ros oncogene 1 (ROS1) with preclinical brain exposure and broad-spectrum potency against ALK-resistant mutations. J Med Chem. 2014;57:4720–44.

51. Katayama R, Sakashita T, Yanagitani N, et al. P-glycoprotein mediates ceritinib resistance in anaplastic lymphoma kinase-rearranged non-small cell lung cancer. EBioMedicine. 2016;3:54–66.
52. Kodama T, Hasegawa M, Takanashi K, et al. Antitumor activity of the selective ALK inhibitor alectinib in models of intracranial metastases. Cancer Chemother Pharmacol. 2014;74:1023–8.
53. Gadgeel SM, Gandhi L, Riely GJ, et al. Safety and activity of alectinib against systemic disease and brain metastases in patients with crizotinib-resistant ALK-rearranged non-small-cell lung cancer (AF-002JG): results from the dose-finding portion of a phase 1/2 study. Lancet Oncol. 2014;15:1119–28.
54. Gadgeel SM, Shaw AT, Govindan R, et al. Pooled analysis of CNS response to alectinib in two studies of pretreated patients with ALK-positive non-small-cell lung cancer. J Clin Oncol. 2016;34:4079–85.
55. Camidge DR, Kim HR, Ahn MJ, et al. Brigatinib versus crizotinib in ALK-positive non-small-cell lung cancer. N Engl J Med. 2018;379:2027–39.
56. Horn L, Infante JR, Reckamp KL, et al. Ensartinib (X-396) in ALK-positive non-small cell lung cancer: results from a first-in-human phase I/II, multicenter study. Clin Cancer Res. 2018;24:2771–9.
57. Drilon A, Siena S, Ou SI, et al. Safety and antitumor activity of the multitargeted pan-TRK, ROS1, and ALK inhibitor entrectinib: combined results from two phase 1 trials (ALKA-372-001 and STARTRK-1). Cancer Discov. 2017;7:400–9.
58. Camidge DR, Pao W, Sequist LV. Acquired resistance to TKIs in solid tumours: learning from lung cancer. Nat Rev Clin Oncol. 2014;11:473–81.
59. Sharma GG, Mota I, Mologni L, et al. Tumor resistance against ALK targeted therapy-where it comes from and where it goes. Cancers (Basel). 2018;10: 1–30.
60. Choi YL, Soda M, Yamashita Y, et al. EML4-ALK mutations in lung cancer that confer resistance to ALK inhibitors. N Engl J Med. 2010;363:1734–9.
61. Doebele RC, Pilling AB, Aisner DL, et al. Mechanisms of resistance to crizotinib in patients with ALK gene rearranged non-small cell lung cancer. Clin Cancer Res. 2012;18:1472–82.
62. Sasaki T, Koivunen J, Ogino A, et al. A novel ALK secondary mutation and EGFR signaling cause resistance to ALK kinase inhibitors. Cancer Res. 2011;71:6051–60.
63. Katayama R, Shaw AT, Khan TM, et al. Mechanisms of acquired crizotinib resistance in ALK rearranged lung cancers. Sci Transl Med. 2012;4:120ra17.
64. Heuckmann JM, Holzel M, Sos ML, et al. ALK mutations conferring differential resistance to structurally diverse ALK inhibitors. Clin Cancer Res. 2011;17:7394–401.
65. Gainor JF, Dardaei L, Yoda S, et al. Molecular mechanisms of resistance to first- and second-generation ALK inhibitors in ALK-rearranged lung cancer. Cancer Discov. 2016;6:1118–33.
66. Toyokawa G, Inamasu E, Shimamatsu S, et al. Identification of a novel ALK G1123S mutation in a patient with ALK-rearranged non-small-cell lung cancer exhibiting resistance to ceritinib. J Thorac Oncol. 2015;10:e55–7.
67. Tchekmedyian N, Ali SM, Miller VA, et al. Acquired ALK L1152R mutation confers resistance to ceritinib and predicts response to alectinib. J Thorac Oncol. 2016;11:e87–8.
68. Katayama R, Friboulet L, Koike S, et al. Two novel ALK mutations mediate acquired resistance to the next-generation ALK inhibitor alectinib. Clin Cancer Res. 2014;20:5686–96.
69. Ou SH, Greenbowe J, Khan ZU, et al. I1171 missense mutation (particularly I1171N) is a common resistance mutation in ALK-positive NSCLC patients who have progressive disease while on alectinib and is sensitive to ceritinib. Lung Cancer. 2015;88:231–4.
70. Lin YT, Yu CJ, Yang JC, et al. Anaplastic lymphoma kinase (ALK) kinase domain mutation following ALK inhibitor(s) failure in advanced ALK positive non-small-cell lung cancer: analysis and literature review. Clin Lung Cancer. 2016;17:e77–94.
71. Toyokawa G, Hirai F, Inamasu E, et al. Secondary mutations at I1171 in the ALK gene confer resistance to both crizotinib and alectinib. J Thorac Oncol. 2014;9:e86–7.
72. Shaw AT, Friboulet L, Leshchiner I, et al. Resensitization to crizotinib by the lorlatinib ALK resistance mutation L1198F. N Engl J Med. 2016;374:54–61.

73. Katayama R, Khan TM, Benes C, et al. Therapeutic strategies to overcome crizotinib resistance in non-small cell lung cancers harboring the fusion oncogene EML4-ALK. Proc Natl Acad Sci U S A. 2011;108:7535–40.
74. Miyawaki M, Yasuda H, Tani T, et al. Overcoming EGFR bypass signal-induced acquired resistance to ALK tyrosine kinase inhibitors in ALK-translocated lung cancer. Mol Cancer Res. 2017;15:106–14.
75. Tanizaki J, Okamoto I, Okabe T, et al. Activation of HER family signaling as a mechanism of acquired resistance to ALK inhibitors in EML4-ALK-positive non-small cell lung cancer. Clin Cancer Res. 2012;18:6219–26.
76. Dong X, Fernandez-Salas E, Li E, et al. Elucidation of resistance mechanisms to second-generation ALK inhibitors alectinib and ceritinib in non-small cell lung cancer cells. Neoplasia. 2016;18:162–71.
77. Toyokawa G, Seto T. Updated evidence on the mechanisms of resistance to ALK inhibitors and strategies to overcome such resistance: clinical and preclinical data. Oncol Res Treat. 2015;38:291–8.
78. Lamouille S, Xu J, Derynck R. Molecular mechanisms of epithelial-mesenchymal transition. Nat Rev Mol Cell Biol. 2014;15:178–96.
79. Kim HR, Kim WS, Choi YJ, et al. Epithelial-mesenchymal transition leads to crizotinib resistance in H2228 lung cancer cells with EML4-ALK translocation. Mol Oncol. 2013;7:1093–102.
80. Caumont C, Veillon R, Gros A, et al. Neuroendocrine phenotype as an acquired resistance mechanism in ALK-rearranged lung adenocarcinoma. Lung Cancer. 2016;92:15–8.
81. Miyamoto S, Ikushima S, Ono R, et al. Transformation to small-cell lung cancer as a mechanism of acquired resistance to crizotinib and alectinib. Jpn J Clin Oncol. 2016;46:170–3.
82. Cha YJ, Cho BC, Kim HR, et al. A case of ALK-rearranged adenocarcinoma with small cell carcinoma-like transformation and resistance to crizotinib. J Thorac Oncol. 2016;11:e55–8.
83. Takegawa N, Hayashi H, Iizuka N, et al. Transformation of ALK rearrangement-positive adenocarcinoma to small-cell lung cancer in association with acquired resistance to alectinib. Ann Oncol. 2016;27:953–5.
84. Fujita S, Masago K, Katakami N, et al. Transformation to SCLC after treatment with the ALK inhibitor alectinib. J Thorac Oncol. 2016;11:e67–72.
85. Levacq D, D'Haene N, de Wind R, et al. Histological transformation of ALK rearranged adenocarcinoma into small cell lung cancer: a new mechanism of resistance to ALK inhibitors. Lung Cancer. 2016;102:38–41.
86. Niederst MJ, Sequist LV, Poirier JT, et al. RB loss in resistant EGFR mutant lung adenocarcinomas that transform to small-cell lung cancer. Nat Commun. 2015;6:6377.
87. Weickhardt AJ, Scheier B, Burke JM, et al. Local ablative therapy of oligoprogressive disease prolongs disease control by tyrosine kinase inhibitors in oncogene-addicted non-small-cell lung cancer. J Thorac Oncol. 2012;7:1807–14.
88. Chaft JE, Oxnard GR, Sima CS, et al. Disease flare after tyrosine kinase inhibitor discontinuation in patients with EGFR-mutant lung cancer and acquired resistance to erlotinib or gefitinib: implications for clinical trial design. Clin Cancer Res. 2011;17:6298–303.
89. Camidge DR, Kono SA, Lu X, et al. Anaplastic lymphoma kinase gene rearrangements in non-small cell lung cancer are associated with prolonged progression-free survival on pemetrexed. J Thorac Oncol. 2011;6:774–80.
90. Lee JO, Kim TM, Lee SH, et al. Anaplastic lymphoma kinase translocation: a predictive biomarker of pemetrexed in patients with non-small cell lung cancer. J Thorac Oncol. 2011;6:1474–80.
91. Kim DW, Mehra R, Tan DS, et al. Activity and safety of ceritinib in patients with ALK-rearranged non-small-cell lung cancer (ASCEND-1): updated results from the multicentre, open-label, phase 1 trial. Lancet Oncol. 2016;17:452–63.
92. Crino L, Ahn MJ, De Marinis F, et al. Multicenter phase II study of whole-body and intracranial activity with ceritinib in patients with ALK-rearranged non-small-cell lung cancer previously treated with chemotherapy and crizotinib: results from ASCEND-2. J Clin Oncol. 2016;34:2866–73.

93. Barlesi F, Dingemans AMC, Yang JCH, et al. Updated efficacy and safety from the global phase II NP28673 study of alectinib in patients (pts) with previously treated ALK+ non-small-cell lung cancer (NSCLC). Ann Oncol. 2016;27:1263P.
94. Novello S, Mazieres J, Oh IJ, et al. Alectinib versus chemotherapy in crizotinib-pretreated anaplastic lymphoma kinase (ALK)-positive non-small-cell lung cancer: results from the phase III ALUR study. Ann Oncol. 2018;29:1409–16.
95. Felip E, Orlov S, Park K, et al. ASCEND-3: a single-arm, open-label, multicenter phase II study of ceritinib in ALKi-naïve adult patients (pts) with ALK-rearranged (ALK+) non-small cell lung cancer (NSCLC). J Clin Oncol. 2015;33:8060.
96. Shaw AT, Solomon BJ, Besse B, et al: ALK Resistance Mutations and Efficacy of Lorlatinib in Advanced Anaplastic Lymphoma Kinase-Positive Non-Small-Cell Lung Cancer. J Clin Oncol:JCO1802236, 2019.

ROS1

Leslie G. Oesterich and Jonathan W. Riess

Abstract ROS1 is a receptor tyrosine kinase with *ROS1* gene fusions identified in 0.9–2.1% of non-small cell lung cancers (NSCLC), as well as a number of other malignancies. These fusions are constitutively activated, leading to significant changes in cell differentiation, proliferation, growth, and survival. The fusions can be identified by a number of methods including fluorescent in situ hybridization, immunohistochemistry, real-time PCR, and next-generation sequencing. The tyrosine kinase inhibitor crizotinib is a potent inhibitor of ROS1 and was approved by the FDA for treatment of metastatic non-small cell lung cancer (NSCLC) with *ROS1* rearrangement in March 2016. However, as with other oncogenes, patients treated with crizotinib eventually develop resistance and progressive disease. A number of different resistance mutations have been discovered, the mechanisms of which can be broken down into two major categories: mutations within the ROS1 kinase domain and bypass signaling pathways. Several additional tyrosine kinase inhibitors are under development with varying degrees of CNS penetration and efficacy against resistance mutations.

Keywords ROS1 rearrangement · ROS1 inhibitor · Lung cancer · Non-small cell lung cancer · Oncogene · Crizotinib · Ceritinib · Tyrosine kinase inhibitor (TKI) resistance · Targeted therapy · Tyrosine kinase inhibitors

Introduction

Though gene fusions in the receptor tyrosine kinase ROS1 are present in only a small percentage of non-small cell lung cancer (NSCLC), it represents a viable therapeutic target with impressive clinical benefit to ROS1 inhibitors. The first ROS1 inhibitor, crizotinib, was approved for advanced NSCLC harboring *ROS1*

L. G. Oesterich · J. W. Riess (✉)
Department of Internal Medicine, Division of Hematology/Oncology, UC Davis School of Medicine and UC Davis Comprehensive Cancer Center, Sacramento, CA, USA
e-mail: jwriess@ucdavis.edu

© Springer Nature Switzerland AG 2019
R. Salgia (ed.), *Targeted Therapies for Lung Cancer*, Current Cancer Research,
https://doi.org/10.1007/978-3-030-17832-1_3

55

fusions in 2016. Subsequently a number of additional ROS1 inhibitors have been in development and seek to overcome resistance mutations that develop in response to crizotinib. In this chapter we provide an overview of the *ROS1* gene including its history, biology, methods of detection, and role of targeted treatment against ROS1-positive NSCLC, including the development and management of resistance mutations with newer agents targeting ROS1.

Structure and Function

Human c-ros oncogene 1 (*ROS1*) was originally discovered as a homolog of the transforming sequence of the UR2 avian sarcoma virus [1, 2] (Fig. 1). *ROS1* is located on chromosome 6q22 [4, 5]. It is a receptor tyrosine kinase that shares structural similarities to the insulin receptor tyrosine kinase, leukocyte tyrosine kinase (LTK), and anaplastic lymphoma kinase (ALK) families [6]. *ROS-1* encodes a receptor tyrosine kinase that consists of a large N-terminal extracellular domain, a hydrophobic single pass transmembrane region, and a C-terminal intracellular tyrosine kinase domain. It is relatively unique, in that its extracellular domain is composed of six repeat motifs that have high homology to the extracellular matrix and plasma protein fibronectin type III repeats, almost resembling a cell adhesion molecule. Unlike most adhesion molecules, however, the intracellular kinase domain enables ROS to directly translate adhesion engagement along intracellular signaling pathways [3].

The *ROS* receptor tyrosine kinase gene is evolutionarily conserved across multiple organisms. In *Drosophila melanogaster*, SEVENLESS (a ROS orthologue) is associated with a seven-transmembrane G-protein-coupled cell called BOSS (bride of sevenless). It is of particular importance in the developing *Drosophila* eye, where BOSS is required for differentiation of cells into photoreceptors [7, 8]. ROS expression has been examined in mouse, chicken, and rat tissue throughout various stages of development, with expression of *c-Ros* found in kidneys, small intestines, heart, lung, and male reproductive cells with restriction seen to epithelial cells [3]. In mice, testicular expression of *c-Ros* was only detected in adults with in situ hybridization of the adult testes showing expression in mature stages of development (spermatids, spermatozoa) only [9, 10]. In addition, *c-Ros* mutated male mice were noted to be infertile, though otherwise healthy. The defect was noted to be in development of the epithelia in the epididymis, especially in regionalization and terminal differentiation. No such impairment in fertility was noted in female mice. This suggests that expression may be linked to male fertility [11]. In humans, however, research has been hindered by the fact that it remains an orphan tyrosine kinase receptor, without a known ligand. Another barrier is the inability to express the full-length wild-type receptor in cellular models. There is some speculation that c-ROS1 expression may be involved in epithelial-mesenchymal interactions as well as in the cellular differentiation cascade of epithelial tissues [3].

Gene Fusion and Cancer

ROS1 gene fusions were first identified in the human glioblastoma cell line U-118 MG [12, 13]. An intra-chromosomal homozygous microdeletion of 240 kilobases on chromosome 6q21 was found to lead to fusion of the 5′ region of the *FIG* gene (fused in glioblastoma; a Golgi apparatus-associated protein) to the 3′ kinase domain of *ROS* [14–16] (Fig. 1). This fusion led to constitutive activation that was dependent on its localization to the Golgi apparatus [16]. This fusion has also been identified in a number of other malignancies, including ovarian cancer [17], cholangiocarcinoma [18], and NSCLC [19]. Additional *ROS1* gene fusions have been found in a number of other malignancies, including inflammatory myofibroblastic tumors [20, 21], gastric adenocarcinoma [22], colorectal cancer [23], angiosarcoma [24], thyroid cancer [25], atypical meningioma [26], and spitzoid melanomas [27].

Following the identification of *ROS1* fusions in glioblastomas, NSCLC was the second solid tumor in which these rearrangements were identified. This landmark study characterized tyrosine kinase signaling across 41 NSCLC cell lines and over 150 NSCLC tumors using a phosphoproteomic approach. High-level ROS kinase activity was noted in one cell line and one tumor sample. When these samples were

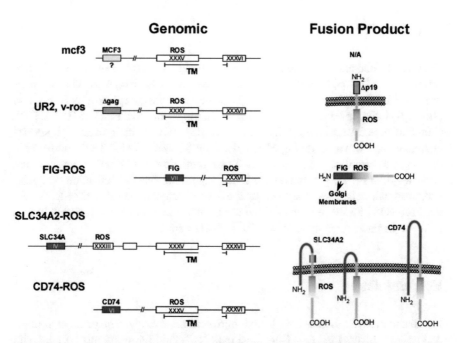

Fig. 1 ROS fusion kinases. Schematic representation of selected ROS fusions and their corresponding protein fusion product. With the exception of FIG-ROS, all of the fusion kinases are predicted to be plasma membrane bound. SLC34A2-ROS and CD740ROS fusion proteins are here illustrated to be bimembrane spanning receptors, though this has not been confirmed experimentally. (Figure from Acquaviva et al. [3])

sequenced, two novel *ROS1* fusions were identified. In the HCC78 cell line, ROS was found to be fused to the transmembrane solute carrier protein SLC34A2. This protein was found to localize to membrane fractions and display a constitutive kinase activity. siRNA against SLC34A2-ROS was found to induce apoptosis, suggesting that ROS signaling is critical for survival of these NSCLC cells. In the solid tumor, c-ROS was found to be fused to the N-terminal half a type II transmembrane protein, CD74 [28] (Fig. 1).

Since this initial publication, multiple other fusion partners have been reported in NSCLC. The *CD74-ROS1* fusion remains the most common, occurring with an estimated frequency of 32% in NSCLC. Other common fusion partners include *SLC34A2-ROS1* (17%), *TMP3-ROS1* (tropomyosin 3; 15%), *SDC4-ROS1* (syndecan 4; 11%), *EZR-ROS1* (ezrin; 6%), and *FIG-ROS1* (3%). Less common fusions, occurring at frequencies of 1% or less, include *CCDC6-ROS1* (coiled-coil domain containing 6), *LRIG3-ROS1* (leucine-rich repeats and immunoglobulin-like domains 3), *KDELR2-ROS1* (KDEL endoplasmic reticulum protein retention receptor 2 gene), *MSN-ROS1* (moesin gene), *CLTC-ROS1* (clathrin heavy chain gene), *TPD5L1-ROS1* (tumor protein D52-like gene), *TMEM106B-ROS1* (transmembrane protein 106B gene), and *LIMA1-ROS* (LIM domain and actin-binding 1 gene) [29].

Signaling Pathway

Once ROS1 becomes activated, either by its (unknown) ligand or via constitutive action from a fusion, a number of signaling pathways are triggered. The key rate-limiting step for this process is thought to be autophosphorylation of ROS1 and phosphorylation of the SH-2 domain-containing phosphatase-2 (SHP-2) [30]. Constitutive activation from a fusion then leads downstream signaling via several oncogenic pathways, including MAPK/ERK, PI3K/AKT, JAK/STAT3, and VAV3; this leads to significant changes in cell differentiation, proliferation, growth, and survival [3] (Fig. 2). Preclinical work has suggested that the activation of downstream signaling pathways depends on the fusion partner of ROS1. CD74-ROS1 but not FIG-ROS1 has been found to lead to phosphorylation of E-Syt1, which in turn led to an invasive phenotype in the CD74-ROS1 cells [31].

Epidemiology

Patients with *ROS1* fusions have been found to be more likely to be younger, female, and never-smokers than *ROS1*-negative patients—a similar profile to patients with *EGFR* activating mutations and *ALK* rearrangements [32–34]. Interestingly, however, the pattern of spread for *ROS1* rearranged disease appears to be different than that for *ALK*; *ROS* fusions are associated with lower rates of extrathoracic disease, including brain metastases, at initial metastatic diagnosis [35]. The vast majority of

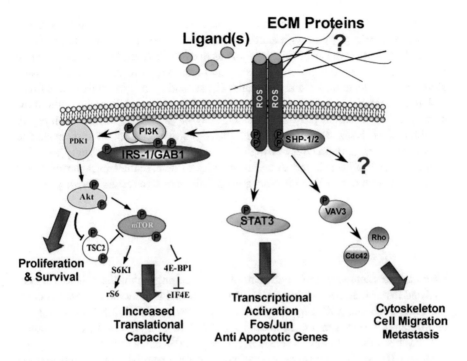

Fig. 2 ROS signaling pathways. (Figure from Acquaviva et al. [3])

cases are adenocarcinoma, although there are rare reports of other histologies such as squamous or large cell [19, 36, 37]. The most common histologic patterns associated with *ROS1* fusion adenocarcinoma are solid growth with hepatoid cytology and acinar growth with cribriform structure. Other pathologic characteristics include mucinous features, signet ring cells, and psammomatous calcifications [38]. The *ROS1* rearrangement usually occurs without other known oncogenic drivers, although there have been rare reported cases of concurrent mutations such as EGFR, KRAS, BRAF, MET, and PIK3CA [19, 27, 39–42].

Prevalence of NSCLC *ROS1* fusion tumor ranges in the literature from 0.9% to 2.1%, though studies are always limited by their screening technique and therefore may miss cases with rare or new fusions. Worldwide prevalence is 1.9% [29].

Detection

FISH

Detection of *ROS1* rearrangements by fluorescence in situ hybridization (FISH) has been considered the gold standard. It was used in the landmark phase I study that resulted in approval of crizotinib for *ROS-1* rearranged NSCLC [42]. The centromeric (3′) part of the fusion breakpoint is labeled with a one fluorochrome and the telomeric (5′) part with another of a different color. The criteria for ROS1 FISH identification in NSCLC is the same as that for ALK rearrangement. The first positive pattern is a classic break-apart pattern, in which there is a single fusion signal and two separated 3′ and 5′ signals. The second is an atypical pattern, with an isolated 3′ signal—usually one fusion signal and one isolated 3′ signal without the corresponding 5′ signal [43]. FISH testing may be performed either on biopsy or cytologic specimens. To be considered FISH positive, at least 15% of evaluated tumor cells must contain split or isolated 3′ signals [44, 45]. Interestingly, a limitation of FISH has been found to be an inability to detect small intrachromasomal deletions, which can lead to false-negative or false-positive results [39, 46].

IHC

Immunohistochemistry (IHC) can be used as a screening technique. It is less expensive and faster than performing FISH. The D4D6 rabbit monoclonal assay is commercially available (Cell Signaling Technology, Danvers, MA, USA). It is applied at different dilutions ranging from 1:50 to 1:1000. In a number of different studies, IHC has been found to have a sensitivity of near 100% and a specificity of between 85% and 100%; specificity varies depending on interpretive cutoffs and method used [19, 43, 45, 47–49].

Unfortunately, ROS1 IHC can be somewhat challenging to interpret. Expression can be seen in osteoclast-like giant cells adjacent to ROS-1 un-mutated tumor cells, as well as in reactive pneumocytes and alveolar macrophages [43, 49]. Staining patterns can vary depending on different intracellular localization of the ROS1 fusions [19, 43]. Results can vary depending on the performing laboratory [50]. Because of this, while it makes for an excellent screening tool, it is important to perform confirmatory testing with FISH or another testing modality.

RT-PCR

Real-time PCR (RT-PCR) utilizes specific primer sets to detect and identify known fusion variants. RT-PCR-based detection of some of the most common *ROS1* fusion genes (*SLC34A2, SDC, CD74, EZR, TPM3, LRIG3, GOPC*) at exons 32, 34, 35, and 36 has been successfully performed with a sensitivity of 100% and specificity of 85–100% with respect to FISH [41, 51]. While this is a relatively easy, rapid, and inexpensive test, it does have some drawbacks. As the list of *ROS1* fusion proteins is large and growing, RT-PCR is likely to miss rare or previously unknown variants. It can also be challenging to obtain sufficient good quality RNA from the formalin-fixed paraffin-embedded tissue samples (FFPE) [52].

In recent years, the nCounter platform (NanoString Technologies; Seattle, WA) has emerged as a clinical option. It is a multiplexed assay that can identify known fusion gene variants via the interrogation of imbalanced 5'/3' expression levels as well as the direct detection of fusion transcript variants. It has shown a good concordance with both IHC and FISH results for *ROS1* fusion detection [53, 54].

NGS

Next-generation sequencing, or NGS, enables sensitive and specific assessments of multiple genomic regions at once, allowing for detection of both known and novel fusions [45]. Several *ROS1* fusions have been identified using NGS [55–59]. A recent study performed next-generation sequencing on 319 FFPE samples and found 100% sensitivity and specificity when compared to reference FISH assays [60]. This method allows for multiplexed detection of molecular aberrations in NSCLC in a single test instead of multiple assays; however, hybrid-based capture NGS methods may have decreased sensitivity in detecting gene fusions [45].

Targeted Therapies

Crizotinib

Crizotinib (previously PF-0234106; brand name Xalkori, Pfizer, New York, USA) is a small molecule multikinase inhibitor (Table 1). It was initially developed as an inhibitor of c-MET but was further explored against a panel of over 120 diverse kinases and was found to be almost 20 times more selective for ALK and MET as compared to other evaluated kinases [61]. Following a phase I trial and initial efficacy results from a phase II trial (PROFILE 1001) that showed 50% response rates, it was approved by the FDA for use in metastatic NSCLC with *ALK* rearrangements in 2011 [62, 63]. Preclinical investigation of NSCLC cell lines, including HCC78 (*SLC34A2-ROS1*), revealed dose-dependent inhibition with crizotinib; inhibition of *ROS1* led to subsequent inhibition of its downstream targets and apoptosis of the cell line [64]. This combined with *ALK* and *ROS1*'s known homology [6] with shared high-binding affinity to crizotinib [65] and case reports of response to crizotinib in patients with *ROS1*-mutated NSCLC [33, 37] led to the incorporation of patients with *ROS-1* rearranged NSCLC into the expansion cohort of the phase I PROFILE 1001 study. This landmark study included 50 patients with *ROS1* rearranged NSCLC. Overall response rate (ORR) to crizotinib was 72% with a median duration of response (DOR) of 17.6 months, median progression-free survival (PFS) of 19.2 months, and a disease control rate (DCR) of 90% [42]. Interestingly DOR to crizotinib in *ALK*-rearranged patients is only 49.1 weeks, with a median PFS of

Table 1 Clinical trials of drugs targeting ROS1

Drug (target kinases)	Trial	Phase	Status	Enrollment: ROS1 (total)	ORR	DOR (mo)	PFS (mo)	DCR	CNS disease control	Enrollment: crizotinib resistant	Response: crizotinib resistant	Trial ID
Crizotinib (ALK, ROS1, MET)	PROFILE 1001	I	Complete	50	72%	17.6	19.2	NR	NR			NCT 585195
	Wu et al.	II	Complete	127	71.70%	19.7	15.9	NR	N = 23; PFS 10.2 mo			NCT 1945021
	ACSé	II	Ongoing	34	63%	NR	NR	88%	NR			NCT 2034981
	EUCROSS	II	Ongoing	34	69%	NR	NR	NR	NR			NCT 2183870
	EUROS1	Retrospective	Complete	32	80%	NR	9.1	86.70%	NR			n/a
	METROS	II	Ongoing	Not yet reported	Not yet reported							NCT 2499614
Ceritinib (ALK, ROS1)	Lim et al.	II	Complete	32	62%	21	9.3	81%	63% (5/8)	2 (6%)	0	NCT 1964157
Entrectinib (ROS1, ALK, TRK A/B/C)	ALKA-372-001	I	Complete	14 (119)	86%	NR	19	NR	100% (2/2)	6 (43%)	0	EudraCT 2012-000148-88
	STARTRK-1											NCT02097810
	STARTRK-2	I/II	Ongoing	32	75%	17.2	19.1	NR	71% (5/7)			NCT 2568267
Lorlatinib (ROS1, ALK)	Shaw et al.	I	Complete	12 (54)	50%	Not reported		NR	60% (3/5)	7 (58%)	2/7 PR or SD	NCT 1970865
	Solomon et al.	II	Ongoing	47 (275)	36%	NR	NR	NR	56% (14/25)	NR	NR	NCT 1970865

Ropotrectinib (ROS1, ALK, TRK A/B/C)	TRIDENT	I	Ongoing	29 (65)	Not yet reported					19 (66%)	NR	NCT 3093116
DS-6051b (ROS1, TRK A/B/C)	Fujiwara et al.	I	Complete	15	58.3%[a]	NR	NR	100%	NR	4 (27%)	ORR 25% (1)	NCT 2675491
	Papadopoulos et al.	I/Ib	Ongoing	9 (35)	4/6 PR or SD	NR	NR	NR	NR	7 (78%)	2 PR, 2 SD	NCT 2279433
Brigatinib (ALK, ROS1)	Gettinger et al.	I/II	Complete	3 (137)	33% (1/3)	NR	NR	NR	NR	2 (66%)	1 SD	NCT 1449461

NR Not reported, *ORR* overall response rate, *DOR* duration of response, *PFS* progression-free survival, *DCR* disease control rate, *OS* overall survival, *CNS* central nervous system, *PR* partial response, *SD* stable disease, *n/a* not applicable

[a]66.7% in crizotinib-naïve patients

9.7 months, suggesting that crizotinib may be a more potent inhibitor of *ROS1* than *ALK* [42, 66]. Toxicities in this study were similar to those previously described; the most common grade 3 events were hypophosphatemia (10%), neutropenia (10%), and an elevated aminotransferase activity (10%). No grade 4 or 5 events were seen [42]. Based on this study, crizotinib was approved by the FDA for treatment of metastatic NSCLC with *ROS1* rearrangement in March 2016.

There have been several other studies that yielded overall similarly promising results. The retrospective EUROS1 study identified 32 patients with advanced NSCLC who had positive ROS1 rearrangement by FISH and who had received crizotinib, 30 of whom were evaluable. ORR was 80% and DCR 86.7%, and median PFS was 9.1 months; PFS at 1 year was 44% [67]. Preliminary results from the French phase II ACSé trial prospectively looked at 34 patients with *ROS1*-rearranged NSCLC who were given crizotinib, 24 of whom were evaluable at the time of preliminary analysis. ORR was 63%, and DCR 88% [68]. Preliminary results from the prospective European phase II EUCROSS study similarly looked at 34 patients with *ROS1*-rearranged NSCLC (by FISH) who were given crizotinib, 29 of whom were eligible for efficacy assessment and 20 of whom had tumor tissue available for further sequencing. Of the patients who underwent additional sequencing, 19 tested positive for the ROS1 fusion. ORR was 69% in the overall trial population and 83% in those *ROS-1* positive by next-generation sequencing [69]. A phase II study in East Asian patients included 127 patients with *ROS1*-rearranged NSCLC who received crizotinib. ORR was 71.7%, with a median PFS of 15.9 months and a median duration of response of 19.7 months [70]. All studies included patients who had received varying numbers of prior therapies and who were overall fairly heavily pretreated, though crizotinib was their first tytyrosine kinase inhibitor (TKI).

Resistance to ROS1 TKI

While ROS-1 mutated tumors initially respond well to targeted therapy with crizotinib, most patients inevitably develop resistance. The mechanism of resistance can be broken down into two major categories: mutations within the ROS1 kinase domain or bypass signaling pathways [35].

There are two major mechanisms by which kinase domain mutations appear to confer crizotinib resistance. The first is by a gatekeeping mechanism that directly interferes with the combination of ROS1 tyrosine kinase and crizotinib, leading to resistance. The second is a solvent front mutation in the kinase domain adjacent to the crizotinib-binding site; these confer resistance via steric interference [71] (Table 2).

The first kinase domain mutation described is also the one that has been most frequently observed. A 48-year-old woman with CD74-ROS1-rearranged NSCLC was started on crizotinib with excellent response. However after 3 months of therapy she was found to have progressive disease. Biopsy upon progression revealed the persistence of the *ROS1* rearrangement by FISH but RT-PCR sequencing

Table 2 Crizotinib-resistant *ROS1* mutations based on preclinical data

	G2032R	L1951R	D2033N	S1986Y/F	L2026M
Mutation type	Solvent front	Solvent front	Solvent front	αC helix	Gatekeeper
Crizotinib	No[a]	No	No[a]	No	No
Ceritinib	No	No	No	No	Yes
Cabozantinib	Yes	Yes	Yes[a]	Unknown	Yes
Entrectinib	No	Unknown	Unknown	Unknown	Unclear
Lorlatinib	Unclear	Unknown	Yes	Yes[a]	Yes
Ropotrectinib	Yes[a]	Yes	Yes	Yes	Yes
DS-6051b	Unknown	Unknown	Unknown	Unknown	Unknown
Brigatinib	No	No	No	Unknown	Yes

Unclear indicates preclinical data for activity has been mixed
[a]Also supported by clinical data

revealed a c6094G→A, p.Gly2032Arg (G2032R) mutation that was not noted on her pretreatment biopsy. This mutation is analogous to the ALK G1202R mutation. Biopsy was repeated at autopsy, and all sites examined harbored this mutation, suggesting that it was an early event in the clonal evolution of resistance [72]. Crizotinib was designed to bind ROS1 at the ATP-binding site that sits within the cleft between the N and C terminal domains of the kinase [73]. Crystal structure analysis revealed that the G2032 residue sits at the solvent front of the kinase hinge (solvent-exposed region of the kinase). G2032R causes steric hindrance with the piperidine ring of crizotinib while still allowing for ATP binding and therefore oncogenic kinase activity [72]. One recent evaluation of 16 patients with *ROS1*-positive advanced NSCLC with a total of 17 repeat biopsies after progression identified G2032R mutations in 41% of the biopsy specimens [35].

Following the identification of this initial resistance mutation, a multitude of others have been identified in clinical samples. A patient with CD74-ROS1-rearranged NSCLC who progressed on crizotinib was found to acquire the solvent-front mutation D2033N. Upon crystal modeling, this mutation was noted to interfere with the favorable interaction of the ATP-binding site with the protonated piperidine region of crizotinib. It is analogous to the *ALK* D1203N mutation. This patient proceeded to respond to cabozantinib; upon crystal modeling, cabozantinib was not found to interact with this altered 2033 residue [74]. Multiple other mutations have been discovered in vitro but not yet been replicated in the clinical setting.

Additional kinase domain mutations have been reported. These include S1986Y/F, which leads to alterations in the alpha C helix of the kinase domain and therefore steric interference with drug binding [35, 75]. It is analogous to the ALK C1156Y substitution [76]. L1951R is a solvent front mutation without an analogous ALK mutation. L2026M is a gatekeeper mutation in the ATP pocket that impedes drug binding and is analogous to *ALK* L1196M [71, 77]. Interestingly when the L2026M, L1951R, and G2032R mutations were evaluated in vivo, the mutations associated with highest crizotinib resistance were those located close to the crizotinib-binding domain—G2032R and L1951 [71].

Less information is available about off-target mechanisms of crizotinib resistance. The best described is a mechanism by which cancer cells achieve resistance via activation of an alternative signaling pathway (bypass pathway). One case report describes the appearance of a *BRAF* V600E mutation in a woman with SDC-*ROS1* fusion NSCLC who had developed resistance to crizotinib; this mutation was not present on her initial biopsy. She was started on dabrafinib and trametinib but died 11 days later [78]. Similarly a new *KIT* p.D816G mutation was found after progression on crizotinib in a patient with *ROS1* fusion NSCLC [79]. Two case reports describe patients with alterations in KRAS; one described a new point mutation in *KRAS* pG12D accompanied by *KRAS* gene amplification found on progression biopsy. Patient was treated with the MEK inhibitor selumetinib as well as pemetrexed and was alive at the time of article submission [80]. The second report only noted focal *KRAS* amplification seen in a *ROS1* fusion tumor biopsy of a patient who had progressed on crizotinib, though this analysis was hampered by the lack of pretreatment sample to see if this was truly a bypass mutation [81]. Another patient with *CD74-ROS1* fusion NSCLC who had progressed on crizotinib was found on next-generation sequencing to have a novel point mutation of the *PIK3CA* gene (pL531P) that led to activation of the *m*TOR signaling pathway; patient was placed on an *m*TOR signaling pathway inhibitor but passed shortly thereafter [82]. One study that performed next-generation sequencing on 12 *ROS1* fusion patients who had progressed on crizotinib identified the same KIT D816G mutation previously characterized. It also noted a HER2 (ERBB2) mutation, though no pre-crizotinib samples were available for comparison. It also noted a β-catenin *CTNNB1* S45F mutation that had previously been hypothesized as a potential oncogenic driver, though they were not able to evaluate pretreatment tissue in this patient to prove its presence as a bypass mutation [77, 83]. Another study created a cell line from a patient who had developed acquired resistance to crizotinib; the cell line revealed a switch in the control of growth and survival signaling pathways from ROS1 to EGFR in the resistant cell line, though this has not yet been verified in the clinic [84, 85].

Less is known about the potential for phenotypic changes leading to resistance. In EGFR and ALK fusion cancers, histologic transformation from adenocarcinoma to small cell cancer has been observed as a mechanism for TKI resistance, but this has yet to be demonstrated in ROS1 fusion NSCLC [86]. One preclinical study that took tumor tissue from NSCLC patients who had progressed on crizotinib noted evidence of epithelial to mesenchymal transition by way of upregulated vimentin and downregulated E-cadherin. A similar finding was noted in HCC78CR1-2 cell clones, though they also harbored a L2155S mutation that had previously been found to confer crizotinib resistance in cell lines [85].

Ceritinib

Ceritinib (previously LDK378l, brand name Zykadia; Novartis Pharmaceuticals) is an oral small molecule tyrosine kinase inhibitor of ALK [87] (Table 1). Preclinical studies suggested that it would inhibit ROS1 as well [88, 89]. A Korean phase II study evaluated 32 patients with advanced NSCLC who tested positive for *ROS1* rearrangement by FISH. All but two of them were crizotinib-naïve. They received ceritinib 750 mg daily. ORR was 62%, with 1 complete response (CR) and 19 partial responses (PR). DOR was 21 months, with a DCR of 81%. Median PFS was 9.3 months overall and 19.3 months in crizotinib-naïve patients. Median overall survival (OS) was 24 months. Eight patients entered the trial with metastases to the brain; intracranial disease control was obtained in five (63%) of them, with an intracranial ORR of 25%. Of note, at the beginning of the trial two patients who had previously received treatment with crizotinib were enrolled. Neither were available for objective response—one passed due to suspected leptomeningeal disease, and one withdrew from the trial 2 weeks after their first dose due to grade 3 weakness and anorexia. However, neither of them showed signs of clinical improvement after initiation of ceritinib, and the protocol was subsequently amended to only enroll crizotinib-naïve patients who had previously been treated with at least one chemo-therapeutic agent [89].

Adverse events in this study were primarily grade 1-2, the most common of which were diarrhea (78%), nausea (59%), and anorexia (56%)—all of which occurred at higher frequencies than with crizotinib [42, 89]. A recent randomized phase I study of 137 patients with metastatic *ALK*-mutated NSCLC found that ceritinib 450 mg taken with a low-fat meal resulted in fewer GI toxicities as compared with the standard 750 mg taken fasting and was associated with comparable plasma levels when assessed pharmacokinetically [90]. Ceritinib is not FDA approved for management of *ROS1*-rearranged advanced NSCLC, but it is noted as an option for front-line therapy per NCCN guidelines.

Cabozantinib

Cabozantinib (PF-06463922; brand name Cabometyx; Exelixis, Alameda, CA) is an oral multikinase inhibitor with CNS penetration (Table 1). It is FDA approved for use in medullary thyroid cancer and as a second-line agent in advanced renal cell carcinoma. In vitro studies found it to exhibit excellent activity against both the wild-type ROS1 fusion and the G2032R and G2026M mutations at concentrations less than 30 nmol/L—a dose much lower than what is clinically achievable [71, 91]. It has been found to inhibit *CD74-ROS1*-transformed Ba/F3 cells with more potency than entrectinib, brigatinib, lorlatinib [92], or foretinib [71].

One case report described a 50-year-old woman with metastatic NSCLC who progressed after platinum-based therapy and was found to have a *ROS1* fusion. She was treated with crizotinib and progressed, at which point she was found to have the *ROS1* D2033N mutation within her ROS1 kinase domain. She was started on crizotinib 60 mg orally daily and achieved PR by 4 weeks and near CR by 12 weeks (92% reduction in disease burden). At the time of paper publication, she remained on therapy (near 8 months duration). In vitro analysis of CD74-ROS1 cells with D2033N mutation found significantly more suppression with cabozantinib than ceritinib, brigatinib, and lorlatinib, though they remained highly sensitive to foretinib [74]. A recent abstract evaluated HCC78R cell lines with SLC34A2-ROS1 and ABC-20 cell lines harboring CD74-ROS1 (resistant to crizotinib). NGS evaluation found both an upregulation of HB-EGF and activation of the EGFR signaling pathway as well as an upregulation of AXL. The combination of cabozantinib and gefitinib was found to inhibit the growth of HCC28R tumors in an in vivo NOG mice model [93].

Unfortunately, cabozantinib is associated with a number of toxicities. The landmark METEOR trial which evaluated its use in renal cell carcinoma noted that 71% of patients experienced grade 3 or 4 events, the most common of which were hypertension (15%), diarrhea (13%), fatigue (11%), and palmar-plantar erythrodysesthesia syndrome (8%). Sixty-two percent of patients required dose reductions [94].

Entrectinib

Entrectinib (RXDX-101, Ignyta Pharmaceuticals, San Diego, CA, USA) is a small molecule that inhibits the tyrosine kinases TRKA/B/C, ROS1, and ALK (Table 1). It has a preclinical median inhibitory concentration (IC50) of 7 nm against ROS1, higher than crizotinib [95, 96]. Entrectinib was specifically designed to cross the blood-brain barrier [95]. Two recent phase I studies (ALKA-372-001 and STARTRK-1) evaluated entrectenib in patients with advanced solid tumors. Fourteen patients with *ROS1*-rearranged solid tumors (all NSCLC except one melanoma) were evaluated. These patients were all crizotinib-naïve. ORR was 86%, with an intracranial ORR of 100% (in the two ROS1 fusion patients evaluated). Median PFS was 19 months. Interestingly, six patients with ROS-1-rearranged disease who had previously received crizotinib were not observed to have any response to entrectinib [97]. Preliminary phase II data was recently reported, in which 32 patients with ROS1 fusion proven NSCLC (by NGS) who were naïve to prior TKI therapy were given 600 mg by mouth of entrectinib daily in 4 weeks cycles. ORR was 75% with three complete responses, intracranial ORR 71%, median PFS 19.1 months. The most common treatment-related adverse events were fatigue/asthenia (34%), dysguisia (34%), and dizziness (24%) [98]. There has been no preclinical activity demonstrated against *ROS1* resistance mutations G2032 or L2026; this combined with the lack of response in crizotinib-pretreated patients as noted above suggests that entrectinib's role in treating crizotinib-resistant disease may be limited unless progression is only in the CNS [92].

Lorlatinib

Lorlatinib (PF-06463922, Pfizer Oncology, Groton, CT, USA) is an oral TKI that targets both ALK and ROS1 with high affinity and good CNS penetration [91] (Table 1). Phase I data has been published looking at lorlatinib in NSCLC with *ALK* or *ROS1* rearrangement; patients were allowed to have both CNS disease and prior TKI therapy. In this study, 12 patients had *ROS1* rearrangements, 7 of whom were pretreated with crizotinib. ORR was 50% [99]. Preliminary data has been presented from the phase II component of this study; the ROS1 cohort contained 47 patients, each of whom was treated with lorlatinib 100 mg daily. Regardless of prior treatment, ORR was 36%, with intracranial ORR 56%. The most common treatment-related adverse events and grade 3/4 adverse events were hypercholesterolemia (81%/16%) and hypertriglyceridemia (60%/16%) [100].

Lorlatinib is intriguing because of its activity against several crizotinib-resistant mutations. Dong et al. published a case report of a 57-year-old gentleman with a history of stage IIIB lung adenocarcinoma who initially went into remission following platinum-based chemotherapy but then relapsed and was found to have an EZR-ROS1 mutation. He initially responded well to crizotinib, with PFS of 6 months. After disease progression, he was started on lorlatinib 100 mg daily with favorable response after 3 months; he remained on drug at time of article publication [101]. Mutation type was not assessed in that publication, but another case report described an excellent response to lorlatinib in a patient who had the crizotinib- and ceritinib-resistant mutations S1986Y/F [75]. Additional cell-based assays have described sensitivity in the setting of D2033N [74] and L2026M [91] mutations. It is less clear what the role of lorlatinib is in the setting of the G2032 mutation; in preclinical studies this mutation has been found to significantly reduce lorlatinib's potency though activity still remained overall robust. *ROS1*-rearranged BA/F3 cells with the G2032 mutation have been found to have an IC50 of 508 nM as compared to 0.5 nM in wild-type *ROS1* [91].

Ropotrectinib

Ropotrectinib (TPX-0005; TP Therapeutics, San Diego, CA, USA) is a next-generation ROS1 inhibitor, a novel three-dimensional macrocyle with a much smaller size (MW <370) than current ROS1 inhibitors (Table 1). It was specifically designed to overcome resistance mutations. Preclinical studies have shown activity against gatekeeper and solvent mutations, including G2032R, D2033N, L2026M, S1986F/Y, L1951R, and kinases involved in bypass signaling such as focal adhesion kinase, SRC proto-oncogene, and non-receptor tyrosine kinase [102, 103]. Preliminary results have been reported from the phase I TRIDENT study. It included patients with *ALK*, *ROS1*, or *NTRK1-3* fusion-positive advanced solid tumors. Patients could be either TKI pretreated or naïve, and brain metastases were allowed. At the time of report of preliminary results, 29 ROS1 patients were enrolled. Confirmed PR have been observed in both TKI-naïve and pre-treated ROS1/NTRK+ patients at all dose levels, including one crizotinib refractory ROS1 G2032R+ patient with untreated CNS metastases. Median duration of clinical PR was 6.7 months with 88% (7 out of 8) responses ongoing. Toxicities have been tolerable, with the majority of adverse events remaining at grade 1–2; most common include dysgusia (38%), dizziness (35%), paresthesia (24%), and nausea (12%) [104].

DS-6051b

DS-6051b (Daiichi Sankyo, Japan) is an oral small molecule tyrosine kinase inhibitor that has demonstrated preclinical activity against *ROS1* and *NTRK1-3* rearrangements [105] (Table 1). A phase I trial evaluated 15 Japanese patients with NSCLC harboring *ROS1* fusions. ORR was 58.3% in the 12 patients with target lesions and 66.7% in the 9 patients who were crizotinib-naïve; DCR was 100%. Common toxicities included transaminitis (80%), diarrhea (53.3%), and nausea (46.7%). Maximal tolerated dose and recommended phase II dose was 600 mg by mouth daily [106]. Preliminary data was recently presented for a phase I trial of DS-6051b in advanced solid tumors conducted in the United States. 35 patients were enrolled, with 31 tumors evaluable. Nine patients had ROS1 fusions, including seven patients who had NSCLC and who had previously received crizotinib. Of the six evaluable NSCLC *ROS1*-rearranged patients who had previously received crizotinib, two patients had PR, and two had stable disease (SD). DS-6051b was noted to be tolerable up to 800 mg by mouth daily, with the primary adverse events being gastrointestinal (89%) [107].

Brigatinib

Brigatinib (AP26113, brand name Alunbrig; ARIAD Pharmaceuticals, Cambridge, MA, USA) is an inhibitor of both *ALK* and *ROS1* fusion NSCLC (Table 1). In preclinical studies, it was found to inhibit viability of *CD4-ROS1*-expressing Ba/F3 cells with an IC50 of 7.5 nM, as compared to a IC50 of 9.8 nM in *EMLA4-ALK* cells [108, 109]. It was FDA approved for use in metastatic crizotinib-resistant *ALK* fusion NSCLC in April 2017. A single armed phase I/II trial evaluated patients with advanced malignancies including *ALK*-rearranged NSCLC refractory to currently available therapies. Three patients in this study had *ROS1*-rearranged NSCLC. Two of these patients had previously received crizotinib; one had progressive disease (PD), and one had SD. The single crizotinib-naïve ROS1-rearranged NSCLC patient experienced a partial response and was continuing to receive brigatinib at the time of data cutoff (21.6 mo of therapy) [110]. In a phase II trial of 222 patients with advanced ALK fusion NSCLC that had progressed on crizotinib, common treatment-related adverse events were noted to be nausea (33/44%), diarrhea (19/38%), headache (28/27%), and cough (13/34%) (brigatinib 90 mg daily/180 mg daily). A subset of patients were noted to have early onset pulmonary events (all grades 6%; grade $\geq$ 3 3%) [111]. Preclinical work examining *CD74-ROS1* transformed BA/F3 cells in vivo has revealed that brigatinib exhibits activity against L2026M [92], but does not fare as well against D2033N [74], G2032R [71, 92, 109], or L1951R [71].

Foretenib

Foretinib (GSK1363089; GlaxoSmithKline) is an oral multikinase inhibitor that targets MET, VEGFR-2, RON, KIT, and AXL kinases. Preclinical data suggested that it was a potent inhibitor of *ROS1* fusions. It also demonstrated effective inhibition against the G2032 mutation at clinically feasible concentrations [112]. However it has been found to be less potent and effective than cabozantinib, and further development of the drug was discontinued [113].

Chemotherapy and Immunotherapy

Pemetrexed (formerly LY231514, brand name Alimta, Eli Lilly, Indianapolis, Indiana, USA) is a folate-based antimetabolite that exerts its activity via inhibition of enzymes critical in purine and pyrimidine synthase. These include thymidine synthase (TS), dihydrofolate reductase, and glycinamine ribonucleotide formyltransferase [114]. Multiple studies have found that patients with *ALK* fusions have improved outcomes as compared to their wild-type colleagues [115]. The same appears to be true for patients with *ROS1* gene rearrangements. One retrospective study of 25 patients who had received pemetrexed (with or without bevacizumab) for 12 months or longer as therapy for their advanced stage non-squamous NSCLC included 5 patients with a *ROS1* gene rearrangement. Median OS was 42.2 months with median PFS of 22.1 months; patients with an oncogenic driver mutation (including but not limited to ROS1) had a statistically significant improvement in their PFS ($p = 0.006$) and OS ($p = 0.001$) compared to wild type [115]. Another retrospective study looked at four patients with metastatic NSCLC and FISH-detected ROS1 rearrangement who received pemetrexed. PFS ranged from 18 to more than 47 months [116]. A different retrospective study evaluated 253 patients with advanced NSCLC who were screened for driver mutations using RT-PCR. 19 patients (7.5%) had *ROS1* fusions. These patients were noted to have a better ORR (57.9%, $p = 0.026$), DCR (89.5%, $p = 0.033$), and PFS (7.5 mo; $p = 0.003$) as compared to patients with other driver mutations. Interestingly, while low levels of TS have historically been considered a favorable marker for pemetrexed efficacy in NSCLC, in this population this effect was not seen [117].

Although, PD(L)1 blockade has revolutionized the treatment of advanced NSCLC both as single agent and in combination with chemotherapy, no clear data currently exists suggesting the efficacy of immunotherapy specifically in patients with *ROS1* gene rearrangements. A phase I/II study evaluating the safety and tolerability of nivolumab plus crizotinib in the treatment of patients with metastatic NSCLC and ALK fusions was stopped early due to the degree of toxicity observed [118]. A recent phase II trial evaluated the use of pembrolizumab in NSCLC patients with both EGFR mutated and PD-L1-positive disease; study was similarly terminated early due to lack of efficacy even in patients with PD-L1 expression ≥50% [119]. Extrapolating from EGFR-mutant NSCLC which, like ROS1, is also associated with patients who have not smoked, a recent meta-analysis evaluating three trials found that the use of single agent PD(L)1 inhibitors failed to improve overall survival in the *EGFR* mutant NSCLC, though survival was improved in wild-type lung cancers [120]. Another meta-analysis similarly revealed that in *EGFR*-mutated patients with metastatic NSCLC, PD-1/PD-L1 therapy is inferior to EGFR TKI in terms of progression-free survival [121]. Malignancies associated with tobacco smoking are frequently associated with a higher tumor mutational load and smoking-associated signatures that may underlie their improved response to immune checkpoint blockade [122]. As patients with driver oncogene mutations such as ROS1 are much less likely to have a history of tobacco smoking and low tumor mutational burden compared to patients with smoking-associated lung cancers, it is possible that this may explain inferior outcomes to single agent immunotherapy in these oncogene-driven tumors.

Interestingly, the recent IMpower150 trial that evaluated the addition of atezolizumab to the combination of carboplatin, paclitaxel, and bevacizumab (BCP) in patients with metastatic non-squamous NSCLC found a significantly improved PFS and OS as compared to the non-atezolizumab arm. This included patients who had received TKIs, irrespective of *ALK* or *EGFR* mutational status [123]. In the subgroup analysis, addition of atezolizumab in patients with *EGFR* exon19 deletion or L858R mutation led to improved PFS (HR 0.41; 95% CI 0.22–0.78) vs BCP alone [124]. Hopefully, one would expect comparable results in ROS1 NSCLC.

Conclusions

With the data currently available, first-line therapy for patients with advanced *ROS1*-rearranged NSCLC should be crizotinib. While resistance mutations such as G2032R can pose a treatment challenge, there are a number of next-generation TKIs that may assist in the management of these patients. Although immunotherapy likely does not appear to provide benefit as a monotherapy, immune therapy combinations warrant further study. Additional studies will need to be performed to fully define the role of next-generation TKIs, combination-targeted therapies against ROS1, and bypass tract mechanisms or resistance in *ROS1*-rearranged NSCLC that become resistant to crizotinib.

References

1. Matsushime H, Wang LH, Shibuya M. Human c-ros-1 gene homologous to the v-ros sequence of UR2 sarcoma virus encodes for a transmembrane receptorlike molecule. Mol Cell Biol. 1986;6(8):3000–4.
2. Birchmeier C, et al. Characterization of an activated human ros gene. Mol Cell Biol. 1986;6(9):3109–16.

3. Acquaviva J, Wong R, Charest A. The multifaceted roles of the receptor tyrosine kinase ROS in development and cancer. Biochim Biophys Acta. 2009;1795(1):37–52.

4. Satoh H, et al. Regional localization of the human c-ros-1 on 6q22 and flt on 13q12. Jpn J Cancer Res. 1987;78(8):772–5.

5. Nagarajan L, et al. The human c-ros gene (ROS) is located at chromosome region 6q16—6q22. Proc Natl Acad Sci U S A. 1986;83(17):6568–72.

6. Robinson DR, Wu YM, Lin SF. The protein tyrosine kinase family of the human genome. Oncogene. 2000;19(49):5548–57.

7. Raabe T. The sevenless signaling pathway: variations of a common theme. Biochim Biophys Acta. 2000;1496(2–3):151–63.

8. Hart AC, et al. Induction of cell fate in the Drosophila retina: the bride of sevenless protein is predicted to contain a large extracellular domain and seven transmembrane segments. Genes Dev. 1990;4(11):1835–47.

9. Sonnenberg E, et al. Transient and locally restricted expression of the ros1 protooncogene during mouse development. EMBO J. 1991;10(12):3693–702.

10. Tessarollo L, Nagarajan L, Parada LF. c-ros: the vertebrate homolog of the sevenless tyrosine kinase receptor is tightly regulated during organogenesis in mouse embryonic development. Development. 1992;115(1):11–20.

11. Sonnenberg-Riethmacher E, et al. The c-ros tyrosine kinase receptor controls regionalization and differentiation of epithelial cells in the epididymis. Genes Dev. 1996;10(10):1184–93.

12. Birchmeier C, et al. Characterization of ROS1 cDNA from a human glioblastoma cell line. Proc Natl Acad Sci U S A. 1990;87(12):4799–803.

13. Birchmeier C, Sharma S, Wigler M. Expression and rearrangement of the ROS1 gene in human glioblastoma cells. Proc Natl Acad Sci U S A. 1987;84(24):9270–4.

14. Charest A, et al. Fusion of FIG to the receptor tyrosine kinase ROS in a glioblastoma with an interstitial del(6)(q21q21). Genes Chromosomes Cancer. 2003;37(1):58–71.

15. Charest A, et al. Association of a novel PDZ domain-containing peripheral Golgi protein with the Q-SNARE (Q-soluble N-ethylmaleimide-sensitive fusion protein (NSF) attachment protein receptor) protein syntaxin 6. J Biol Chem. 2001;276(31):29456–65.

16. Charest A, et al. Oncogenic targeting of an activated tyrosine kinase to the Golgi apparatus in a glioblastoma. Proc Natl Acad Sci. 2003;100(3):916–21.

17. Birch AH, et al. Chromosome 3 anomalies investigated by genome wide SNP analysis of benign, low malignant potential and low grade ovarian serous tumours. PLoS One. 2011;6(12):e28250.

18. Gu TL, et al. Survey of tyrosine kinase signaling reveals ROS kinase fusions in human cholangiocarcinoma. PLoS One. 2011;6(1):e15640.

19. Rimkunas VM, et al. Analysis of receptor tyrosine kinase ROS1-positive tumors in non-small cell lung cancer: identification of a FIG-ROS1 fusion. Clin Cancer Res. 2012;18(16):4449–57.

20. Lovly CM, et al. Inflammatory myofibroblastic tumors harbor multiple potentially actionable kinase fusions. Cancer Discov. 2014;4(8):889–95.

21. Yamamoto H, et al. ALK, ROS1 and NTRK3 gene rearrangements in inflammatory myofibroblastic tumours. Histopathology. 2016;69(1):72–83.

22. Lee J, et al. Identification of ROS1 rearrangement in gastric adenocarcinoma. Cancer. 2013;119(9):1627–35.

23. Aisner DL, et al. ROS1 and ALK Fusions in colorectal cancer, with evidence of intratumoral heterogeneity for molecular drivers. Mol Cancer Res. 2014;12(1):111–8.

24. Giacomini CP, et al. Breakpoint analysis of transcriptional and genomic profiles uncovers novel gene fusions spanning multiple human cancer types. PLoS Genet. 2013;9(4):e1003464.

25. Ritterhouse LL, et al. ROS1 rearrangement in thyroid cancer. Thyroid. 2016;26(6):794–7.

26. Rossing M, et al. Genomic diagnostics leading to the identification of a TFG-ROS1 fusion in a child with possible atypical meningioma. Cancer Genet. 2017;212–213:32–7.

27. Wiesner T, et al. Kinase fusions are frequent in Spitz tumours and spitzoid melanomas. Nat Commun. 2014;5:3116.

28. Rikova K, et al. Global survey of phosphotyrosine signaling identifies oncogenic kinases in lung cancer. Cell. 2007;131(6):1190–203.
29. Pal P, Khan Z. Ros1-1. J Clin Pathol. 2017;70(12):1001–9.
30. Charest A, et al. ROS fusion tyrosine kinase activates a SH2 domain-containing phosphatase-2/phosphatidylinositol 3-kinase/mammalian target of rapamycin signaling axis to form glioblastoma in mice. Cancer Res. 2006;66(15):7473–81.
31. Jun HJ, et al. The oncogenic lung cancer fusion kinase CD74-ROS activates a novel invasiveness pathway through E-Syt1 phosphorylation. Cancer Res. 2012;72(15):3764–74.
32. Wu S, et al. Clinicopathological characteristics and outcomes of ROS1-rearranged patients with lung adenocarcinoma without EGFR, KRAS mutations and ALK rearrangements. Thorac Cancer. 2015;6(4):413–20.
33. Bergethon K, et al. ROS1 rearrangements define a unique molecular class of lung cancers. J Clin Oncol. 2012;30(8):863–70.
34. Marchetti A, et al. ROS1 gene fusion in advanced lung cancer in women: a systematic analysis, review of the literature, and diagnostic algorithm. JCO Precis Oncol. 2017;1:1–9.
35. Gainor JF, et al. Patterns of metastatic spread and mechanisms of resistance to crizotinib in ROS1-positive non-small-cell lung cancer. JCO Precis Oncol. 2017;1:1–13.
36. Davies KD, Doebele RC. Molecular pathways: ROS1 fusion proteins in cancer. Clin Cancer Res. 2013;19(15):4040–5.
37. Davies KD, et al. Identifying and targeting ROS1 gene fusions in non-small cell lung cancer. Clin Cancer Res. 2012;18(17):4570–9.
38. Zhao J, et al. Advanced lung adenocarcinomas with ROS1-rearrangement frequently show hepatoid cell. Oncotarget. 2016;7(45):74162–70.
39. Lin JJ, et al. ROS1 fusions rarely overlap with other oncogenic drivers in non-small cell lung cancer. J Thorac Oncol. 2017;12(5):872–7.
40. Scheffler M, et al. ROS1 rearrangements in lung adenocarcinoma: prognostic impact, therapeutic options and genetic variability. Oncotarget. 2015;6(12):10577–85.
41. Cao B, et al. Detection of lung adenocarcinoma with ROS1 rearrangement by IHC, FISH, and RT-PCR and analysis of its clinicopathologic features. Onco Targets Ther. 2016;9:131–8.
42. Shaw AT, et al. Crizotinib in ROS1-rearranged non-small-cell lung cancer. N Engl J Med. 2014;371(21):1963–71.
43. Bubendorf L, et al. Testing for ROS1 in non-small cell lung cancer: a review with recommendations. Virchows Arch. 2016;469(5):489–503.
44. Yoshida A, et al. ROS1-rearranged lung cancer: a clinicopathologic and molecular study of 15 surgical cases. Am J Surg Pathol. 2013;37(4):554–62.
45. Lindeman NI, et al. Updated molecular testing guideline for the selection of lung cancer patients for treatment with targeted tyrosine kinase inhibitors: guideline from the College of American Pathologists, the International Association for the Study of Lung Cancer, and the Association for Molecular Pathology. Arch Pathol Lab Med. 2018;142(3):321–46.
46. Savic S, Bubendorf L. Role of fluorescence in situ hybridization in lung cancer cytology. Acta Cytol. 2012;56(6):611–21.
47. Su Y, et al. Immunohistochemical detection of ROS1 fusion. Am J Clin Pathol. 2017;147(1):77–82.
48. Yoshida A, et al. Immunohistochemical detection of ROS1 is useful for identifying ROS1 rearrangements in lung cancers. Mod Pathol. 2014;27(5):711–20.
49. Sholl LM, et al. ROS1 immunohistochemistry for detection of ROS1-rearranged lung adenocarcinomas. Am J Surg Pathol. 2013;37(9):1441–9.
50. Fischer AH, et al. Immunohistochemistry practices of cytopathology laboratories: a survey of participants in the College of American Pathologists Nongynecologic Cytopathology Education Program. Arch Pathol Lab Med. 2014;138(9):1167–72.
51. Shan L, et al. Detection of ROS1 gene rearrangement in lung adenocarcinoma: comparison of IHC, FISH and real-time RT-PCR. PLoS One. 2015;10(3):e0120422.

52. Ribeiro-Silva A, Zhang H, Jeffrey SS. RNA extraction from ten year old formalin-fixed paraffin-embedded breast cancer samples: a comparison of column purification and magnetic bead-based technologies. BMC Mol Biol. 2007;8:118.
53. Lira ME, et al. A single-tube multiplexed assay for detecting ALK, ROS1, and RET fusions in lung cancer. J Mol Diagn. 2014;16(2):229–43.
54. Reguart N, et al. Identification of *ALK, ROS1*, and *RET* fusions by a multiplexed mRNA-based assay in formalin-fixed, paraffin-embedded samples from advanced non–small-cell lung cancer patients. Clin Chem. 2017;63(3):751–60.
55. Zhu VW, et al. TPD52L1-ROS1, a new ROS1 fusion variant in lung adenosquamous cell carcinoma identified by comprehensive genomic profiling. Lung Cancer. 2016;97:48–50.
56. Zhu YC, et al. CEP72-ROS1: a novel ROS1 oncogenic fusion variant in lung adenocarcinoma identified by next-generation sequencing. Thorac Cancer. 2018;9(5):652–5.
57. Hartmaier RJ, et al. High-throughput genomic profiling of adult solid tumors reveals novel insights into cancer pathogenesis. Cancer Res. 2017;77(9):2464–75.
58. Ou SH, et al. Identification of a novel TMEM106B-ROS1 fusion variant in lung adenocarcinoma by comprehensive genomic profiling. Lung Cancer. 2015;88(3):352–4.
59. Govindan R, et al. Genomic landscape of non-small cell lung cancer in smokers and never-smokers. Cell. 2012;150(6):1121–34.
60. Zheng Z, et al. Anchored multiplex PCR for targeted next-generation sequencing. Nat Med. 2014;20(12):1479–84.
61. Christensen JG, et al. Cytoreductive antitumor activity of PF-2341066, a novel inhibitor of anaplastic lymphoma kinase and c-Met, in experimental models of anaplastic large-cell lymphoma. Mol Cancer Ther. 2007;6(12 Pt 1):3314–22.
62. Kwak EL, et al. Clinical activity observed in a phase I dose escalation trial of an oral c-met and ALK inhibitor, PF-02341066. J Clin Oncol. 2009;27(15S):3509.
63. Crinò L, et al. Initial phase II results with crizotinib in advanced ALK-positive non-small cell lung cancer (NSCLC): PROFILE 1005. J Clin Oncol. 2011;29(15_suppl):7514.
64. Yasuda H, et al. Preclinical rationale for use of the clinically available multitargeted tyrosine kinase inhibitor crizotinib in ROS1-translocated lung cancer. J Thorac Oncol. 2012;7(7):1086–90.
65. Huber KVM, et al. Stereospecific targeting of MTH1 by (S)-crizotinib as an anticancer strategy. Nature. 2014;508:222.
66. Camidge DR, et al. Activity and safety of crizotinib in patients with ALK-positive non-small-cell lung cancer: updated results from a phase 1 study. Lancet Oncol. 2012;13(10):1011–9.
67. Mazières J, et al. Crizotinib therapy for advanced lung adenocarcinoma and a ROS1 rearrangement: results from the EUROS1 cohort. J Clin Oncol. 2015;33(9):992–9.
68. Moro-Sibilot D, et al. Crizotinib in patients with advanced ROS1-rearranged non-small cell lung cancer (NSCLC). Preliminary results of the ACSé phase II trial. J Clin Oncol. 2015;33(15_suppl):8065.
69. Michels S, et al. MA07.05 EUCROSS: a european phase II trial of crizotinib in advanced adenocarcinoma of the lung harboring ROS1 rearrangements – preliminary results. J Thorac Oncol. 2017;12(1):S379–80.
70. Wu YL, et al. Phase II study of crizotinib in East Asian patients with ROS1-positive advanced non-small-cell lung cancer. J Clin Oncol. 2018;36(14):1405–11.
71. Katayama R, et al. Cabozantinib overcomes crizotinib resistance in ROS1 fusion-positive cancer. Clin Cancer Res. 2015;21(1):166–74.
72. Awad MM, et al. Acquired resistance to crizotinib from a mutation in CD74-ROS1. N Engl J Med. 2013;368(25):2395–401.
73. Cui JJ, et al. Structure based drug design of crizotinib (PF-02341066), a potent and selective dual inhibitor of mesenchymal–epithelial transition factor (c-MET) kinase and anaplastic lymphoma kinase (ALK). J Med Chem. 2011;54(18):6342–63.
74. Drilon A, et al. A novel crizotinib-resistant solvent-front mutation responsive to cabozantinib therapy in a patient with ROS1-rearranged lung cancer. Clin Cancer Res. 2016;22(10):2351–8.

75. Facchinetti F, et al. Crizotinib-resistant ROS1 mutations reveal a predictive kinase inhibitor sensitivity model for ROS1- and ALK-rearranged lung cancers. Clin Cancer Res. 2016;22(24):5983–91.

76. Friboulet L, et al. The ALK inhibitor ceritinib overcomes crizotinib resistance in non-small cell lung cancer. Cancer Discov. 2014;4(6):662–73.

77. McCoach CE, et al. Resistance mechanisms to targeted therapies in ROS1(+) and ALK(+) non-small cell lung cancer. Clin Cancer Res. 2018;24(14):3334–47.

78. Watanabe J, Furuya N, Fujiwara Y. Appearance of a BRAF mutation conferring resistance to crizotinib in non-small cell lung cancer harboring oncogenic ROS1 fusion. J Thorac Oncol. 2018;13(4):e66–9.

79. Dziadziuszko R, et al. An activating KIT mutation induces crizotinib resistance in ROS1-positive lung cancer. J Thorac Oncol. 2016;11(8):1273–81.

80. Zhu YC, et al. Concurrent ROS1 gene rearrangement and KRAS mutation in lung adenocarcinoma: a case report and literature review. Thorac Cancer. 2018;9(1):159–63.

81. Cargnelutti M, et al. Activation of RAS family members confers resistance to ROS1 targeting drugs. Oncotarget. 2015;6(7):5182–94.

82. Xu CW, et al. Patient harboring a novel PIK3CA point mutation after acquired resistance to crizotinib in an adenocarcinoma with ROS1 rearrangement: a case report and literature review. Thorac Cancer. 2017;8(6):714–9.

83. Shigemitsu K, et al. Genetic alteration of the beta-catenin gene (CTNNB1) in human lung cancer and malignant mesothelioma and identification of a new 3p21.3 homozygous deletion. Oncogene. 2001;20(31):4249–57.

84. Davies KD, et al. Resistance to ROS1 inhibition mediated by EGFR pathway activation in non-small cell lung cancer. PLoS One. 2013;8(12):e82236.

85. Song A, et al. Molecular changes associated with acquired resistance to crizotinib in ROS1-rearranged non-small cell lung cancer. Clin Cancer Res. 2015;21(10):2379–87.

86. Lin JJ, Shaw AT. Resisting resistance: targeted therapies in lung cancer. Trends Cancer. 2016;2(7):350–64.

87. Shaw AT, et al. Ceritinib in ALK-rearranged non–small-cell lung cancer. N Engl J Med. 2014;370(13):1189–97.

88. Kim HR, et al. The frequency and impact of ROS1 rearrangement on clinical outcomes in never smokers with lung adenocarcinoma. Ann Oncol. 2013;24(9):2364–70.

89. Lim SM, et al. Open-label, multicenter, phase II study of ceritinib in patients with non-small-cell lung cancer harboring ROS1 rearrangement. J Clin Oncol. 2017;35(23):2613–8.

90. Cho BC, et al. ASCEND-8: a randomized phase 1 study of ceritinib, 450 mg or 600 mg, taken with a low-fat meal versus 750 mg in fasted state in patients with anaplastic lymphoma kinase (ALK)-rearranged metastatic non-small cell lung cancer (NSCLC). J Thorac Oncol. 2017;12(9):1357–67.

91. Zou HY, et al. PF-06463922 is a potent and selective next-generation ROS1/ALK inhibitor capable of blocking crizotinib-resistant ROS1 mutations. Proc Natl Acad Sci U S A. 2015;112(11):3493–8.

92. Chong CR, et al. Identification of existing drugs that effectively target NTRK1 and ROS1 rearrangements in lung cancer. Clin Cancer Res. 2017;23(1):204–13.

93. Kato Y, et al. Combined effect of cabozantinib and gefitinib in crizotinib-resistant lung tumors harboring ROS1 fusions. Cancer Sci. 2018;109:3149.

94. Choueiri TK, et al. Cabozantinib versus everolimus in advanced renal cell carcinoma (METEOR): final results from a randomised, open-label, phase 3 trial. Lancet Oncol. 2016;17(7):917–27.

95. Ardini E, et al. Entrectinib, a Pan–TRK, ROS1, and ALK inhibitor with activity in multiple molecularly defined cancer indications. Mol Cancer Ther. 2016;15(4):628–39.

96. Menichincheri M, et al. Discovery of entrectinib: a new 3-aminoindazole as a potent anaplastic lymphoma kinase (ALK), c-ros Oncogene 1 Kinase (ROS1), and pan-tropomyosin receptor kinases (Pan-TRKs) inhibitor. J Med Chem. 2016;59(7):3392–408.

97. Drilon A, et al. Safety and antitumor activity of the multitargeted Pan-TRK, ROS1, and ALK inhibitor entrectinib: combined results from two phase I trials (ALKA-372-001 and STARTRK-1). Cancer Discov. 2017;7(4):400–9.

98. Ahn M, et al. OA 14.06 entrectinib in patients with locally advanced or metastatic ROS1 fusion-positive non-small cell lung cancer (NSCLC). J Thorac Oncol. 2017;12(11):S1783.

99. Shaw AT, et al. Lorlatinib in non-small-cell lung cancer with ALK or ROS1 rearrangement: an international, multicentre, open-label, single-arm first-in-man phase 1 trial. Lancet Oncol. 2017;18(12):1590–9.

100. Solomon B, et al. OA 05.06 phase 2 study of lorlatinib in patients with advanced ALK⁺/ROS1⁺ non-small-cell lung cancer. J Thorac Oncol. 2017;12(11):S1756.

101. Dong L, et al. Long-term progression-free survival in an advanced lung adenocarcinoma patient harboring EZR-ROS1 rearrangement: a case report. BMC Pulm Med. 2018;18(1):13.

102. Cui JJ, et al. TPX-0005, a novel ALK/ROS1/TRK inhibitor, effectively inhibited a broad spectrum of mutations including solvent front ALK G1202R, ROS1 G2032R and TRKA G595R mutants. Eur J Cancer. 2016;69:S32.

103. Cui JJ, et al. Abstract B185: TPX-0005, a supreme ROS1 inhibitor, overcomes crizotinib-resistant ROS1 mutations including solvent front mutation G2032R and gatekeeper mutation L2026M. Mol Cancer Ther. 2018;17(1 Supplement):B185.

104. Drilon AE, et al. A phase 1 study of the next-generation ALK/ROS1/TRK inhibitor ropotrectinib (TPX-0005) in patients with advanced ALK/ROS1/NTRK+ cancers (TRIDENT-1). J Clin Oncol. 2018;36(15_suppl):2513.

105. Kiga M, et al. Preclinical characterization and antitumor efficacy of DS-6051b, a novel, orally available small molecule tyrosine kinase inhibitor of ROS1 and NTRKs. Eur J Cancer. 2016;69:S35–6.

106. Fujiwara Y, et al. Safety and pharmacokinetics of DS-6051b in Japanese patients with non-small cell lung cancer harboring ROS1 fusions: a phase I study. Oncotarget. 2018;9(34):23729–37.

107. Kyriakos P, Papadopoulos LG, Janne PA, Ou S-HI, Shaw A, Goldberg TR, Greenberg J, Gu X, Tachibana M, Senaldi G, Shiga R, Zahir H, Nakamaru K, Borazanci E. First-in-human study of DS-6051b in patients (pts) with advanced solid tumors (AST) conducted in the US. J Clin Oncol. 2018;36(15_suppl):abstr 2514.

108. Squillace RM, et al. Abstract 5655: AP26113 possesses pan-inhibitory activity versus crizotinib-resistant ALK mutants and oncogenic ROS1 fusions. Cancer Res. 2013;73(8 Supplement):5655.

109. Davare MA, et al. Structural insight into selectivity and resistance profiles of ROS1 tyrosine kinase inhibitors. Proc Natl Acad Sci U S A. 2015;112(39):E5381–90.

110. Gettinger SN, et al. Activity and safety of brigatinib in ALK-rearranged non-small-cell lung cancer and other malignancies: a single-arm, open-label, phase 1/2 trial. Lancet Oncol. 2016;17(12):1683–96.

111. Kim D-W, et al. Brigatinib in patients with crizotinib-refractory anaplastic lymphoma kinase–positive non–small-cell lung cancer: a randomized, multicenter phase II trial. J Clin Oncol. 2017;35(22):2490–8.

112. Davare MA, et al. Foretinib is a potent inhibitor of oncogenic ROS1 fusion proteins. Proc Natl Acad Sci U S A. 2013;110(48):19519–24.

113. Sgambato A, et al. Targeted therapies in non-small cell lung cancer: a focus on ALK/ROS1 tyrosine kinase inhibitors. Expert Rev Anticancer Ther. 2018;18(1):71–80.

114. Shih C, et al. LY231514, a pyrrolo[2,3-d]pyrimidine-based antifolate that inhibits multiple folate-requiring enzymes. Cancer Res. 1997;57(6):1116–23.

115. Liang Y, Wakelee HA, Neal JW. Relationship of driver oncogenes to long-term pemetrexed response in non–small-cell lung cancer. Clin Lung Cancer. 2015;16(5):366–73.

116. Riess JW, et al. A case series of lengthy progression-free survival with pemetrexed-containing therapy in metastatic non–small-cell lung cancer patients harboring ROS1 gene rearrangements. Clin Lung Cancer. 2013;14(5):592–5.

117. Chen YF, et al. Efficacy of pemetrexed-based chemotherapy in patients with ROS1 fusion-positive lung adenocarcinoma compared with in patients harboring other driver mutations in East Asian populations. J Thorac Oncol. 2016;11(7):1140–52.
118. Spigel DR, et al. Phase 1/2 study of the safety and tolerability of nivolumab plus crizotinib for the first-line treatment of anaplastic lymphoma kinase translocation positive advanced nonsmall cell lung cancer (CheckMate 370). J Thorac Oncol. 2018;13(5):682–8.
119. Lisberg A, et al. A phase II study of pembrolizumab in EGFR-mutant, PD-L1+, Tyrosine kinase inhibitor Naïve patients with advanced NSCLC. J Thorac Oncol. 2018;13(8):1138–45.
120. Lee CK, et al. Checkpoint inhibitors in metastatic EGFR-mutated non–small cell lung cancer—a meta-analysis. J Thorac Oncol. 2017;12(2):403–7.
121. Sheng Z, et al. The efficacy of anti-PD-1/PD-L1 therapy and its comparison with EGFR-TKIs for advanced non-small-cell lung cancer. Oncotarget. 2017;8(34):57826–35.
122. Kim JH, Kim HS, Kim BJ. Prognostic value of smoking status in non-small-cell lung cancer patients treated with immune checkpoint inhibitors: a meta-analysis. Oncotarget. 2017;8(54):93149–55.
123. Socinski MA, et al. Atezolizumab for first-line treatment of metastatic nonsquamous NSCLC. N Engl J Med. 2018;378(24):2288–301.
124. Kowanetz M, et al. Abstract CT076: IMpower150: efficacy of atezolizumab (atezo) plus bevacizumab (bev) and chemotherapy (chemo) in 1L metastatic nonsquamous NSCLC (mNSCLC) across key subgroups. Cancer Res. 2018;78(13 Supplement):CT076.

BRAF: Novel Therapies for an Emerging Target

Nathaniel J. Myall and Sukhmani K. Padda

Abstract Driver mutations in the *BRAF* oncogene occur in 2–4% of non-small cell lung cancers (NSCLC). Approximately half of these *BRAF* mutations are characterized by a glutamic acid substitution for valine at position 600 within the BRAF kinase domain (V600E or class I). The remaining non-V600E mutations are a heterogeneous group that can be further subdivided into mutations that activate BRAF kinase activity (class II) and mutations that remain dependent on upstream signaling through Ras-GTPase (class III). In normal cells, the BRAF kinase functions as an intermediary within the MAPK/ERK signaling pathway. Activating mutations in the *BRAF* oncogene lead to downstream signaling through the MAPK/ERK pathway, resulting in an increased risk of malignant transformation in preclinical models. Based on these findings, as well as the need for more effective treatment options for patients with *BRAF*-mutated NSCLC, there has been a significant interest in developing targeted therapies to inhibit the MAPK/ERK pathway. In a series of phase 2 clinical trials enrolling patients with metastatic *BRAF* V600E-mutated NSCLC, Planchard et al. established a role for combined BRAF and MEK tyrosine kinase inhibition (TKI) with dabrafenib and trametinib, respectively. While this represents an important new treatment strategy, a number of questions still remain including how best to sequence targeted therapy with other available treatment options and how to effectively overcome acquired resistance to TKI therapy.

Keywords BRAF · Non-small cell lung cancer · MAPK/ERK signaling pathway · MEK · Targeted therapy · Dabrafenib · Trametinib

N. J. Myall · S. K. Padda (✉)
Department of Medicine, Division of Medical Oncology, Stanford University School of Medicine/Stanford Cancer Institute, Stanford, CA, USA
e-mail: padda@stanford.edu

© Springer Nature Switzerland AG 2019   79
R. Salgia (ed.), *Targeted Therapies for Lung Cancer*, Current Cancer Research,
https://doi.org/10.1007/978-3-030-17832-1_4

Introduction

Following the earliest description of *BRAF* mutations in human cancer nearly two decades ago, an improved understanding of the pathogenesis of these mutations has enabled the development of targeted therapies [1]. Although *BRAF* mutations occur infrequently in non-small cell lung cancer (NSCLC), the recent approval of targeted therapies for patients with metastatic disease represents an important milestone [2, 3]. With new therapeutic options to choose from, it is becoming increasingly important to understand the biology and clinical behavior of *BRAF*-mutated NSCLC. In this chapter, we aim to provide a comprehensive review of this topic, focusing on (1) the molecular mechanisms involved in tumorigenesis, (2) clinical features and outcomes associated with *BRAF* mutations, and (3) the role of targeted therapies. We conclude by describing what questions still remain in the field and how answers to these questions might improve the future management of patients with *BRAF*-mutated NSCLC.

Molecular Foundations

MAPK Signaling Pathways

BRAF-mutated cancers rely on signaling through the mitogen-activated protein kinase/extracellular signal-related kinase (MAPK/ERK) pathway, which regulates the differentiation, growth, and survival of normal cells [4, 5]. It is one of four related signaling pathways, each of which is driven by a specific group of serine-threonine kinases from the MAPK family, including ERK, JNK (c-Jun N-terminal kinase), p38, and ERK5/BMK1 (extracellular signal-related kinase 5/Big MAP kinase 1). Although MAPK signaling pathways have gained attention for their role in cancer, they have also been linked in preclinical models to a number of normal biological processes ranging from cytokine production to embryonic development [6–8]. The function and specific molecular players vary from one MAPK pathway to another but the basic structure of the signaling cascade is highly conserved [9]. At the center of each pathway is a MAPK enzyme that phosphorylates and activates a series of downstream targets through its serine/threonine kinase activity. Two additional kinase families lie upstream of MAPK: the dual-specificity MAPK serine/threonine and tyrosine kinase (MAPKK) and the MAPKK serine/threonine kinase (MAPKKK). Each of these kinases is activated sequentially, beginning with MAPKKK which activates MAPKK and ending with MAPK which is activated by MAPKK [10].

The structure of the MAPK/ERK signaling pathway has been particularly well described (Fig. 1). In its simplest form, the pathway begins upstream with extracel-

Fig. 1 (continued) homolog protein, Src homology 2 domain containing protein (Shc), and others not shown. When bound to GTP, Ras-GTPases recruit rapidly accelerated fibrosarcoma (RAF) proteins such as BRAF to the membrane surface. RAF proteins phosphorylate and activate MEK, which, in turn, activates ERK. ERK then activates numerous downstream targets, including transcription factors and repressors that regulate cellular growth and differentiation

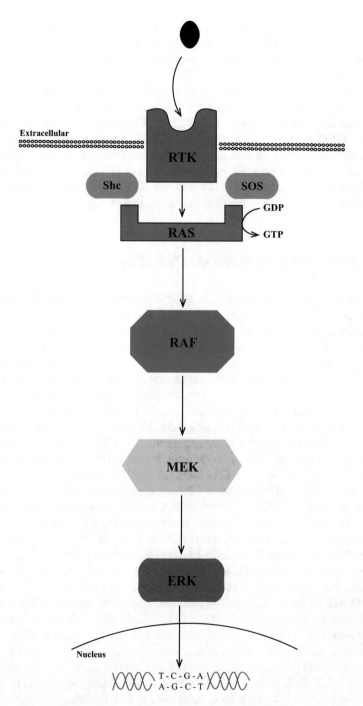

Fig. 1 A schematic representation of the MAPK/ERK signaling pathway is shown. Activation of upstream receptor tyrosine kinases (e.g., EGFR, PDGFR) by extracellular growth signals results in the recruitment of multiple intracellular proteins including Ras-GTPase, son of sevenless (SOS)

lular growth signals that bind to and activate transmembrane receptor tyrosine kinases [11]. Once activated, these receptor tyrosine kinases recruit multiple intracellular proteins to the membrane surface including Ras-GTPases (KRAS, NRAS, HRAS). When bound to GTP, Ras-GTPases are capable of activating proteins of the rapidly accelerated fibrosarcoma (RAF) family, which belong to the MAPKKK group of kinases. RAF in turn phosphorylates downstream MAPK/ERK kinase (MEK), which is a member of the MAPKK group of kinases. The activated form of MEK then phosphorylates ERK, which has numerous terminal targets including transcription factors (e.g., c-Myc), transcription repressors (e.g., ERF), and components of the cytoskeleton (e.g., myosin light chain kinase) [12–14]. Like other signaling pathways, the MAPK/ERK pathway is also tightly regulated at multiple levels by a series of negative feedback loops and inhibitory proteins [11, 15, 16].

Molecular Biology of Wild-Type RAF Kinase

The RAF family is comprised of three serine-threonine kinases: ARAF, BRAF, and CRAF, also known as Raf-1 [17, 18]. BRAF is encoded by the *V-raf murine sarcoma oncogene homolog B1 (BRAF)* gene located on chromosome 7q34 [19]. Expression of the wild-type *BRAF* gene is fairly ubiquitous across multiple organs and tissues, with highest expression found in the testis, thyroid, bone marrow, and brain [20]. The BRAF protein is 766 amino acids long, and, like other RAF kinases, it is arranged into three highly conserved regions (CR1, CR2, and CR3), each of which serves a distinct function (Fig. 2a) [21]. CR1 resides closest to the N-terminus and is comprised of both a cysteine-rich domain and a Ras-binding domain. The cysteine-rich domain coordinates translocation of RAF kinases from the cytoplasm to the membrane surface where they interact with Ras-GTPase via the Ras-binding domain [22, 23]. CR2 links the CR1 and CR3 domains and also contains a binding site for the 14-3-3 inhibitory protein. CR3, which resides closest to the C-terminus, contains a kinase domain that phosphorylates and activates downstream targets.

In addition to containing important binding sites, the CR1 domain also plays a role in regulating RAF kinase activity. Prior to activation by Ras-GTPases, cytoplasmic RAF kinases exist in an auto-inhibited state in which CR1 binds to CR3 and prevents phosphorylation of the kinase domain (Fig. 2b) [24–26]. When the MAPK/ERK pathway is activated, binding of RAF to Ras-GTPases at the cellular membrane interrupts the inhibitory interaction between CR1 and CR3. This, in turn, enables phosphorylation of key residues (e.g., T598, S601) that are necessary for kinase activation (Fig. 2c) [27]. Once activated in this manner, BRAF forms homodimers with itself and heterodimers with other RAF kinases, both of which are then capable of phosphorylating and activating a limited set of downstream targets, primarily MEK [28]. Eventually, phosphorylation and dephosphorylation of other key residues within BRAF by ERK-mediated negative feedback facilitates the dissociation of BRAF from Ras-GTPase, loss of RAF dimerization, and downregulation of kinase activity [29].

a

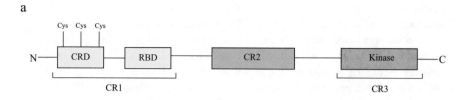

b   c

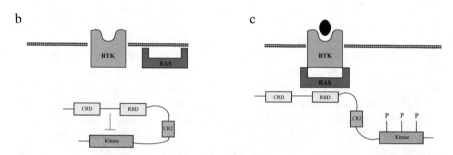

Fig. 2 (**a**) The structure of all RAF kinases is highly conserved and consists of three conserved regions (CR1, CR2, and CR3). CR1 contains both a cysteine-rich domain (CRD) and a Ras-binding domain (RBD). CR3 contains the active kinase domain. (**b**) In the inactive state, RAF kinases exist in an auto-inhibitory conformation whereby CR1 blocks key phosphorylation sites within CR3 that are responsible for activating the kinase. (**c**) When bound to Ras-GTPases at the intracellular cell surface via the Ras-binding domain, CR1 dissociates from CR3, enabling activation of the kinase and phosphorylation of downstream targets

Oncogenic Potential of *BRAF* Mutations

Although multiple effectors along the MAPK/ERK signaling pathway have been implicated in tumorigenesis, the oncogenic potential of *BRAF* mutations was first described in 2002 [30]. In their seminal report, Davis et al. initially sequenced three *BRAF* mutations from a limited number of melanoma and NSCLC cell lines. Two of the mutations occurred in exon 15, which encodes the kinase domain of the BRAF protein. This included both a T1796A substitution, which led to glutamic acid in the place of valine at position 599 (V599E), and a C1786G substitution, which led to valine in the place of leucine at position 596 (L596 V). A third G1403C substitution was found in exon 11, leading to the replacement of glycine with alanine at position 468 within the glycine-rich pocket of the ATP-binding domain (G468A). To confirm these findings, the authors performed a larger follow-up screen, which identified *BRAF* mutations in 59% of melanoma cell lines, 18% of colorectal cancer cell lines, and a smaller minority of cell lines derived from glioma, sarcoma, ovarian cancer, and NSCLC, among others. As the majority of *BRAF* mutations in melanoma involved a T1796A substitution, which is now known to result in the replacement of valine with glutamic acid at position 600 within the BRAF kinase domain, these mutations came to be known as V600E. On the other hand, mutations affecting other sites within the BRAF kinase were subsequently termed non-V600E. Davis et al. showed that mutations from both groups were capable of activating the MAPK/ERK pathway. Specifically, transfecting either *BRAF* V599E (now known as V600E) or G468A mutations into cell culture resulted in increased activity of the BRAF kinase as well as downstream phosphorylation of ERK.

Following this initial report from Davis et al., it became clear from subsequent studies that *BRAF* V600E mutations transform the BRAF protein into a constitutively active kinase that functions independently of upstream activation. Brummer et al. demonstrated this by engineering *BRAF* genes to co-express both V600E (T1796A) and R188L mutations, the latter of which renders BRAF ineffective at binding to upstream Ras-GTPases [31]. While R188L mutations alone prevented BRAF-mediated MAPK/ERK pathway activation, the presence of a concomitant *BRAF* V600E mutation restored phosphorylation of ERK, suggesting that BRAF V600E mutant kinases act independently of upstream Ras-GTPases. This conclusion was further supported by the finding that EGFR inhibition was not effective against lung cancer cell lines harboring *BRAF* mutations, despite EGFR being identified as an upstream activator of the MAPK/ERK pathway [32]. Although *BRAF* V600E mutations have gained more attention due to their frequent occurrence in melanoma, several *BRAF* non-V600E mutations (e.g., G468A, L596 V) have also been associated with increased kinase activity compared to wild-type *BRAF* [33]. However, this may not be true of all non-V600E mutations, as we discuss in greater detail below.

After establishing that many *BRAF* mutations activate the MAPK/ERK pathway, in vivo studies were then conducted to determine the potential association between *BRAF* mutations, MAPK/ERK pathway activation, and tumorigenesis. In one of these studies, Ji et al. engineered mice to express *BRAF* V600E mutations in the lung epithelium [34]. These mice developed lung adenomas at 6 weeks followed by adenocarcinomas at 16 weeks. Subsequent silencing of *BRAF* gene expression led to dephosphorylation of ERK, decreased expression of cyclin D, and decreased tumor burden. This suggested that BRAF activity and downstream MAPK/ERK signaling were the link between *BRAF* V600E mutations and the ongoing survival of lung tumors.

In other mouse models, however, *BRAF* mutations have been found to be necessary but not sufficient for the induction of malignant tumorigenesis. Dankort et al., for example, found that while expression of *BRAF* V600E in the lung parenchyma of mice led to increased phosphorylation of MEK and ERK as well as the development of lung adenomas, these adenomas entered a state of growth arrest, and very few progressed to adenocarcinoma unless a tumor suppressor gene such as *TP53* was also mutated [35]. A two-hit process was also suggested by a second mouse model in which co-expression of both *BRAF* V600E and *PIK3CA* H1047R mutations was associated with increased tumor burden, higher risk of developing malignant tumors, and shorter overall survival (OS) compared to mice with *BRAF* V600E mutations alone [36]. Malignant tumorigenesis in these mice was further enhanced when *TP53* mutations were also introduced. Interestingly, in vivo models of melanoma have similarly suggested that *BRAF* mutations may predispose to the growth of benign nevi but not malignant melanomas [37]. Taken together, these findings suggest that while *BRAF* mutations predispose to benign, premalignant tumors, other concomitant mutations may be necessary for the full induction of malignancy.

Regardless of the complex molecular interactions by which *BRAF* mutations initiate tumorigenesis, ongoing survival of *BRAF*-mutated tumors appears to rely strongly on signaling through the MAPK/ERK pathway. In multiple preclinical studies, inhibition of mutant BRAF V600E itself or its downstream targets such as MEK has been shown to lead to tumor regression in patient-derived xenografts and other mouse models of melanoma and lung cancer [35, 38, 39]. These results suggest that continued activation of the MAPK/ERK pathway is necessary for sustained tumor growth and that use of targeted therapies to block this pathway in *BRAF*-mutated tumors represents a promising treatment strategy.

Classification of BRAF *Mutations*

As described above, *BRAF* mutations have traditionally been classified as either V600E or non-V600E. However, our understanding of the varied mechanisms by which different *BRAF* mutations activate the MAPK/ERK pathway has evolved. A newer classification system has now been proposed that divides *BRAF* mutations into three classes (class I, II, or III) based on their effect on BRAF kinase activity and their interaction with upstream Ras-GTPases (Table 1).

In the first of two studies, Yao et al. highlighted the differences between what would become known as class I and class II *BRAF* mutations. They initially demonstrated that expression of either *BRAF* V600E mutations or certain *BRAF* non-V600E mutations (e.g., G469A, L597 V, K601E) in cell culture was associated with increased phosphorylation of MEK, decreased phosphorylation of CRAF, and reduced expression of Ras-GTPase [40]. The authors concluded that these *BRAF* mutations function in a Ras-independent manner to facilitate both downstream MAPK/ERK activation and upstream feedback inhibition of CRAF and Ras-GTPase. Despite these common endpoints, the authors found that the mechanisms

Table 1 Classification of *BRAF* mutations in cancer

	Kinase activity	Ras-independent	Monomer vs. Dimer	Vemurafenib sensitive[a]	Common mutations
Class I	Increased	Yes	Monomer	Yes	V600E
Class II	Increased	Yes	Dimer	No	G469A
Class III	Impaired	No	Dimer	No	G466 V

[a]Based on preclinical data reported in Yao et al. [40, 41] (see references for full citations).

by which different *BRAF* mutations induced downstream signaling were not the same. Whereas *BRAF* V600E/K/D/R (V600) mutations produced constitutively active BRAF kinases that functioned as Ras-independent monomers, *BRAF* mutations affecting sites other than position 600 (non-V600) produced active BRAF kinases that formed Ras-independent dimers. From a treatment perspective, this designation was important, as only BRAF V600 monomers but not BRAF non-V600 mutant dimers were sensitive to vemurafenib in vitro. Based on these findings, the authors defined two groups of *BRAF* mutations according to their mechanisms of Ras-independent signaling: V600 mutations that signal as constitutively active BRAF monomers (class I) and non-V600 mutations that signal as constitutively active BRAF dimers (class II).

In a second study, Yao et al. broadened their classification system to include a third class of *BRAF* mutations (class III) [41]. The authors identified a subset of non-V600 mutations, including D594G/N and G466 V/E, that encode for "kinase dead" or "kinase impaired" versions of the BRAF protein. Although these mutations were still capable of activating the MAPK/ERK pathway in vitro through their strong interaction with Ras-GTPase, they were less active than class I or II *BRAF* mutations, and they remained dependent on upstream Ras-GTPase. The authors proposed that class III *BRAF* mutations are oncogenic when paired synergistically with upstream activation of Ras-GTPase. Consistent with this hypothesis, the authors found that class III *BRAF* mutations in melanoma cell lines were often accompanied by activating mutations in *RAS* or *NF1* while class III *BRAF* mutations in NSCLC and colorectal cancer cell lines had high levels of phosphorylated receptor tyrosine kinases such as EGFR, ERBB2, and MET. As class III *BRAF* mutations activate the MAPK/ERK pathway in a Ras-dependent manner, the authors also found that patient-derived xenografts of class III *BRAF*-mutated colorectal cancer were not responsive to BRAF inhibition with vemurafenib. However, they were sensitive to cetuximab (EGFR monoclonal antibody) and, to a lesser degree, trametinib (MEK inhibitor), suggesting dependency on the MAPK/ERK pathway.

The value of the novel class I–III classification system is that it shifts focus away from the structural amino acid changes that characterize different mutations and toward the functional significance of the mutations instead. In the era of targeted therapy, acknowledging the heterogeneous mechanisms by which different *BRAF* mutations activate the MAPK/ERK pathway is arguably more important and has the potential to shed light on targets beyond BRAF and MEK that may be therapeutically relevant. The distinction between different types of *BRAF* non-V600 mutations is especially important, given that these mutations had been previously grouped together into a heterogeneous category. Clinical trials for patients with *BRAF* non-V600 mutations are clearly needed, and drug development as well as clinical trial designs should consider class II and class III *BRAF* non-V600 mutations separately, given the different functional mechanisms by which these mutations regulate the MAPK/ERK pathway.

BRAF Mutations in Non-small Cell Lung Cancer

BRAF mutations occur most commonly in melanoma, where the incidence of V600E mutations is >50% in metastatic disease [42, 43]. Other cancers in which *BRAF* is recurrently mutated include papillary thyroid carcinoma, hairy cell leukemia, and microsatellite unstable colorectal cancer [44–46]. The biological significance of *BRAF* mutations in these different tumor types likely varies, which is clear when considering the utility of targeted therapy in different cancers. At one extreme, BRAF inhibition alone with vemurafenib was highly efficacious in small cohorts of relapsed, refractory hairy cell leukemia [47]. At the other extreme, BRAF targeted monotherapy was ineffective when studied in colorectal cancer and has no current role in the disease [48]. These different susceptibilities to BRAF targeted therapy suggest that while the downstream MAPK/ERK pathway is targetable in *BRAF*-mutated tumors in general, the development of resistance and reliance on other bypass growth pathways likely varies from one tumor type to the other.

In lung cancer, *BRAF* mutations are relatively uncommon but represent an early, clonal event in cancer development, suggesting that they are an important oncogenic driver in this setting [49]. While they have also been described as secondary resistance mutations arising in previously treated *EGFR*-mutated NSCLC, it is their role as primary driver mutations that has garnered the most attention [50].

Pathologic and Clinical Characteristics

The overall incidence of *BRAF* mutations in NSCLC is approximately 2–4% [51–53]. Although the distribution of *BRAF* V600E versus *BRAF* non-V600E mutations varies between studies, *BRAF* non-V600E mutations appear to represent nearly half of all *BRAF* mutations occurring in NSCLC [52, 54–56].

Consistent with their role as drivers in NSCLC, *BRAF* mutations are usually found independently of mutations in *EGFR* or rearrangements in *ALK* [57]. Identifying other co-occurring mutations in *BRAF*-mutated NSCLC has been limited by (1) the relative infrequency with which *BRAF* mutations occur in lung cancer and (2) sequencing panels that test only for mutations in a select number of driver genes. However, the advent of next-generation sequencing has allowed for broader mutational testing. In one study of 1007 patients with metastatic or recurrent lung adenocarcinoma whose tumors were genotyped using multiplexed assays of up to 10 genes, 2 of the 14 patients whose tumors harbored *BRAF* V600E mutations also had co-occurring *PIK3CA* E542K mutations [53]. In another cohort of 174 patients with *BRAF*-mutated NSCLC, next-generation sequencing of 17 genes identified co-mutations in *TP53* in 89 cases (51%) [58]. Findings such as this are potentially consistent with the preclinical studies described previously that suggested that co-occurring mutations contribute to the malignant differentiation of *BRAF*-mutated tumors.

It remains unclear as to how co-occurring mutations affect survival or response to treatment in patients with *BRAF*-mutated NSCLC. In our own single-center study of 18 patients with *BRAF*-mutated NSCLC, we found that those patients with metastatic disease whose tumors harbored co-occurring *TP53* mutations ($n = 4$) had a numerically worse OS compared to patients without *TP53* mutations ($n = 12$) (37.7 vs. 13.7 months; $P = 0.23$) [59]. Conclusions are limited by the very small sample size, although the suggestion of worse outcomes in patients harboring co-mutations in *TP53* is consistent with studies of other driver-mutated lung cancers. For example, shorter OS has been reported in patients with NSCLC whose tumors harbor *TP53* mutations alongside driver mutations in *EGFR, ALK,* or *ROS1* [60]. On the other hand, *TP53* mutations in *KRAS*-mutated NSCLC have been associated with increased somatic mutation burden and an enhanced response to immunotherapy [61, 62]. As molecular tumor testing expands and more patients with *BRAF*-mutated NSCLC are identified, further prognostic and predictive studies of patients with co-occurring *TP53* mutations are warranted.

Given the fact that other driver mutations are known to be enriched in particular patients with NSCLC, there has been a strong interest in identifying clinicopathologic features that associate with *BRAF* mutations. Across multiple studies, *BRAF* mutations have been primarily found in NSCLC with adenocarcinoma histology [52, 55, 56, 59, 63, 64]. As pointed out by Cardarella et al., genomic testing in clinical practice may be more routinely performed for adenocarcinomas compared to other histologic subtypes, which could reflect a source of bias [52]. However, two studies performed genomic sequencing in resected lung cancers from 1046 (37 *BRAF*-positive) and 2001 (26 *BRAF*-positive) patients with primarily early stage disease who otherwise might not have undergone routine molecular testing. In both of these studies, *BRAF* mutations occurred more commonly in adenocarcinoma than in squamous cell cancer, suggesting that histology is closely associated with *BRAF* mutation status [55, 64].

With respect to demographic characteristics, including age, sex, and smoking history, Cardarella et al. found no differences in 36 patients with *BRAF*-mutated NSCLC compared to those with wild-type NSCLC as determined by Sanger sequencing [52]. In contrast, it has been difficult to draw conclusions about associations with ethnicity from individual retrospective studies, as many them have been conducted in ethnically homogenous cohorts. In multiple reports consisting primarily of Asian patients, *BRAF* mutations have been reported in 0.7–1.7% of cases, which is similar to the 0.4% rate reported in an African American cohort but lower than the 4% rate described in a predominantly Caucasian cohort [52, 65–67]. It may be tempting to conclude from these numbers that *BRAF* mutations occur more commonly in certain ethnic groups but comparing results across studies requires a certain degree of caution. In addition, prior studies have suggested that tumor mutation testing may not be performed equally in patients of different ethnic backgrounds, which reflects a potential source of bias [68].

Within the group of patients with *BRAF*-mutated NSCLC, there may be more significant demographic differences between those with *BRAF* V600E versus *BRAF* non-V600E mutations. Sex differences have been reported in two studies that each found *BRAF* V600E mutations to be more common in females [55, 69]. A more consistent finding has been that patients with *BRAF* V600E mutations are more likely to have been never or light smokers compared to patients with *BRAF* non-V600E mutations [52, 54, 55, 59, 69]. Given the potential relationship between smoking, tumor mutation burden, and response to immunotherapy, this difference between patients with *BRAF* V600E versus *BRAF* non-V600E mutations may have important therapeutic implications [70]. Of note, fewer studies have evaluated demographic characteristics in patients with *BRAF*-mutated NSCLC using the newer class I–III classification system. However, one retrospective study that did evaluate *BRAF* mutations according to this classification system similarly found that patients with class I *BRAF* V600-mutated NSCLC were more commonly never-smokers than patients with class II or III *BRAF* non-V600-mutated NSCLC [71].

Outcomes and Prognosis

BRAF-mutated NSCLC was originally thought to have a more aggressive phenotype given its association with papillary and micropapillary histologic features [72]. However, retrospective studies suggest that the outcomes of patients with *BRAF*-mutated NSCLC compare favorably to the outcomes of patients whose tumors harbor other driver mutations or are wild-type for known drivers. In one of the earlier studies of *BRAF*-mutated NSCLC, for example, 739 resected adenocarcinomas from patients with primarily early stage disease were sequenced to identify *BRAF* mutations in exons 11 and 15 [55]. The median OS of 36 patients with *BRAF*-mutated adenocarcinoma (21 V600E and 15 non-V600E) was not statistically different than that of patients with *BRAF* wild-type adenocarcinoma (data not reported). In a separate cohort of patients with metastatic or recurrent adenocarcinoma from the Lung Cancer Mutation Consortium, Villaruz et al. reported a median OS of 56 months for 15 patients with *BRAF*-mutated NSCLC, which was not statistically different than the median OS reported for patients with *EGFR* mutations (43 months), *KRAS* mutations (33 months), *ALK* rearrangements (52 months), or no oncogenic driver (25 months) ($P > 0.20$) [73]. Notably, only three patients with *BRAF*-mutated NSCLC in this study had received MEK-directed targeted therapy (selumetinib), and none received BRAF-directed targeted therapy. In a third study of French patients, Tissot et al. similarly found that the median OS of 80 patients with *BRAF*-mutated NSCLC (42 V600E, 57.5% stage IV) was not statistically different than that of patients whose tumors were wild-type in *EGFR, KRAS, HER2, PI3K*, and *ALK* (22.1 vs. 14.5 months; $P = 0.095$) [56]. Only a small number of patients in this study ($n = 9$; 11%) received BRAF or combined BRAF-MEK targeted therapy.

Although all *BRAF* mutations were analyzed together in the above studies, subgroup analyses from these and other studies suggest that not all *BRAF* mutations behave the same. Marchetti et al. found that 21 patients with *BRAF* V600E-mutated early stage disease undergoing resection had a shorter median disease-free survival (DFS) (15.2 vs. 52.1 months; $P < 0.001$) and OS (29.3 vs. 72.4 months; $P < 0.001$)

compared to those with *BRAF* V600E wild-type disease [55]. In contrast, 15 patients with *BRAF* non-V600E mutations had similar DFS (42.8 vs. 43.2 months; $P = 0.84$) and OS (56.4 vs. 65.1 months; $P = 0.42$) compared to those with *BRAF* non-V600E wild-type disease. In a cohort of patients with stage IV NSCLC, Cardarella et al. similarly reported a non-significantly lower response rate to platinum-based chemo-therapy (29% vs. 71%; $P = 0.286$) and shorter progression-free survival (PFS) (4.1 vs. 8.9 months; $P = 0.297$) in patients with metastatic NSCLC harboring *BRAF* V600E ($n = 7$) versus *BRAF* non-V600E ($n = 7$) mutations [52]. A few additional patients with metastatic disease were available for the survival analysis, which revealed non-significantly shortened OS (10.8 vs. 15.2 months; $P = 0.726$) in patients with *BRAF* V600E-mutated NSCLC ($n = 12$) versus *BRAF* non-V600E-mutated NSCLC ($n = 12$). In contrast to these studies, Litvak et al. found that the 3-year OS rate for patients with stage IIIB/IV *BRAF* V600E-mutated NSCLC ($n = 20$) was 24% compared to 0% for patients with non-V600E mutations ($n = 9$) ($P < 0.001$) [54]. The 3-year OS rate of patients with *BRAF* V600E-mutated NSCLC was not statistically different than that of patients with unresectable *EGFR*-mutated NSCLC (38%). However, 94% of patients with *EGFR*-mutated NSCLC in this study received EGFR-directed targeted therapy compared to only 50% of patients with *BRAF*-mutated NSCLC receiving BRAF-directed targeted therapy.

In conjunction with these conflicting findings are multiple case reports that have described long-term survival lasting several years in select patients with metastatic *BRAF* V600E-mutated NSCLC [74, 75]. However, the small patient numbers in these reports as well as in the retrospective studies described above have limited conclu-sions regarding the differential effect of *BRAF* V600E versus *BRAF* non-V600E mutations on outcomes. A recent study from Dagogo-Jack et al. begins to overcome this limitation by describing one of the largest cohorts of *BRAF*-mutated NSCLC to date [71]. Using the newer class I–III classification system, the authors identified 236 patients at their center whose tumors had a *BRAF* mutation detected by either next-generation sequencing or multiplex polymerase chain reaction. This included 107 patients with class I *BRAF* V600 mutations and 129 patients with class II or III *BRAF* non-V600 mutations. Among the 139 patients with metastatic disease at diagnosis, 62 of them received first-line carboplatin plus pemetrexed. The median PFS was longer in patients with class I *BRAF* mutations compared to patients with class II or III *BRAF* mutations (6.2 vs. 3.3 months, $P = 0.069$ for class I vs. class II and 6.2 vs. 4.9 months, $P = 0.034$ for class I vs. class III). Overall survival for the entire group of 139 patients with metastatic disease was also longer in those with class I *BRAF* mutations com-pared to class II or III *BRAF* mutations (40.1 vs. 13.9 months, $P < 0.001$ for class I vs. class II and 40.1 vs. 15.6 months, $P = 0.023$ for class I vs. class III).

Interestingly, the authors found that patients with class I *BRAF* mutations were less likely to have brain metastases at diagnosis than patients with class II or III *BRAF* mutations. They were also more likely to have intrathoracic metastases alone than patients with class II *BRAF* mutations. When survival analyses were limited to patients with extra-thoracic metastases who did not receive targeted therapy, median OS between the mutation classes was not significantly different (9.4 months for class I vs. 7.9 months for class II vs. 9.7 months for class III), suggesting that extent of disease and response to targeted therapy are prognostically important. Although additional studies are needed for confirmation, these results suggest that favorable outcomes may be achieved in a subset of patients with *BRAF*-mutated NSCLC and that patients with class I *BRAF* mutations in particular may have a better prognosis due to the different clinical behavior of these mutations compared to class II or III *BRAF* non-V600E mutations.

A Changing Therapeutic Landscape

Efficacy of Targeted Therapy

Despite long-term survival in some cases of *BRAF*-mutated NSCLC, additional advances are required to improve outcomes. Furthermore, prior to the approval of targeted therapies for *BRAF*-mutated NSCLC, more than half of patients with these tumors received only best supportive care in the second-line setting, suggesting a need for additional therapeutic options for this patient population [76].

Targeted therapies inhibiting the MAPK/ERK signaling pathway have been most extensively studied in melanoma, due to the frequency of *BRAF* mutations in this disease. Initial front-line trials in melanoma evaluated reversible BRAF kinase inhibitors (dabrafenib or vemurafenib) as monotherapy in the treatment of patients with metastatic or unresectable *BRAF* V600E-mutated disease. In this setting, dabrafenib was associated with an overall response rate (ORR) of 50% (95% CI 42.4–57.1) compared to 6% (95% CI 1.8–15.5) with dacarbazine [77]. Single-agent vemurafenib was similarly effective with an ORR of 57% (95% CI NR) versus 9% (95% CI NR) for dacarbazine [78]. Vemurafenib was also associated with an OS benefit of 13.6 months versus 9.7 months (HR 0.70, 95% CI 0.57–0.87, $P = 0.0008$). As resistance to BRAF targeted therapies developed quickly in these patients, subsequent studies focused on the combination of reversible MEK kinase inhibitors (trametinib or cometinib) with BRAF kinase inhibitors in untreated metastatic melanoma. Combined therapy in this setting was associated with significantly improved response rates and longer PFS and OS compared to BRAF kinase inhibitors alone, thus establishing dual inhibition as the standard of care [79–82].

Support for using BRAF targeted therapy in lung cancer initially came from case reports that described responses in individual patients [83–85]. This was supported by a retrospective study of 35 patients with *BRAF*-mutated NSCLC (29 V600E, 6 non-V600E) who were treated with a BRAF kinase inhibitor (dabrafenib, vemurafenib, or sorafenib) outside of the clinical trial setting. The response rate among all patients, the majority of whom received targeted therapy in the later-line setting, was 53% (95% CI 35–70) [86].

The earliest prospective studies evaluating BRAF targeted therapy in lung cancer were basket trials that included not only NSCLC but also multiple other cancers harboring *BRAF* V600E mutations as well. The first was a phase 1 trial of dabrafenib that enrolled one patient with *BRAF* V600E-mutated NSCLC who achieved a partial response with an 83% reduction in tumor size [87]. In a phase 2 trial enrolling 20 patients with *BRAF* V600E-mutated NSCLC, most of whom had received prior systemic therapy, the response rate to vemurafenib was 42% (95% CI 20–67), consisting entirely of partial responses [88].

Based on these encouraging results, Planchard et al. conducted three phase 2 multicenter, open-label trials evaluating the use of targeted therapy in patients with metastatic *BRAF* V600E-mutated NSCLC (Table 2) [89–91]. In the first trial, previously treated patients received BRAF targeted therapy alone with dabrafenib 150 mg twice daily. Treatment was active in a subset of patients, with an overall response rate of 33% (95% CI 23–45) and a median PFS of 5.5 months (95% CI 3.4–7.3). In the second trial enrolling another cohort of previously treated patients, combination BRAF and MEK targeted therapy was administered with dabrafenib 150 mg twice daily and trametinib 2 mg once daily, respectively. Outcomes in response to combination therapy were better than those reported in the dabrafenib monotherapy cohort, although the two groups were enrolled separately and not intended for direct comparison. Nonetheless, the response rate to combination therapy was 63.2% (95% CI 49.3–75.6) with a median PFS of 9.7 months (95% CI 6.9–19.6). This led to a third study evaluating combination dabrafenib plus trametinib in patients with previously untreated metastatic *BRAF* V600E-mutated NSCLC. Combination therapy in the frontline setting was active, with an overall response rate of 64% (95% CI 46–79) that included two complete responses and a median PFS of 10.9 months (95% CI 7.0–16.6). Only 5 patients (14%) in this cohort had a best response of progressive disease.

The most common grade 3 or higher adverse events in patients receiving dabrafenib monotherapy were asthenia, squamous cell carcinoma of the skin, and basal cell carcinoma. The side effect profile of dabrafenib plus trametinib was slightly different with fever and cytopenias occurring more commonly but basal and squamous cell carcinoma of the skin occurring less commonly. In patients with previously treated NSCLC, dabrafenib plus trametinib was also associated with higher rates of treatment discontinuation (12% vs. 6%), treatment interruption (61% vs.

Table 2 Consecutive phase 2 trials of dabrafenib with or without trametinib in *BRAF* V600E-mutated non-small cell lung cancer

	Therapy	Setting	ORR[a]	PFS[b] (months)	OS[c] (months)
Cohort A (*n* = 78)	Dabrafenib	Relapsed[d]	33%	5.5	12.7
Cohort B (*n* = 57)	Dabrafenib/trametinib	Relapsed	63.2%	9.7	–[e]
Cohort C (*n* = 36)	Dabrafenib/trametinib	Untreated	64%	10.9	24.6

[a]*ORR* investigator-assessed overall response rate
[b]*PFS* median progression free survival
[c]*OS* median overall survival
[d]Cohort A included primarily patients with relapsed disease receiving targeted therapy in the second- or later-line setting (*n* = 78). The study also enrolled six previously untreated patients, but the results presented here are for the cohort with relapsed disease only
[e]Survival data was not mature at the time of publication

43%), and dose reduction (35% vs. 18%) compared to patients receiving dabrafenib alone. However, side effects in both groups were ultimately felt to be manageable overall. Based on the acceptable safety profile and potential benefit associated with targeted therapy, dabrafenib 150 mg twice daily plus trametinib 2 mg once daily is now approved as of 2017 for patients with untreated or previously treated, advanced *BRAF* V600E-mutated NSCLC, making it the only combination targeted therapy regimen that is approved in lung cancer [92].

As described above, NSCLC is unique in that approximately half of *BRAF* mutations are non-V600E. However, clinical trials of BRAF targeted therapies have excluded patients with *BRAF* non-V600E mutations. It has been reasonable to assume that *BRAF* non-V600E mutations may be less responsive to BRAF-directed targeted therapy given that the mechanisms by which they activate MAPK/ERK signaling are different than those of V600E mutations [40, 41]. However, further studies are needed for confirmation. The hope is that by further exploring the signaling mechanisms that underlie different *BRAF* mutations, new targets for the treatment of *BRAF* non-V600E-mutated NSCLC will emerge that can be tested in the clinical trial setting.

Mechanisms of Resistance to Targeted Therapy

Although BRAF-directed targeted therapies are effective, the development of resistance and eventual disease progression are inevitable. Much more is known about secondary resistance in *BRAF*-mutated melanoma given that targeted therapy for metastatic *BRAF* V600E-mutated NSCLC was only recently approved. As a result, our current understanding of secondary resistance in NSCLC is limited primarily to case reports.

Studies of melanoma have identified mechanisms of both innate and acquired resistance to BRAF-directed targeted therapy. With respect to innate resistance, the tumor microenvironment is thought to play an important role. In a study by Straussman et al., extracellular hepatocyte growth factor (HGF) secreted by stromal cells was shown to activate the MAPK and PIK3CA pathways in melanoma cells via binding to the MET receptor [93]. In a series of experiments, the authors showed that while PLX4720, a BRAF kinase inhibitor, effectively inhibited proliferation of melanoma cells in vitro, the addition of increasing concentrations of HGF resulted in resistance and sustained melanoma cell growth. Notably, when HGF expression was then measured by immunohistochemistry in 34 melanoma biopsy samples derived from patients enrolled in clinical trials, HGF positivity pretreatment was associated with a lower response to BRAF inhibition with or without dual inhibition of MEK.

On the other hand, acquired resistance in melanoma has been attributed to multiple secondary mutations that induce either upregulation of the MAPK/ERK signaling pathway or activation of bypass pathways. In the case of other driver-mutated cancers, acquired gatekeeper mutations occurring in the same driver genes can confer resistance and pathway reactivation. In the classic example of *EGFR*-mutated

NSCLC, for example, a gatekeeper T790 M mutation arises in a subset of patients treated with erlotinib or gefitinib. The T790 M mutation renders the EGFR kinase resistant to binding by first- and second-generation EGFR tyrosine kinase inhibitors, thus restoring EGFR-mediated growth signaling and cancer progression [94]. In the case of *BRAF*-mutated melanoma, gatekeeper mutations producing an amino acid substitution for threonine at residue 529 within the BRAF kinase have been successfully introduced into cell lines and confer resistance in vitro to PLX4720 [95]. However, the spontaneous occurrence of gatekeeper mutations in *BRAF*-mutated melanoma cell lines or patient tumor samples has not been described, with multiple studies demonstrating instead that secondary *BRAF* mutations are uncommon and that V600E mutations are preserved [96–98]. Retention of the original *BRAF* mutation suggests that treatment after the development of resistance might benefit not only from additional therapy to target the mechanism of resistance but also ongoing inhibition of the MAPK/ERK pathway since the mutant BRAF kinase could be a source of continued signaling.

The MAPK/ERK pathway is commonly reactivated in *BRAF*-mutated melanoma by secondary mutations in upstream Ras-GTPases. Across multiple studies of melanoma resistant to BRAF inhibition alone, mutations have been identified in both *NRAS* (G12D/R, G13R, Q61K/R/L) and *KRAS* (G12C/R, Q61H, K117 N) [96–98]. Reactivation of the MAPK/ERK pathway may also occur secondary to *BRAF* amplification, increased expression of the CRAF kinase, and activating C121S mutations in *MEK1* [97, 99, 100]. Resistance mutations have also been identified in the PI3K pathway, including *AKT* (E17K and Q79K), *PIK3CA, PIK3CG*, and *PTEN*, suggesting that PI3K may act as a bypass pathway [97].

A certain number of these resistance mutations occurring secondary to BRAF inhibitor monotherapy might be expected to be less effective at conferring resistance to combination BRAF plus MEK inhibition. *RAS* mutations, for example, have been shown to mediate resistance to BRAF inhibition by activating CRAF, which initiates signaling through the MAPK/ERK pathway at the level of MEK [96, 98]. In one study using a resistant *KRAS* K117 N-mutated melanoma xenograft, tumor growth was effectively inhibited by the combination of vemurafenib plus a MEK inhibitor, confirming that the effectiveness of MEK inhibition was maintained in the setting of an upstream *RAS* activating mutation. Nonetheless, *NRAS* G12D and Q61K mutations have been identified in melanoma samples derived from patients who had progressed on combination dabrafenib plus trametinib, which raises the possibility that upstream Ras activation might confer resistance by mechanisms other than CRAF-mediated MEK activation alone [101]. Interestingly, *BRAF* amplification has also been observed in melanoma samples resistant to combination targeted therapy, similar to what has been described for melanomas resistant to BRAF inhibition alone. However, the increase in *BRAF* copy number has been noted to be significantly higher in those cells that are resistant to dabrafenib plus trametinib compared to cells resistant to BRAF inhibition alone. Thus, while there is clearly some degree of overlap with respect to the targets of resistance in melanomas treated with BRAF inhibition alone compared to those treated with combination BRAF plus MEK inhibition, the mechanisms by which these targets confer resistance likely vary.

Furthermore, downstream mutations in the MAPK/ERK pathway appear to be more common in melanomas treated with combination dabrafenib plus trametinib. In addition to identifying *NRAS* mutations and *BRAF* amplification, Long et al. discovered *MEK1/2* mutations in 27% of patient melanoma samples with acquired resistance to dabrafenib plus trametinib, which is higher than the 3–5% incidence reported in studies of melanomas treated with BRAF inhibitor therapy alone [101]. Mutations in *MEK2* were more common than mutations in *MEK1*, and only the *MEK2* C125S mutation was associated with increased colony growth in the presence of dabrafenib plus trametinib. Together, these findings suggest that particular isoforms of MEK may be more capable of mediating resistance to targeted therapy combinations than others [100].

Case reports of patients with *BRAF*-mutated NSCLC progressing on targeted therapy suggest that upstream activation of Ras-GTPase may be a mediator of resistance in lung cancer as well. In two reports of single patients with *BRAF* V600E-mutated NSCLC who progressed on third-line dabrafenib plus trametinib and later-line dabrafenib monotherapy, respectively, re-biopsy at the time of progression identified a new *NRAS* Q61K mutation in the first patient and a new *KRAS* G12D mutation in the second patient [102, 103]. In both cases, the original *BRAF* V600E mutation was maintained at the time of progression, which is consistent with studies from melanoma. In a third report, the tumor of a patient with *BRAF* V600E NSCLC receiving vemurafenib did not have a *RAS* mutation at the time of progression but did have increased chromosomal instability, suggesting that multiple pathways of resistance are possible [104].

Future Directions

Overcoming resistance to targeted therapy represents just one of the ongoing challenges in the treatment of *BRAF* V600E-mutated NSCLC. Another unanswered question is how best to sequence therapies now that multiple treatment options exist for metastatic *BRAF* V600E-mutated NSCLC, including targeted therapy, chemotherapy, and immunotherapy. Even in melanoma, for which BRAF targeted therapy has been approved for longer, the optimal sequence is not clear, with recommendations drawn primarily from retrospective studies. Previous reviews have suggested that OS may be better in patients with metastatic melanoma who are treated with ipilimumab prior to BRAF targeted therapy [105]. However, BRAF and MEK inhibitors may increase the expression of PD-1 on melanoma cells, which raises the question as to whether outcomes may be improved by using targeted therapy followed by PD-L1 axis-directed therapy [106]. In the case of NSCLC, it is also currently unclear as to how well *BRAF*-mutated NSCLC responds to immunotherapy. In a recent study, high PD-L1 expression, defined as ≥50%, was seen in nearly half of patients with either *BRAF* V600E or non-V600E mutations [107]. Tumor mutation burden, on the other hand, was low to intermediate in both groups, and the overall response rate to immunotherapy in primarily the later-line setting was 25%

in patients with *BRAF* V600E mutations and 33% in patients with *BRAF* non-V600E mutations. As pointed out by the authors, these response rates are comparable to those of second-line immunotherapy in unselected patients with NSCLC. While this suggests that immunotherapy may be more effective in *BRAF*-mutated NSCLC than it is in NSCLC harboring other driver mutations (e.g., *EGFR, ALK*), larger studies are needed.

Conclusion

Although *BRAF* mutations occur infrequently in NSCLC, their ability to constitutively activate the MAPK/ERK signaling pathway has proven to be an important mechanism of cancer cell survival. Understanding this molecular link between *BRAF* mutations and malignancy has led to the approval of targeted therapy (dabrafenib plus trametinib) in both untreated and relapsed, refractory *BRAF* V600E-mutated metastatic NSCLC. While *BRAF* mutations are distinguished from one another in part based on their susceptibility to targeted therapy, it is becoming increasingly clear that other inherent biological differences likely contribute to variability in clinical behavior and prognosis. In addition, much remains unknown regarding the effect of co-occurring mutations on prognosis or response to therapy. More routine use of next-generation sequencing and collaboration between centers specializing in thoracic malignancies should be encouraged, with the goal of addressing ongoing gaps in our knowledge and improving the management of patients with *BRAF*-mutated NSCLC.

References

1. Flaherty KT, McArthur G. BRAF, a target in melanoma: implications for solid tumor drug development. Cancer. 2010;116(21):4902–13.
2. Baik CS, Myall NJ, Wakelee HA. Targeting BRAF-mutant non-small cell lung cancer: from molecular profiling to rationally designed therapy. Oncologist. 2017;22(7):786–96.
3. Odogwu L, et al. FDA approval summary: dabrafenib and trametinib for the treatment of metastatic non-small cell lung cancers harboring BRAF V600E mutations. Oncologist. 2018;23(6):740–5.
4. Santarpia L, Lippman SL, El-Naggar AK. Targeting the MAPK-RAS-RAF signaling pathway in cancer therapy. Expert Opin Ther Targets. 2012;16(1):103–19.
5. Yang SH, Sharrocks AD, Whitmarsh AJ. MAP kinase signalling cascades and transcriptional regulation. Gene. 2013;513(1):1–13.
6. Lee JC, et al. A protein kinase involved in the regulation of inflammatory cytokine biosynthesis. Nature. 1994;372(6508):739–46.
7. Lu HT, et al. Defective IL-12 production in mitogen-activated protein (MAP) kinase kinase 3 (Mkk3)-deficient mice. EMBO J. 1999;18(7):1845–57.
8. Yang D, et al. Targeted disruption of the MKK4 gene causes embryonic death, inhibition of c-Jun NH2-terminal kinase activation, and defects in AP-1 transcriptional activity. Proc Natl Acad Sci U S A. 1997;94(7):3004–9.

9. Burotto M, et al. The MAPK pathway across different malignancies: a new perspective. Cancer. 2014;120(22):3446–56.
10. Cargnello M, Roux PP. Activation and function of the MAPKs and their substrates, the MAPK-activated protein kinases. Microbiol Mol Biol Rev. 2011;75(1):50–83.
11. McCubrey JA, et al. Mutations and deregulation of Ras/Raf/MEK/ERK and PI3K/PTEN/Akt/mTOR cascades which alter therapy response. Oncotarget. 2012;3(9):954–87.
12. Chang F, et al. Signal transduction mediated by the Ras/Raf/MEK/ERK pathway from cytokine receptors to transcription factors: potential targeting for therapeutic intervention. Leukemia. 2003;17(7):1263–93.
13. Klemke RL, et al. Regulation of cell motility by mitogen-activated protein kinase. J Cell Biol. 1997;137(2):481–92.
14. Le Gallic L, et al. Transcriptional repressor ERF is a Ras/mitogen-activated protein kinase target that regulates cellular proliferation. Mol Cell Biol. 1999;19(6):4121–33.
15. Mischak H, et al. Negative regulation of Raf-1 by phosphorylation of serine 621. Mol Cell Biol. 1996;16(10):5409–18.
16. Sasaki A, et al. Mammalian Sprouty4 suppresses Ras-independent ERK activation by binding to Raf1. Nat Cell Biol. 2003;5(5):427–32.
17. Dankner M, et al. Classifying BRAF alterations in cancer: new rational therapeutic strategies for actionable mutations. Oncogene. 2018;37(24):3183–99.
18. Roskoski R Jr. RAF protein-serine/threonine kinases: structure and regulation. Biochem Biophys Res Commun. 2010;399(3):313–7.
19. Eychene A, et al. Chromosomal assignment of two human B-raf(Rmil) proto-oncogene loci: B-raf-1 encoding the p94Braf/Rmil and B-raf-2, a processed pseudogene. Oncogene. 1992;7(8):1657–60.
20. Fagerberg L, et al. Analysis of the human tissue-specific expression by genome-wide integration of transcriptomics and antibody-based proteomics. Mol Cell Proteomics. 2014;13(2):397–406.
21. Sithanandam G, et al. Complete coding sequence of a human B-raf cDNA and detection of B-raf protein kinase with isozyme specific antibodies. Oncogene. 1990;5(12):1775–80.
22. Ghosh S, et al. The cysteine-rich region of raf-1 kinase contains zinc, translocates to liposomes, and is adjacent to a segment that binds GTP-ras. J Biol Chem. 1994;269(13):10000–7.
23. Mott HR, et al. The solution structure of the Raf-1 cysteine-rich domain: a novel ras and phospholipid binding site. Proc Natl Acad Sci U S A. 1996;93(16):8312–7.
24. Chong H, Guan KL. Regulation of Raf through phosphorylation and N terminus-C terminus interaction. J Biol Chem. 2003;278(38):36269–76.
25. Cutler REJ, et al. Autoregulation of the Raf-1 serine/threonine kinase. Proc Natl Acad Sci U S A. 1998;95(16):9214–9.
26. Tran NH, Wu X, Frost JA. B-Raf and Raf-1 are regulated by distinct autoregulatory mechanisms. J Biol Chem. 2005;280(16):16244–53.
27. Zhang BH, Guan KL. Activation of B-Raf kinase requires phosphorylation of the conserved residues Thr598 and Ser601. EMBO J. 2000;19(20):5429–39.
28. Desideri E, Cavallo AL, Baccarini M. Alike but different: RAF paralogs and their signaling outputs. Cell. 2015;161(5):967–70.
29. Ritt DA, et al. Impact of feedback phosphorylation and Raf heterodimerization on normal and mutant B-Raf signaling. Mol Cell Biol. 2010;30(3):806–19.
30. Davies H, et al. Mutations of the BRAF gene in human cancer. Nature. 2002;417(6892):949–54.
31. Brummer T, et al. Functional analysis of the regulatory requirements of B-Raf and the B-Raf(V600E) oncoprotein. Oncogene. 2006;25(47):6262–76.
32. Pratilas CA, et al. Genetic predictors of MEK dependence in non-small cell lung cancer. Cancer Res. 2008;68(22):9375–83.
33. Wan PT, et al. Mechanism of activation of the RAF-ERK signaling pathway by oncogenic mutations of B-RAF. Cell. 2004;116(6):855–67.
34. Ji H, et al. Mutations in BRAF and KRAS converge on activation of the mitogen-activated protein kinase pathway in lung cancer mouse models. Cancer Res. 2007;67(10):4933–9.

35. Dankort D, et al. A new mouse model to explore the initiation, progression, and therapy of BRAFV600E-induced lung tumors. Genes Dev. 2007;21(4):379–84.
36. Trejo CL, et al. Mutationally activated PIK3CA(H1047R) cooperates with BRAF(V600E) to promote lung cancer progression. Cancer Res. 2013;73(21):6448–61.
37. Chudnovsky Y, et al. Use of human tissue to assess the oncogenic activity of melanoma-associated mutations. Nat Genet. 2005;37(7):745–9.
38. Hoeflich KP, et al. Antitumor efficacy of the novel RAF inhibitor GDC-0879 is predicted by BRAFV600E mutational status and sustained extracellular signal-regulated kinase/mitogen-activated protein kinase pathway suppression. Cancer Res. 2009;69(7):3042–51.
39. Micel LN, et al. Antitumor activity of the MEK inhibitor TAK-733 against melanoma cell lines and patient-derived tumor explants. Mol Cancer Ther. 2015;14(2):317–25.
40. Yao Z, et al. BRAF mutants evade ERK-dependent feedback by different mechanisms that determine their sensitivity to pharmacologic inhibition. Cancer Cell. 2015;28(3):370–83.
41. Yao Z, et al. Tumours with class 3 BRAF mutants are sensitive to the inhibition of activated RAS. Nature. 2017;548(7666):234–8.
42. Kumar R, et al. BRAF mutations in metastatic melanoma: a possible association with clinical outcome. Clin Cancer Res. 2003;9(9):3362–8.
43. Shinozaki M, et al. Incidence of BRAF oncogene mutation and clinical relevance for primary cutaneous melanomas. Clin Cancer Res. 2004;10(5):1753–7.
44. Tiacci E, et al. BRAF mutations in hairy-cell leukemia. N Engl J Med. 2011;364(24):2305–15.
45. Nikiforova MN, et al. BRAF mutations in thyroid tumors are restricted to papillary carcinomas and anaplastic or poorly differentiated carcinomas arising from papillary carcinomas. J Clin Endocrinol Metab. 2003;88(11):5399–404.
46. Saridaki Z, et al. BRAF mutations, microsatellite instability status and cyclin D1 expression predict metastatic colorectal patients' outcome. Br J Cancer. 2010;102(12):1762–8.
47. Tiacci E, et al. Targeting mutant BRAF in relapsed or refractory hairy-cell leukemia. N Engl J Med. 2015;373(18):1733–47.
48. Kopetz S, et al. Phase II pilot study of vemurafenib in patients with metastatic BRAF-mutated colorectal cancer. J Clin Oncol. 2015;33(34):4032–8.
49. Jamal-Hanjani M, et al. Tracking the evolution of non-small-cell lung cancer. N Engl J Med. 2017;376(22):2109–21.
50. Ohashi K, et al. Lung cancers with acquired resistance to EGFR inhibitors occasionally harbor BRAF gene mutations but lack mutations in KRAS, NRAS, or MEK1. Proc Natl Acad Sci U S A. 2012;109(31):E2127–33.
51. Brose MS, et al. BRAF and RAS mutations in human lung cancer and melanoma. Cancer Res. 2002;62(23):6997–7000.
52. Cardarella S, et al. Clinical, pathologic, and biologic features associated with BRAF mutations in non-small cell lung cancer. Clin Cancer Res. 2013;19(16):4532–40.
53. Kris MG, et al. Using multiplexed assays of oncogenic drivers in lung cancers to select targeted drugs. JAMA. 2014;311(19):1998–2006.
54. Litvak AM, et al. Clinical characteristics and course of 63 patients with BRAF mutant lung cancers. J Thorac Oncol. 2014;9(11):1669–74.
55. Marchetti A, et al. Clinical features and outcome of patients with non-small-cell lung cancer harboring BRAF mutations. J Clin Oncol. 2011;29(26):3574–9.
56. Tissot C, et al. Clinical characteristics and outcome of patients with lung cancer harboring BRAF mutations. Lung Cancer. 2016;91:23–8.
57. Dearden S, et al. Mutation incidence and coincidence in non small-cell lung cancer: meta-analyses by ethnicity and histology (mutMap). Ann Oncol. 2013;24(9):2371–6.
58. Kron A, et al. Impact of co-occurring genomic alterations on overall survival of BRAF V600E and non-V600E mutated NSCLC patients: results of the network genomic medicine. Ann Oncol. 2017;28(Suppl_5):mdx380.003.
59. Myall NJ, et al. Natural disease history, outcomes, and co-mutations in a series of patients with BRAF-mutated non-small cell lung cancer. Clin Lung Cancer. 2018;20(2):e208–17.

60. Aisner DL, et al. The impact of smoking and TP53 mutations in lung adenocarcinoma patients with targetable mutations-the Lung Cancer Mutation Consortium (LCMC2). Clin Cancer Res. 2018;24(5):1038–47.
61. Dong ZY, et al. Potential predictive vaue of TP53 and KRAS mutation status for response to PD-1 blockade immunotherapy in lung adenocarcinoma. Clin Cancer Res. 2017;23(12):3012–24.
62. Skoulidis F, et al. Co-occurring genomic alterations define major subsets of KRAS-mutant lung adenocarcinoma with distinct biology, immune profiles, and therapeutic vulnerabilities. Cancer Discov. 2015;5(8):860–77.
63. Brustugun OT, et al. BRAF-mutations in non-small cell lung cancer. Lung Cancer. 2014;84(1):36–8.
64. Kinno T, et al. Clinicopathological features of nonsmall cell lung carcinomas with BRAF mutations. Ann Oncol. 2014;25(1):138–42.
65. Araujo LH, et al. Somatic mutation spectrum of non-small-cell lung cancer in African Americans: a pooled analysis. J Thorac Oncol. 2015;10(10):1430–6.
66. Ding X, et al. Clinicopathologic characteristics and outcomes of Chinese patients with non-small-cell lung cancer and BRAF mutation. Cancer Med. 2017;6(3):555–62.
67. Serizawa M, et al. Assessment of mutational profile of Japanese lung adenocarcinoma patients by multitarget assays: a prospective, single-institute study. Cancer. 2014;120(10):1471–81.
68. Lynch JA, et al. Underutilization and disparities in access to EGFR testing among Medicare patients with lung cancer from 2010 - 2013. BMC Cancer. 2018;18(1):306.
69. Chen D, et al. BRAF mutations in patients with non-small cell lung cancer: a systematic review and meta-analysis. PLoS One. 2014;9(6):e101354.
70. Davis AA, et al. Association of tumor mutational burden with smoking and mutation status in non-small cell lung cancer (NSCLC). J Clin Oncol. 2017;35(7_suppl):24–24.
71. Dagogo-Jack I, et al. Impact of BRAF mutation class on disease characteristics and clinical outcomes in BRAF-mutant lung cancer. Clin Cancer Res. 2019;25(1):158–65.
72. Yousem SA, Nikiforova M, Nikiforov Y. The histopathology of BRAF-V600E-mutated lung adenocarcinoma. Am J Surg Pathol. 2008;32(9):1317–21.
73. Villaruz LC, et al. Clinicopathologic features and outcomes of patients with lung adeno-carcinomas harboring BRAF mutations in the Lung Cancer Mutation Consortium. Cancer. 2015;121(3):448–56.
74. Myall NJ, et al. Long-term survival of a patient with non-small-cell lung cancer harboring a V600E mutation in the BRAF oncogene. Clin Lung Cancer. 2016;17(2):e17–21.
75. Nakanishi Y, et al. Favorable outcome with pemetrexed treatment for advanced BRAF-V600E-positive lung adenocarcinoma in a patient followed up over 8 years. J Thorac Oncol. 2018;13(10):e199–202.
76. Barlesi F, et al. Routine molecular profiling of patients with advanced non-small-cell lung cancer: results of a 1-year nationwide programme of the French Cooperative Thoracic Intergroup (IFCT). Lancet. 2016;387(10026):1415–26.
77. Hauschild A, et al. Dabrafenib in BRAF-mutated metastatic melanoma: a multicentre, open-label, phase 3 randomised controlled trial. Lancet. 2012;380(9839):358–65.
78. McArthur GA, et al. Safety and efficacy of vemurafenib in BRAFV600E and BRAFV600K mutation-positive melanoma (BRIM-3): extended follow-up of a phase 3, randomised, open-label study. Lancet Oncol. 2014;15(3):323–32.
79. Flaherty KT, et al. Combined BRAF and MEK inhibition in melanoma with BRAF V600 mutations. N Engl J Med. 2012;367(18):1694–703.
80. Larkin J, et al. Combined vemurafenib and cobimetinib in BRAF-mutated melanoma. N Engl J Med. 2014;371(20):1867–76.
81. Long GV, et al. Combined BRAF and MEK inhibition versus BRAF inhibition alone in melanoma. N Engl J Med. 2014;371(20):1877–88.
82. Robert C, et al. Improved overall survival in melanoma with combined dabrafenib and trametinib. N Engl J Med. 2015;372(1):30–9.

83. Gautschi O, et al. A patient with BRAF V600E lung adenocarcinoma responding to vemurafenib. J Thorac Oncol. 2012;7(10):e23–4.
84. Peters S, Micheielin O, Zimmermann S. Dramatic response induced by vemurafenib in a BRAF V600E-mutated lung adenocarcinoma. J Clin Oncol. 2013;31(20):e341–4.
85. Robinson SD, et al. BRAF V600E-mutated lung adenocarcinoma with metastases to the brain responding to treatment with vemurafenib. Lung Cancer. 2014;85(2):326–30.
86. Gautschi O, et al. Targeted therapy for patients with BRAF-mutant lung cancer: results from the European EURAF cohort. J Thorac Oncol. 2015;10(10):1451–7.
87. Falchook GS, et al. Dabrafenib in patients with melanoma, untreated brain metastases, and other solid tumours: a phase 1 dose-escalation trial. Lancet. 2012;379(9829):1893–901.
88. Hyman DM, et al. Vemurafenib in multiple nonmelanoma cancers with BRAF V600 mutations. N Engl J Med. 2015;373(8):726–36.
89. Planchard D, et al. Dabrafenib plus trametinib in patients with previously treated BRAF V600E -mutant metastatic non-small cell lung cancer: an open-label, multicentre phase 2 trial. Lancet Oncol. 2016;17(7):984–93.
90. Planchard D, et al. Dabrafenib in patients with BRAFV600E-positive advanced non-small-cell lung cancer: a single-arm, multicentre, open-label, phase 2 trial. Lancet Oncol. 2016;17(5):642–50.
91. Planchard D, et al. Dabrafenib plus trametinib in patients with previously untreated BRAF V600E -mutant metastatic non-small-cell lung cancer: an open-label, phase 2 trial. Lancet Oncol. 2017;18(10):1307–16.
92. National Comprehensive Cancer Network. Non-small cell lung cancer (Version 6.2018). https://www.nccn.org/professionals/physician_gls/pdf/nscl.pdf. Accessed 22 Oct 2018.
93. Straussman R, et al. Tumour micro-environment elicits innate resistance to RAF inhibitors through HGF secretion. Nature. 2012;487(7408):500–4.
94. Pao W, et al. Acquired resistance of lung adenocarcinomas to gefitinib or erlotinib is associated with a second mutation in the EGFR kinase domain. PLoS Med. 2005;2(3):e73.
95. Whittaker S, et al. Gatekeeper mutations mediate resistance to BRAF-targeted therapies. Sci Transl Med. 2010;2(35):35–41.
96. Nazarian R, et al. Melanomas acquire resistance to B-RAF(V600E) inhibition by RTK or N-RAS upregulation. Nature. 2010;468(7326):973–7.
97. Shi H, et al. Acquired resistance and clonal evolution in melanoma during BRAF inhibitor therapy. Cancer Discov. 2014;4(1):80–93.
98. Su F, et al. Resistance to selective BRAF inhibition can be mediated by modest upstream pathway activation. Cancer Res. 2012;72(4):969–78.
99. Montagut C, et al. Elevated CRAF as a potential mechanism of acquired resistance to BRAF inhibition in melanoma. Cancer Res. 2008;68(12):4853–61.
100. Wagle N, et al. Dissecting therapeutic resistance to RAF inhibition in melanoma by tumor genomic profiling. J Clin Oncol. 2011;29(22):3085–96.
101. Long GV, et al. Increased MAPK reactivation in early resistance to dabrafenib/trametinib combination therapy of BRAF-mutant metastatic melanoma. Nat Commun. 2014;5:5694.
102. Abravanel DL, et al. An acquired NRAS Q61K mutation in BRAF V600E-mutant lung adenocarcinoma resistant to dabrafenib plus trametinib. J Thorac Oncol. 2018;13(8):e131–3.
103. Rudin CM, Hong K, Streit M. Molecular characterization of acquired resistance to the BRAF inhibitor dabrafenib in a patient with BRAF-mutant non-small-cell lung cancer. J Thorac Oncol. 2013;8(5):e41–2.
104. Lucchesi C, et al. Molecular determinants of acquired resistance to BRAF inhibition in human lung cancer. Lung Cancer. 2018;126:227.
105. Atkins MB, Larkin J. Immunotherapy combined or sequenced with targeted therapy in the treatment of solid tumors: current perspectives. J Natl Cancer Inst. 2016;108(6):djv414.
106. Sanlorenzo M, et al. BRAF and MEK inhibitors increase PD-1-positive melanoma cells leading to a potential lymphocyte-independent synergism with anti-PD-1 antibody. Clin Cancer Res. 2018;24(14):3377–85.
107. Dudnik E, et al. BRAF mutant lung cancer: programmed death ligand 1 expression, tumor mutational burden, microsatellite instability status, and response to immune check-point inhibitors. J Thorac Oncol. 2018;13(8):1128–37.

MET as a Therapeutic Target: Have Clinical Outcomes Been "MET" in Lung Cancer?

Arin Nam and Ravi Salgia

Abstract Targeted therapy is an especially attractive approach for treating lung cancer since overactivation of oncogenic proteins often drives disease progression. In particular, dysregulation of the MET receptor tyrosine kinase (RTK) pathway via genetic mechanisms, such as gene amplification and exon 14 skipping mutations, has been identified. With significant advancements made in the realm of targeted therapeutics, such as small molecules and antagonistic antibodies, developing novel strategies to target MET is at the forefront of lung cancer treatment. This chapter will introduce the MET signaling pathway and various genetic abnormalities implicated in lung cancer. Then, the currently used MET-targeted therapies and investigative agents will be highlighted along with their status in clinical trials. The final section will shed light on preclinical data revealing possible mechanisms of resistance to MET-targeted therapy.

Keywords Targeted therapy · MET · Receptor tyrosine kinase · Lung cancer · Exon 14 skipping

Introduction

Lung cancer remains to be the most commonly diagnosed and fatal cancer type among both men and women in the United States and worldwide [1, 2]. Lung cancer is typically classified as non-small cell lung cancer (NSCLC) and small cell lung cancer (SCLC), which account for 85% and 15% of cases, respectively. NSCLC diagnoses can be further identified based on subtypes, such as adenocarcinoma,

A. Nam
Department of Medical Oncology and Experimental Therapeutics,
City of Hope National Medical Center, Duarte, CA, USA

R. Salgia (✉)
Department of Medical Oncology and Therapeutics Research,
City of Hope National Medical Center, Duarte, CA, USA
e-mail: rsalgia@coh.org

© Springer Nature Switzerland AG 2019   101
R. Salgia (ed.), *Targeted Therapies for Lung Cancer*, Current Cancer Research,
https://doi.org/10.1007/978-3-030-17832-1_5

squamous cell carcinoma, and large cell carcinoma. Current treatment for early-stage NSCLC is surgical removal of the tumor and sometimes treated with adjuvant chemotherapy alone or in combination with radiation. Late-stage NSCLC is usually treated with conventional chemotherapy, targeted therapy, immunotherapy, alone or in a combined regimen. Treatment options for SCLC remain quite limited to traditional chemotherapy alone or in combination with radiation [1]. Although patients may initially respond to these therapeutic regimens, often times, tumors acquire resistance to these agents, and the disease progresses as reflected by a dismal 18% five-year survival rate [1]. Developing additional targeted therapies is particularly an attractive approach for lung cancer because overactivation of certain proteins plays a key role in lung tumorigenesis.

Several receptor tyrosine kinases (RTKs), which constitute the largest family of tyrosine kinases [3], have been identified to be upregulated in lung cancer, contributing as important drivers of disease progression. RTKs are a subclass of tyrosine kinases that mediate cell-to-cell communication and control a wide range of biological functions, including cell growth, motility, differentiation, and metabolism [4]. All RTKs share a similar protein structure comprised of an extracellular ligand-binding domain, a single transmembrane helix, and an intracellular region that contains a juxtamembrane regulatory region, a tyrosine kinase domain (TKD), and a carboxyl (C-) terminal tail [5]. The extracellular domain of the RTKs binds specific ligands, such as growth factors, cytokines, and hormones, that can activate various intracellular signal transduction cascades including survival and migration [6]. However, abnormal expression and/or signaling of RTKs are implicated in many types of cancer that fuel its progression via unregulated proliferation and invasion through surrounding tissue [7]. Ninety unique kinase genes can be identified in the human genome of which 58 are of the receptor type, distributed into 20 subfamilies [3].

This chapter will focus on one member of the RTK family namely MET or hepatocyte growth factor receptor (HGFR) that plays an important role in lung cancer [8, 9]. First, the structure and function of MET will be described together with its normal function within the cell. The following section will outline various abnormalities in lung cancer that have been frequently identified in patients. The remaining sections will discuss various therapeutic approaches targeting MET signaling in lung cancer as well as the more recent developments regarding mechanism(s) of resistance to these agents.

Structure and Function

Gene

The human gene encoding MET is ~126 kilobases and is located on chromosome 7, locus 7q21–q31. MET was originally discovered in 1984 as a partner in the fusion oncogene TPR-MET of an immortalized cell line derived from osteosarcoma [10].

Upon treatment of this cell line with the carcinogenic compound N-methyl-N'-nitronitrosoguanidine, genetic fusion was induced between the TPR gene on locus 1q25 and the MET gene on locus 7q31 [10]. At least three different isoforms are reported. The most commonly expressed isoform encodes for the protein precursor that is 1390 amino acids long.

Protein

When the precursor is posttranslationally cleaved and glycosylated, a 50-kDa alpha chain and a 140-kDa beta chain are produced. The alpha chain is linked via disulfide bonds to the extracellular portion of the beta chain, which also includes the transmembrane and intracellular portions of the receptor. Sharing domain homology with other protein structures, the beta chain is comprised of: the semaphorin domain, plexin-semaphorin-integrin (PSI) domain, four immunoglobulin-plexin-transcription (IPT) repeats, transmembrane domain, juxtamembrane domain, tyrosine kinase domain, and the C-terminal region (Fig. 1).

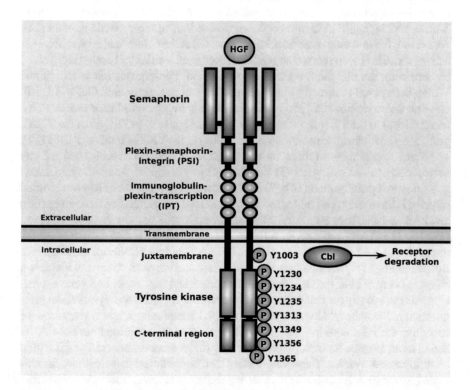

Fig. 1 MET structure, domains, and phosphorylation sites

Ligand HGF

Hepatocyte growth factor (HGF), also known as scatter factor (SF), is the only known natural ligand that binds to the MET receptor and activates it. It resembles other growth factors in the plasminogen-related growth factor family [11] and is secreted by mesenchymal cells as a precursor that is proteolytically cleaved by HGF activator (HGFA). Active HGF is produced in the form of a disulfide-linked heterodimer. HGF has six domains: the N-terminal domain, four kringle domains, and the C-terminal domain. The ligand binds to the receptor at the semaphorin domain, a seven beta-propeller structure where blades 2 and 3 form the active binding site for HGF [12].

Signaling

Like other RTK activation pathways, such as RON and Sea [13], ligand binding induces receptor dimerization and activation of the tyrosine kinase. In the active state, MET autophosphorylation and recruitment of a number of signal transducer molecules initiate several signaling cascades as seen in Fig. 2. Phosphorylation at Y1230, Y1234, and Y1235 turn on the activation loop at the catalytic domain [14]. As a result, the multisubstrate docking site located at the C-terminal region becomes activated and is able to recruit intracellular adaptor molecules that can be recognized by certain motifs like the Src homology-2 domain. Phosphorylation at Y1349 and Y1356 is required to directly bind Src and Shc and indirectly bind Gab1 [15, 16]. Only phosphorylation at Y1356 is required for binding growth factor receptor protein 2 (Grb2) to the YXN motif at Y1349, phospholipase C-γ (PLC-γ) to the YXXL motif at Y1365, phosphoinositol 3-kinase (PI3K) to the YXXM motif at Y1313 [17], and Shp2. Recruitment of these various signal transduction molecules can activate several downstream pathways: (1) Ras/Raf pathway is activated and involved in cell scattering and proliferation [18]; (2) PI3K pathway, downstream of Ras or recruited directly, is involved in cell migration via cytoskeletal reorganization through paxillin and FAK and also triggers a survival signal through AKT recruitment and activation [19, 20]; (3) MAPK pathway is activated through recruitment of Gab1/Grb2/SOS molecules as well as Ras/Raf to prompt cell survival and proliferation [21]. From ligand binding to activation of several signal transduction cascades, many biological changes occur within the cell, such as transcriptional regulation and gene expression, in order to trigger cell growth, differentiation, survival, and cytoskeletal reorganization. Phosphorylation at Y1003 in the juxtamembrane domain is required for recruiting the E3 ubiquitin ligase, Cbl. Cbl facilitates the ubiquitination of MET by acting as an adaptor for endophilin in order to direct receptor internalization within clathrin-coated vesicles. These vesicles can then be trafficked to endosomes for ultimate lysosomal degradation [22]. Aberrant signaling at any or multiple points from ligand binding to downstream changes in cellular function can give rise to cancer cell differentiation, progression, and/or metastasis [23].

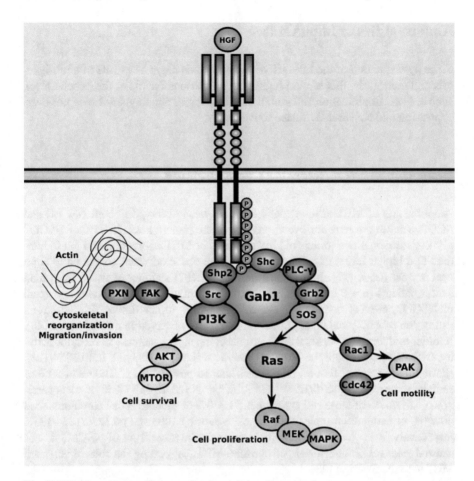

Fig. 2 MET downstream effector molecules and signaling cascades

Normal Function

Activation by MET of the various downstream pathways initiate the regulation of normal cellular processes, such as cell survival, differentiation, and migration. MET also plays an essential role in embryonic development, specifically migration of mesenchymal cells and neuronal precursors for muscle and nervous tissue organogenesis [24]. In adults, MET can be activated to prompt wound healing and tissue remodeling [25]. Hematopoietic cells can also utilize MET activation for differentiation and proliferation to generate mature blood cells [26].

Abnormalities in Lung Cancer

Since dysregulation of the MET/HGF signaling axis plays a key role in tumorigenesis and metastasis, this section highlights the various factors at the genetic level, such as gene amplification and mutations, resulting in phenotypes of receptor overexpression and constitutive kinase activation.

Gene Amplification/Receptor Overexpression

Amplification of MET at the genetic level has been observed in both NSCLC and SCLC, resulting in receptor overexpression at the protein level. In 25% of NSCLC primary tumors, a two to ten-fold higher levels of MET expression and ten to hundred fold higher levels of HGF expression were observed when compared to adjacent normal tissue [27]. Immunohistochemical (IHC) staining of tissue from lung cancer patients (n = 32) showed MET expression in all samples. Sixty-one percent of NSCLC, 60% of carcinoids, and 25% of SCLC tumor tissues showed strong expression of MET, and no significant staining was observed in normal tissue [28]. In order to determine whether there is an accompanying increase in receptor activity, IHC staining for phospho-MET at catalytic residues Y1003 or Y1230/1234/1235 showed that in SCLC tissues, all samples stained positive for pY1003 and 50% of samples expressed pY1230/1234/1235 [28]. For NSCLC, 44%/33% of adenocarcinoma, 86%/57% of large cell carcinoma, 71%/0% of squamous cell carcinoma, and 40%/0% of carcinoid samples stained positive for pY1003 and pY1230/1234/1235, respectively. It is also worth mentioning that the invasive front of NSCLC tissues showed relatively higher levels of phospho-MET, suggesting the role of activated MET in tissue invasion [28].

MET Overexpression and Correlation with Paxillin

MET is able to affect cell motility by regulating cytoskeletal reorganization through actin polymerization and depolymerization. Upon phosphorylation of key focal adhesion molecules, such as paxillin, FAK, and Pyk2, by the MET kinase, filopodia and lamellipodia formation and retraction were observed [29]. Activated paxillin by MET induces an interaction with the cytoskeleton, resulting in cell motility and migration [30]. It has been shown that the correlated activity between MET and paxillin coincide with their expression in tumor tissue. An increase in paxillin expression with higher NSCLC disease stage has been observed as well as a correlation between high paxillin expression and copy number of the MET gene [31]. In contrast, SCLC has relatively low levels of paxillin [32]. Thus, this correlation is not observed in this lung cancer type.

MET Overexpression and Mitochondrial Dynamics

Lung cancer cells with MET overexpression are highly dependent on receptor signaling to sustain viability. These overexpressing cells are more sensitive to MET inhibitor (MGCD 516) than cells with lower MET expression [33]. Interestingly, signaling of dynamin-related protein-1 (DRP1), a mitochondrial protein involved in the fission process, is attenuated when treated with this MET inhibitor [33]. As a result, mitochondrial morphology appears to be more elongated.

Missense Mutations in the Juxtamembrane and Semaphorin Domain

The MET gene is a target for several missense mutations that cause dysregulation of receptor function. Mutations are primarily found within the juxtamembrane region and semaphorin domain for lung cancer. Although mutations can be found in the MET tyrosine kinase domain in head and neck cancers [34], glioblastomas [35], and hereditary papillary renal carcinomas [36], none are found in lung cancer. Missense mutations in the juxtamembrane domain cause aberrant receptor signaling due to this region's key role as a regulator site for catalytic function of tyrosine kinases. In NSCLC, R988C, T1010I, and S1058P mutations increase phosphorylation of MET and downstream signal transduction molecules, enhance tumorigenicity, cell motility, and alter cellular morphology. These mutations also contribute to a stronger response to inhibition with small molecule compounds targeting MET [28]. Missense mutations can also be found in the semaphorin region, E168D, which can alter the binding of HGF and subsequent receptor dimerization and activation [37]. Another missense mutation found in the semaphorin domain, N375S, conferred resistance to MET inhibitors and was most frequently detected in tumor tissues of East Asians (13%) and not detected in that of African Americans (0%) [38].

Modeling Mutations in Caenorhabditis elegans

Modeling a cancer phenotype in a multicellular organism can be achieved with *Caenorhabditis elegans,* especially in a high-throughput manner. The phenotype of the nematode's vulva reflects any developmental abnormalities. In wild-type N2 adult worms, a "normal" vulva is apparent, however, the cancer phenotype exhibits a multivulval characteristic [39]. Various transgenic worms with MET missense mutations have been used as a model for determining phenotypic changes and developmental abnormalities. For example, transgenic worms expressing wild-type human MET genes exhibited ectopic hypodermal growth in the posterior region, but transgenic worms expressing the R988C mutant MET construct exhibited a tumor-like growth of vulva-forming cells [40]. Using these transgenic worms as a model, exposure to nicotine and other smoke toxins resulted in a multivulval-resembling phenotype, suggesting synergy between MET and nicotine. [40] This model system may be useful to study other environmental toxins as well as dysregulation of other oncogenes.

Exon 14 Skipping Mutation

A shorter variant of the MET receptor was first discovered in mice in 1994 that led to tumorigenicity in vivo [41]. We were the first to identify exon 14 splicing mutation in NSCLC and SCLC [28, 37]. This variant lacked a portion of the juxtamembrane domain, which is a key regulatory site for kinase activity. In patients' genomic data, mutations were found to occur near splice sites that cause exon skipping within the MET gene in multiple tumor types, including lung cancer [42]. Primarily found in lung adenocarcinomas, exon 14 of the MET gene is susceptible to mutations near the splice site. This mutation results in exon 14 skipping during the splicing process from pre-mRNA to the mature mRNA. Because exon 14 encodes for the juxtamembrane portion of the protein that includes residue Y1003, mutations that cause exon 14 skipping produces a protein lacking this key domain and kinase regulatory site [43]. Phosphorylation at Y1003 is required for binding the E3 ubiquitin ligase, Cbl, which promotes MET ubiquitination, internalization, and degradation. However, if the MET protein product lacks this site as a result of exon 14 skipping, the receptor half-life is prolonged, resulting in MET overexpression and extended catalytic function within the cell [43]. Cbl mutations have also been found to be highly prevalent in MET-mutated NSCLC that enhance cell viability and motility [44]. Altered Cbl in NSCLC cells have higher MET expression than wild-type cells and are more sensitive to MET inhibitor SU11274. [45]

Modeling Mutations with DNA Walks and Their Fractal Patterns

DNA walks depict nucleotide sequence patterns that can be used to model wild-type genes and mutated counterparts. In particular for the MET gene, point mutations create larger gaps in the pattern, generating an increase in self-similarity or fractal dimension. On the other hand, MET deletion mutations, as seen in exon 14 skipping, decrease fractal dimension in the pattern because of a reduction in nucleotide variance [46]. This type of modeling has potential predictive capabilities for exon 14 deletions. One can introduce unknown exon 14 alterations to the genetic sequence, generate a DNA walk, and compare the fractal dimension to known patterns that lead to exon skipping [46].

Various Therapeutic Approaches and Outcomes

The shift from traditional cytotoxic chemotherapy to a more targeted approach has given clinicians and researchers insight into biomarker-based therapies and drug development. Because abnormal signaling in the MET axis can be implicated in lung cancer as well as other types of solid cancers, it represents an attractive target for developing small molecule compounds and biological antagonists, such as antibodies, that block HGF-binding and/or MET activation as seen in Fig. 3. Screening for patients with genetic alterations in MET, as well as EGFR, has allowed clinicians to treat patients with targeted therapies and improve overall survival, since often times, patients with EGFR mutations develop resistance to EGFR inhibitors due to MET overexpression/amplification. In this section, several small molecule inhibitors and biological antagonists will be described in addition to their mechanisms of action and current status in clinical trials.

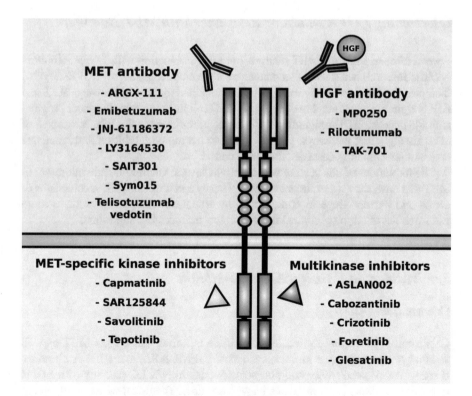

Fig. 3 Current therapeutic approaches targeting MET

Small Molecule Inhibitors Against MET

Small molecule kinase inhibitors or tyrosine kinase inhibitors (TKIs) that block receptor activation have shown promise in clinical settings where dysregulated signaling of these receptors drive cancer progression. When these agents bind to the receptor, activation of downstream signaling events is prevented and thus, tumor cells are directed to apoptosis. These types of inhibitors are an appealing strategy for developing targeted therapies because of their small size (<500 Da), cost-effectiveness, and availability, as compared to monoclonal antibodies. First generation TKIs, such as crizotinib and cabozantinib, also target other types of RTKs and hence, they are classified as a multikinase inhibitor. The primary drawback to inhibitors that target a wider range of receptor kinases is toxicity, drawing attention toward the need for more specific RTK inhibitors. Recently developed small molecule inhibitors against MET, such as capmatinib, have exhibited more potent activity and selective binding for the MET receptor than other kinases [47]. These MET-specific inhibitors have shown promise in clinical trials especially for patients with MET amplification and/or exon 14 skipping mutations. [42]

Overcoming EGFR Inhibitor Resistance with MET Inhibitors

Several clinical trials for MET inhibitors are in combination with EGFR inhibitors because research has shown that cancer cells develop resistance to EGFR-targeted therapies via MET overactivation [48]. Crosstalk and synergism between MET and EGFR signaling was found to occur in NSCLC cell lines to promote cancer progression [49]. When EGFR signaling is blocked, tumorigenic cells take advantage of alternate signaling pathways, such as MET, to overcome inhibition and reactivate downstream signaling cascades that drive cancer progression.

The remainder of this section will highlight several small molecule inhibitors of MET that have shown significant clinical efficacy and describe their mechanisms of action and current stage in clinical trial investigations. Table 1 presents a more extensive list of ongoing clinical trials with the various MET inhibitors.

Small Molecule Tyrosine Kinase Inhibitors

Cabozantinib (XL184)

Cabozantinib is a small molecule multikinase inhibitor that targets MET as well as other receptor tyrosine kinases, such as VEGFR2, AXL, and RET. A phase Ib/II study investigated safety and pharmacokinetics in NSCLC patients with EGFR mutations that were previously treated with erlotinib. Treatment with a combination

Table 1 Current status of MET-targeted agents in clinical trials

Drug	Manufacturer	Conditions	Combination	Phase	NCT	Study Start Date
Small molecule inhibitors against MET						
ASLAN002 (BMS-777607) *Small molecule inhibitor against MET and RON*	Bristol-Myers Squibb	Malignant solid tumor	–	I, completed	NCT01721148	October 2012
Cabozantinib (XL184) *Multikinase small molecule inhibitor against MET, VEGFR2, AXL, RET*	Exelixis	NSCLC with brain metastases	–	II, recruiting	NCT02132598	December 2015
Capmatinib (INC280) *MET small molecule inhibitor*	Novartis	NSCLC	–	II, recruiting	NCT02414139	June 11, 2015
			Erlotinib	Ib, recruiting	NCT02468661	September 23, 2015
			EGFR TKI Nazartinib (EGF816)	I/II, recruiting	NCT02335944	January 13, 2015
			PD-1 antibody Nivolumab	II, recruiting	NCT02323126	February 9, 2015
		Recurrent NSCLC	Erlotinib	I, recruiting	NCT01911507	July 2013
		Solid tumors, MET dysregulated	–	I, completed	NCT02925104	December 14, 2016
		NSCLC, METex14 skipping alterations	–	II, recruiting	NCT02750215	May 2016
Crizotinib (PF-02341066) *Multikinase small molecule inhibitor against MET, ALK, ROS1*	Pfizer	NSCLC	–	II, recruiting	NCT03088930	December 13, 2017
			Erlotinib	I, completed	NCT00965731	January 2010
			Rifampin, Itraconazole	I, recruiting	NCT00585195	April 19, 2006

(continued)

Table 1 (continued)

Drug	Manufacturer	Conditions	Combination	Phase	NCT	Study Start Date
Foretinib (GSK1363089) *Small molecule inhibitor against MET and VEGFR2*	GlaxoSmithKline	Lung cancer	Erlotinib	I/II, completed	NCT01068587	December 2009
Glesatinib (MGCD265) *Small molecule inhibitor against MET and AXL*	Mirati Therapeutics	NSCLC	Nivolumab	II, recruiting	NCT02954991	November 2016
SAR125844 *MET small molecule inhibitor*	Sanofi	Malignant neoplasm	–	II, completed	NCT02435121	November 2015
Savolitinib (AZD6094) *MET small molecule inhibitor*	AstraZeneca	NSCLC	Gefitinib	I, not yet recruiting	NCT02374645	April 2015
			Osimertinib (AZD9291)	I, recruiting	NCT02143466	August 5, 2014
		Tumors	–	I, recruiting	NCT01985555	May 2013
Tepotinib (MSC2156119J) *MET small molecule inhibitor*	Merck	NSCLC	Gefitinib	I/II, not yet recruiting	NCT01982955	December 23, 2013
		NSCLC, METex14 skipping alterations	–	II, recruiting	NCT02864992	September 13, 2016
Antibodies against MET/HGF						
ARGX-111 *MET antibody*	argenx	Cancer, overexpressing MET	–	I, completed	NCT02055066	January 2014
Emibetuzumab (LY2875358) *MET monoclonal antibody*	Eli Lilly	Solid tumors	Ramucirumab	I/II, completed	NCT02082210	March 7, 2014
		NSCLC	Erlotinib	II, not yet recruiting	NCT01897480	August 28, 2013

INJ-61186372 Bispecific antibody against MET and EGFR	Johnson & Johnson	NSCLC	—	I, recruiting	NCT02609776	May 24, 2016
LY3164530 Bispecific antibody against MET and EGFR	Eli Lilly	Solid tumors	—	I, completed	NCT02221882	August 2014
MP0250 HGF antibody mimetic, also targets VEGF	Molecular Partners	Advanced solid tumors	—	I/II, completed	NCT02194426	February 20, 2018
Rilotumumab (AMG 102) HGF monoclonal antibody	Amgen	SCLC	Etoposide and cisplatin/carboplatin	I/II, completed	NCT00791154	December 2008
SAIT301 MET antibody	Samsung	Solid tumors	—	I, completed	NCT02296879	January 20, 2015
Sym015 MET antibody	Symphogen	NSCLC	—	I/II, recruiting	NCT02648724	March 2016
TAK-701 HGF monoclonal antibody	Takeda	Advanced solid tumors	—	I, completed	NCT00831896	March 2009
Telisotuzumab vedotin (ABBV-399) MET monoclonal antibody	AbbVie	Recurrent squamous cell lung carcinoma	—	II, recruiting	NCT03574753	February 5, 2018
		NSCLC	—	II, recruiting	NCT03539536	October 10, 2018
		Advanced solid tumors, with MET amplification or overexpression	Docetaxel or FOLFIRI/cetuximab or erlotinib	I, completed	NCT01472016	October 6, 2011

Accessed from ClinicalTrials.gov on January 21, 2019

of cabozantinib and erlotinib failed to show response in phase II and cabozantinib did not resensitize these tumors to erlotinib [50]. In a patient harboring a MET exon 14 skipping mutation, intracranial progression was observed with crizotinib treatment. Upon switching therapies to cabozantinib, rapid intracranial response to this small molecule was observed underscoring the potential of this strategy to overcome metastasis to the brain with MET-altered NSCLC [51]. Clinical studies with cabozantinib are currently recruiting for phase II in NSCLC patients with brain metastases.

Capmatinib (INC280)

Capmatinib is a competitive inhibitor with very potent and selective activity against MET compared to other kinases. It has been shown in vitro that cell lines made resistant to erlotinib, an EGFR inhibitor, could be resensitized after capmatinib treatment [52]. Results from a phase Ib/II study of patients with EGFR-mutated, MET-dysregulated NSCLC have shown promising responses to a combination of capmatinib and gefitinib (EGFR TKI) following disease progression from an only EGFR TKI treatment regimen. Recommended phase II dose was determined to be capmatinib 400 mg twice/day and gefitinib 250 mg once/day. Most common adverse events were nausea, peripheral edema, decreased appetite, rash, and increased amylase and lipase levels [53].

Crizotinib (PF-02341066)

Crizotinib is a small molecule inhibitor that competitively binds to the ATP-binding pocket of MET. Patients with MET amplification have shown remarkable response to this drug. Originally developed as a MET inhibitor, this compound also exhibited activity against anaplastic lymphoma kinase (ALK) [54] and ROS proto-oncogene 1 (ROS) rearrangements, leading to clinical trials targeting patients with this mutation. More recent studies have shown that patients with MET amplification and no ALK rearrangement treated with crizotinib have responded well in NSCLC [55] and squamous cell lung carcinoma [56]. We were the first to identify MET exon 14 skipping in patients and demonstrate that this variant can serve as a biomarker. Such biomarkers can aid clinical decisions by correctly identifying patients that would most likely benefit from MET-targeted therapies of differing class. Earlier this year, the US Food and Drug Administration (FDA) granted crizotinib a breakthrough therapy designation for the treatment of patients with metastatic NSCLC harboring MET exon 14 alterations that progress after receiving platinum-based chemotherapy. An expansion cohort of 21 patients from the PROFILE 1001 study with MET exon 14-altered NSCLC were treated with crizotinib 250 mg twice/day for 0.5–9.1+ months. Among 18 evaluable patients, 8 patients had partial responses and 9 patients had stable disease. None had progressive disease. Most adverse events were grade 1 and 2 with one case of grade 3 edema and one case of grade 3 bradycardia. No grade 4 adverse events occurred [57]. This significant designation underscores the urgency for identifying additional biomarkers and our commitment to delivering personalized medicine for patients that carry these genomic alterations.

Foretinib (GSK1363089)

Foretinib is a multikinase inhibitor that targets MET and VEGFR2 and also exhibits an inhibitory effect against KIT, Flt-3, PDGFRb, and Tie-2. In vitro, foretinib blocks activation of MET and VEGFR2-induced signaling pathways. In vivo experiments show a dose-dependent decrease in tumor burden in a lung metastasis experimental model [58]. Foretinib has also shown to be effective against ROS1 mutations especially when acquired with crizotinib resistance. A clinical trial investigating the dosing and safety profile of combining foretinib and erlotinib was designed for advanced pretreated NSCLC patients. This regimen demonstrated response in an unselected group, but also some toxicity, suggesting future trial designs to select patients based on molecular profiling [59].

Glesatinib (MGCD265)

Glesatinib is a TKI that targets tumors with MET and AXL alterations. Nonclinical models have shown glesatinib to be effective in MET exon 14 skipping mutations [60]. It is currently being evaluated in phase II trials in NSCLC patients with MET alterations.

Savolitinib (AZD6094)

Savolitinib selectively inhibits the MET receptor, blocking the PI3K/AKT/MAPK-signaling pathway as well as downregulating MYC [61]. It is currently being evaluated in phase I clinical trials in combination with EGFR TKIs in NSCLC patients.

Tepotinib (MSC2156119J)

Tepotinib is a highly selective inhibitor against MET. In xenograft models, acquired resistance to EGFR TKIs via secondary EGFR T790 M mutations can be overcome with tepotinib treatment [62]. Tepotinib is currently being evaluated in combination with EGFR TKI gefitinib and also a separate trial in NSCLC patients with MET exon 14 skipping mutation and MET amplification.

Monoclonal Antibodies Against MET/HGF

Biological antagonists such as monoclonal antibodies can prevent ligand-receptor activation by either binding to the ligand or the receptor itself. As a result, downstream signaling events cannot be activated via this receptor. Several antibodies have been developed that target the extracellular portion of MET to block HGF binding as well as antibodies that target HGF to inhibit normal ligand binding to its receptor. Although monoclonal antibodies are larger in size (150 kDa) and more expensive to produce as compared to small molecule inhibitors, their target specificity is an advantage as it lessens the likelihood of toxicity to the patient.

This section will highlight several antibodies against HGF/MET that are currently under clinical investigation. Table 1 includes a more extensive list of the ongoing clinical trials with antibodies targeting HGF/MET.

Emibetuzumab (LY2875358)

Emibetuzumab is a bivalent antibody that blocks HGF- and MET-receptor interaction, leading to MET internalization and degradation [47]. A phase I study determined a tolerable dose for emibetuzumab to be 700–2000 mg as a monotherapy and in combination with erlotinib in NSCLC patients [63]. It is currently being investigated in phase II in combination with erlotinib.

Onartuzumab (MetMAb)

Onartuzumab is a monoclonal antibody that blocks the binding of HGF to the MET receptor. However, results from clinical trials in NSCLC patients show that onartuzumab is ineffective in improving clinical outcomes in (i) combination with current first-line chemotherapy in advanced nonsquamous cell NSCLC [64], (ii) combination with erlotinib in previously treated stage IIIB or IV NSCLC patients (Phase III) [65], and (iii) combination with platinum-doublet chemotherapy in advanced squamous cell NSCLC (Phase II) [66]. Patients enrolled in this trial were biomarker unselected.

Rilotumumab (AMG 102)

Rilotumumab is an anti-HGF antibody that prevents ligand binding to MET and its activation. A phase I/II trial of rilotumumab in combination with erlotinib was evaluated in previously treated NSCLC patients with metastatic disease. The results indicated a favorable safety profile and success in terms of disease control rate [67]. A phase Ib/II trial of rilotumumab or ganitumab in combination with etoposide and carboplatin or cisplatin was evaluated in extensive-stage SCLC patients. This combination was determined to be tolerable, but overall outcomes in treating the disease were dismal [68].

Telisotuzumab Vedotin (ABBV-399)

Telisotuzumab vedotin (Teliso-V) is an antibody drug conjugate that targets the MET receptor. In the first in-human phase I trial for Teliso-V, NSCLC patients with MET-overexpressing tumors received monotherapy. The results of this innovative trial indicated favorable safety and tolerability responses and also showed promising antitumor activity in NSCLC patients with MET overexpression [69]. Current clinical investigations are now in phase II recruiting.

Mechanisms of Resistance

Inhibition of a specific kinase with small molecule inhibitors and/or biological antagonists adds selective pressure for tumor cells to acquire resistance through genetic mutations and nongenetic mechanisms [70]. For example, EGFR-mutated NSCLC tumors initially treated with EGFR TKIs can develop resistance to these agents through a secondary genetic mutation in the EGFR gene, activation of another receptor signaling axis, such as MET, and/or dysregulation of downstream pathways [71]. Although how lung cancer patients develop resistance to MET-targeting agents is not fully understood, this section will highlight the ongoing preclinical research to uncover the mechanisms of resistance to current MET therapeutics in solid tumors.

Genetic Mechanisms Contributing to Resistance

Acquiring a mutation at residue Y1230 in the MET activation loop was one mechanism that was observed to render MET TKI resistance in initially drug-sensitive gastric cells, in vitro and in vivo. As a result of this mutation, the interaction with the MET inhibitor is hindered and cells are able to bypass drug treatment [72]. It has also been shown in "MET-addicted" gastric cell lines that are initially sensitive to MET TKIs can acquire resistance through MET and KRAS gene amplification after incremental increases in drug concentrations. Resistant cells first acquired MET gene amplification and overexpression. Cells that subsequently harbored KRAS amplification lost dependence to MET and became dependent on wild-type KRAS as a way to become resistant to a MET TKI [73]. Although these preclinical data were observed in gastric cell lines, these findings may guide future studies investigating genetic mechanisms of resistance in "MET-addicted" lung cancer cells.

Alternative Pathways Contributing to Resistance

Various cell lines that are dependent on the MET pathway and are initially sensitive to MET TKIs, can develop resistance via kinase reprogramming. It has been shown that c-Myc is dissociated from the MET axis and overtaken by a variety of other kinases. As a result, this kinase reprogramming to take over c-Myc signaling provides a way for MET-addicted cancer cells to become resistant to agents targeting the MET axis [74]. Another mechanism by which gastric cells can become resistant to MET inhibitors is by utilizing the EGFR-signaling pathway to activate downstream effectors. This type of resistance was able to be overcome by dual inhibition of combined EGFR- and MET-targeted agents [72]. In MET-amplified NSCLC cell lines, it was found that alternative signaling pathways and downstream effectors, such as EGFR and PIK3CA were utilized to acquire resistance to capmatinib. A combination of EGFR, PIK3CA, and MET inhibitors could be an effective strategy to circumvent acquired resistance to capmatinib in MET-amplified NSCLC [75]. Lastly, in MET exon 14-mutated NSCLC, amplification and activation of KRAS was observed to mediate resistance to MET-targeted therapy in a patient-derived cell line [76] and genomic data from lung cancer patients [77]. In a patient with MET exon 14 skipping treated with crizotinib, a mutation in the MET kinase domain, D1228N, was acquired that conferred resistance to the inhibitor [78]. Other second-site mutations in the MET gene and mechanisms of resistance to MET inhibitors remain to be elucidated.

Future Directions

Much progress has been made in understanding the MET signaling axis and developing novel therapeutics to target this receptor with high specificity. However, as the landscape of precision medicine is constantly evolving, there is always more progress to be made for better and more effective clinical strategies. For example, despite the great advancements made with targeted therapies, clinical success can be out of reach for those patients that encounter severe side effects and toxicity, which remains to be a common issue among many. Furthermore, the affordability of these innovative drugs is also a challenge that impedes patients from being able to receive targeted treatments [79]. Managing these two factors is imperative as new therapeutic agents are discovered, designed, and brought into the market [79].

Inhibiting the MET/HGF signaling axis in novel ways are currently being investigated especially in the field of HGFA inhibitors and other serine protease inhibitors. These enzymes that are involved in the proteolytic cleavage of pro-HGF to active HGF can be blocked with antibodies and/or small molecules [80, 81]. Disabling the formation of active HGF may have therapeutic benefits in MET-addicted cancers since the ligand would not be able to activate the receptor. Currently, preclinical studies are extensively investigating optimal strategies for drug design [80].

As mechanisms of resistance to MET-targeted agents are continually being investigated, developing agents to overcome this resistance is crucial. Deciphering signaling pathways that are dysregulated when treated with certain agents will aid researchers and clinicians to bridge the translational gap between in vitro and in vivo models and strategies used in the clinic. Investigating novel and more effective combinatorial strategies to target MET and other RTKs can potentially attenuate the mechanisms of resistance that is acquired after MET-targeted therapy. It will also be interesting to see whether novel preclinical findings will come to clinical fruition. For example, a study that investigated simultaneously inhibiting MET and mitochondrial dynamics showed to be effective in MET-amplified NSCLC and mesothelioma cell lines. Targeting this crosstalk could possibly be an effective clinical strategy in MET-amplified NSCLC patients [33]. Lastly, a combination of MET inhibitors with immunotherapy could potentially be effective for lung cancer patients with MET exon 14 alterations since a considerable number of tumor samples were shown to express PD-L1 [82].

Discovering the MET exon 14 skipping mutation in patients and their remarkable response to MET TKIs demonstrates the need to determine additional biomarkers that will indicate good response to these agents. Equipped with the knowledge of potential biomarkers, clinicians will be able to make more effective decisions for their patients to achieve better responses to MET TKIs and monoclonal antibodies. As novel biomarkers that can be used to monitor MET-targeted agents with high specificity and sensitivity, and effective combinatorial strategies to overcome resistance are discovered, the ultimate purpose of precision medicine to guide clinical decision-making can be realized, bringing us closer to having clinical outcomes truly being "MET" in lung cancer.

References

1. Siegel RL, Miller KD, Jemal A. Cancer statistics, 2018. CA Cancer J Clin. 2018;68(1):7–30.
2. Bray F, et al. Global cancer statistics 2018: GLOBOCAN estimates of incidence and mortality worldwide for 36 cancers in 185 countries. CA Cancer J Clin. 2018;68(6):394–424.
3. Robinson DR, Wu YM, Lin SF. The protein tyrosine kinase family of the human genome. Oncogene. 2000;19(49):5548–57.
4. Du Z, Lovly CM. Mechanisms of receptor tyrosine kinase activation in cancer. Mol Cancer. 2018;17(1):58.
5. Hubbard SR. Structural analysis of receptor tyrosine kinases. Prog Biophys Mol Biol. 1999;71(3–4):343–58.
6. Lemmon MA, Schlessinger J. Cell signaling by receptor tyrosine kinases. Cell. 2010;141(7):1117–34.
7. Zwick E, Bange J, Ullrich A. Receptor tyrosine kinase signalling as a target for cancer intervention strategies. Endocr Relat Cancer. 2001;8(3):161–73.
8. Lawrence RE, Salgia R. MET molecular mechanisms and therapies in lung cancer. Cell Adhes Migr. 2010;4(1):146–52.
9. Gelsomino F, et al. Targeting the MET gene for the treatment of non-small-cell lung cancer. Crit Rev Oncol Hematol. 2014;89(2):284–99.

10. Cooper CS, et al. Molecular cloning of a new transforming gene from a chemically transformed human cell line. Nature. 1984;311(5981):29–33.
11. Stoker M, et al. Scatter factor is a fibroblast-derived modulator of epithelial cell mobility. Nature. 1987;327(6119):239–42.
12. Gherardi E, et al. Structural basis of hepatocyte growth factor/scatter factor and MET signalling. Proc Natl Acad Sci U S A. 2006;103(11):4046–51.
13. Maestrini E, et al. A family of transmembrane proteins with homology to the MET-hepatocyte growth factor receptor. Proc Natl Acad Sci U S A. 1996;93(2):674–8.
14. Rodrigues GA, Park M. Autophosphorylation modulates the kinase activity and oncogenic potential of the Met receptor tyrosine kinase. Oncogene. 1994;9(7):2019–27.
15. Ponzetto C, et al. A multifunctional docking site mediates signaling and transformation by the hepatocyte growth factor/scatter factor receptor family. Cell. 1994;77(2):261–71.
16. Furge KA, Zhang YW, Vande Woude GF. Met receptor tyrosine kinase: enhanced signaling through adapter proteins. Oncogene. 2000;19(49):5582–9.
17. Maulik G, et al. Activated c-Met signals through PI3K with dramatic effects on cytoskeletal functions in small cell lung cancer. J Cell Mol Med. 2002;6(4):539–53.
18. Marshall CJ. Specificity of receptor tyrosine kinase signaling: transient versus sustained extracellular signal-regulated kinase activation. Cell. 1995;80(2):179–85.
19. Gentile A, Trusolino L, Comoglio PM. The Met tyrosine kinase receptor in development and cancer. Cancer Metastasis Rev. 2008;27(1):85–94.
20. Birchmeier C, et al. Met, metastasis, motility and more. Nat Rev Mol Cell Biol. 2003;4(12):915–25.
21. Boccaccio C, et al. Induction of epithelial tubules by growth factor HGF depends on the STAT pathway. Nature. 1998;391(6664):285–8.
22. Abella JV, et al. Met/Hepatocyte growth factor receptor ubiquitination suppresses transformation and is required for Hrs phosphorylation. Mol Cell Biol. 2005;25(21):9632–45.
23. Sadiq AA, Salgia R. MET as a possible target for non-small-cell lung cancer. J Clin Oncol Off J Am Soc Clin Oncol. 2013;31(8):1089–96.
24. Birchmeier C, Gherardi E. Developmental roles of HGF/SF and its receptor, the c-Met tyrosine kinase. Trends Cell Biol. 1998;8(10):404–10.
25. Chmielowiec J, et al. c-Met is essential for wound healing in the skin. J Cell Biol. 2007;177(1):151–62.
26. Mizuno K, et al. Hepatocyte growth factor stimulates growth of hematopoietic progenitor cells. Biochem Biophys Res Commun. 1993;194(1):178–86.
27. Olivero M, et al. Overexpression and activation of hepatocyte growth factor/scatter factor in human non-small-cell lung carcinomas. Br J Cancer. 1996;74(12):1862–8.
28. Ma PC, et al. Functional expression and mutations of c-met and its therapeutic inhibition with SU11274 and small interfering RNA in non–small cell lung cancer. Cancer Res. 2005;65(4):1479.
29. Sattler M, et al. A novel small molecule met inhibitor induces apoptosis in cells transformed by the oncogenic TPR-MET tyrosine kinase. Cancer Res. 2003;63(17):5462.
30. Ma PC, et al. c-Met: structure, functions and potential for therapeutic inhibition. Cancer Metastasis Rev. 2003;22(4):309–25.
31. Jagadeeswaran R, et al. Paxillin is a target for somatic mutations in lung cancer: implications for cell growth and invasion. Cancer Res. 2008;68(1):132–42.
32. Salgia R, et al. Expression of the focal adhesion protein paxillin in lung cancer and its relation to cell motility. Oncogene. 1999;18(1):67–77.
33. Wang J, et al. Inhibiting crosstalk between MET signaling and mitochondrial dynamics and morphology: a novel therapeutic approach for lung cancer and mesothelioma. Cancer Biol Ther. 2018:1–10.
34. Seiwert TY, et al. The MET receptor tyrosine kinase is a potential novel therapeutic target for head and neck squamous cell carcinoma. Cancer Res. 2009;69(7):3021–31.
35. Sattler M, Salgia R. c-Met and hepatocyte growth factor: potential as novel targets in cancer therapy. Curr Oncol Rep. 2007;9(2):102–8.

36. Schmidt L, et al. Germline and somatic mutations in the tyrosine kinase domain of the MET proto-oncogene in papillary renal carcinomas. Nat Genet. 1997;16(1):68–73.
37. Ma PC, et al. c-MET mutational analysis in small cell lung cancer: novel juxtamembrane domain mutations regulating cytoskeletal functions. Cancer Res. 2003;63(19):6272–81.
38. Krishnaswamy S, et al. Ethnic differences and functional analysis of MET mutations in lung cancer. Clin Cancer Res. 2009;15(18):5714–23.
39. Salgia R. Role of c-Met in cancer: emphasis on lung cancer. Semin Oncol. 2009;36:S52–8.
40. Siddiqui SS, et al. *C. elegans* as a model organism for in vivo screening in cancer: effects of human c-Met in lung cancer affect *C. elegans* vulva phenotypes. Cancer Biol Ther. 2008;7(6):856–63.
41. Lee CC, Yamada KM. Identification of a novel type of alternative splicing of a tyrosine kinase receptor. Juxtamembrane deletion of the c-met protein kinase C serine phosphorylation regulatory site. J Biol Chem. 1994;269(30):19457–61.
42. Frampton GM, et al. Activation of MET via diverse exon 14 splicing alterations occurs in multiple tumor types and confers clinical sensitivity to MET inhibitors. Cancer Discov. 2015;5(8):850–9.
43. Kong-Beltran M, et al. Somatic mutations Lead to an oncogenic deletion of met in lung cancer. Cancer Res. 2006;66(1):283.
44. Tan YH, et al. CBL is frequently altered in lung cancers: its relationship to mutations in MET and EGFR tyrosine kinases. PLoS One. 2010;5(1):e8972.
45. Tan YC, et al. Differential responsiveness of MET inhibition in non-small-cell lung cancer with altered CBL. Sci Rep. 2017;7(1):9192.
46. Hewelt B, et al. The DNA walk and its demonstration of deterministic Chaos- relevance to genomic alterations in lung cancer. Bioinformatics. 2019. (in press)
47. Miranda O, Farooqui M, Siegfried JM. Status of agents targeting the HGF/c-Met axis in lung cancer. Cancers. 2018;10(9):280.
48. Engelman JA, et al. MET amplification leads to gefitinib resistance in lung cancer by activating ERBB3 signaling. Science. 2007;316(5827):1039–43.
49. Puri N, Salgia R. Synergism of EGFR and c-Met pathways, cross-talk and inhibition, in non-small cell lung cancer. J Carcinog. 2008;7:9.
50. Wakelee HA, et al. A phase Ib/II study of cabozantinib (XL184) with or without erlotinib in patients with non-small cell lung cancer. Cancer Chemother Pharmacol. 2017;79(5):923–32.
51. Klempner SJ, et al. Intracranial activity of cabozantinib in MET exon 14-positive NSCLC with brain metastases. J Thorac Oncol. 2017;12(1):152–6.
52. Lara MS, et al. Preclinical evaluation of MET inhibitor INC-280 with or without the epidermal growth factor receptor inhibitor erlotinib in non-small-cell lung cancer. Clin Lung Cancer. 2017;18(3):281–5.
53. Wu YL, et al. Phase Ib/II study of capmatinib (INC280) plus gefitinib after failure of Epidermal Growth Factor Receptor (EGFR) inhibitor therapy in patients with EGFR-mutated, MET factor-dysregulated non-small-cell lung cancer. J Clin Oncol. 2018:JCO2018777326.
54. Nwizu T, et al. Crizotinib (PF02341066) as a ALK /MET inhibitor- special emphasis as a therapeutic drug against lung cancer. Drugs Future. 2011;36(2):91–9.
55. Ou SH, et al. Activity of crizotinib (PF02341066), a dual mesenchymal-epithelial transition (MET) and anaplastic lymphoma kinase (ALK) inhibitor, in a non-small cell lung cancer patient with de novo MET amplification. J Thorac Oncol. 2011;6(5):942–6.
56. Schwab R, et al. Major partial response to crizotinib, a dual MET/ALK inhibitor, in a squamous cell lung (SCC) carcinoma patient with de novo c-MET amplification in the absence of ALK rearrangement. Lung Cancer. 2014;83(1):109–11.
57. Drilon AE, et al. Efficacy and safety of crizotinib in patients (pts) with advanced MET exon 14-altered non-small cell lung cancer (NSCLC). J Clin Oncol. 2016;34(15_suppl):108–108.
58. Qian F, et al. Inhibition of tumor cell growth, invasion, and metastasis by EXEL-2880 (XL880, GSK1363089), a novel inhibitor of HGF and VEGF receptor tyrosine kinases. Cancer Res. 2009;69(20):8009–16.

59. Leighl NB, et al. A phase I study of foretinib plus erlotinib in patients with previously treated advanced non-small cell lung cancer: Canadian cancer trials group IND.196. Oncotarget. 2017;8(41):69651–62.
60. Engstrom LD, et al. Glesatinib exhibits antitumor activity in lung cancer models and patients harboring MET exon 14 mutations and overcomes mutation-mediated resistance to type I MET inhibitors in nonclinical models. Clin Cancer Res. 2017;23(21):6661.
61. Henry RE, et al. Acquired savolitinib resistance in non-small cell lung cancer arises via multiple mechanisms that converge on MET-independent mTOR and MYC activation. Oncotarget. 2016;7(36):57651–70.
62. Friese-Hamim M, et al. The selective c-Met inhibitor tepotinib can overcome epidermal growth factor receptor inhibitor resistance mediated by aberrant c-Met activation in NSCLC models. Am J Cancer Res. 2017;7(4):962–72.
63. Rosen LS, et al. A first-in-human phase I study of a bivalent MET antibody, emibetuzumab (LY2875358), as monotherapy and in combination with erlotinib in advanced cancer. Clin Cancer Res. 2017;23(8):1910.
64. Wakelee H, et al. Efficacy and safety of onartuzumab in combination with first-line bevacizumab- or pemetrexed-based chemotherapy regimens in advanced non-squamous non-small-cell lung cancer. Clin Lung Cancer. 2017;18(1):50–9.
65. Spigel DR, et al. Results from the phase III randomized trial of onartuzumab plus erlotinib versus erlotinib in previously treated stage IIIB or IV non–small-cell lung cancer: METLung. J Clin Oncol. 2016;35(4):412–20.
66. Hirsch FR, et al. Efficacy and safety results from a phase II, placebo-controlled study of onartuzumab plus First-line platinum-doublet chemotherapy for advanced squamous cell non-small-cell lung cancer. Clin Lung Cancer. 2017;18(1):43–9.
67. Tarhini AA, et al. Phase 1/2 study of rilotumumab (AMG 102), a hepatocyte growth factor inhibitor, and erlotinib in patients with advanced non-small cell lung cancer. Cancer. 2017;123(15):2936–44.
68. Glisson B, et al. A randomized, placebo-controlled, phase 1b/2 study of rilotumumab or ganitumab in combination with platinum-based chemotherapy as first-line treatment for extensive-stage small-cell lung cancer. Clin Lung Cancer. 2017;18(6):615–625 e8.
69. Strickler JH, et al. Dose-escalation and -expansion study of telisotuzumab vedotin, an antibody-drug conjugate targeting c-Met, in patients with advanced solid tumors. J Clin Oncol. 2018:JCO2018787697.
70. Salgia R, Kulkarni P. The genetic/non-genetic duality of drug 'resistance' in cancer. Trends Cancer. 2018;4(2):110–8.
71. Morgillo F, et al. Mechanisms of resistance to EGFR-targeted drugs: lung cancer. ESMO Open. 2016;1(3).
72. Qi J, et al. Multiple mutations and bypass mechanisms can contribute to development of acquired resistance to MET inhibitors. Cancer Res. 2011;71(3):1081.
73. Cepero V, et al. MET and KRAS gene amplification mediates acquired resistance to MET tyrosine kinase inhibitors. Cancer Res. 2010;70(19):7580.
74. Shen A, et al. c-Myc alterations confer therapeutic response and acquired resistance to c-met inhibitors in MET-addicted cancers. Cancer Res. 2015;75(21):4548.
75. Kim S, et al. Acquired resistance of MET-amplified non-small cell lung cancer cells to the MET inhibitor capmatinib. J Korean Cancer Assoc. 2018. (in press).
76. Bahcall M, et al. Amplification of wild-type KRAS imparts resistance to crizotinib in MET exon 14 mutant non–small cell lung cancer. Clin Cancer Res. 2018;24(23):5963–76.
77. Suzawa K, et al. Activation of KRAS mediates resistance to targeted therapy in MET exon 14 mutant non-small cell lung cancer. Clin Cancer Res. 2019;25(4):1248–60.
78. Heist RS, et al. Acquired resistance to crizotinib in NSCLC with MET exon 14 skipping. J Thorac Oncol. 2016;11(8):1242–5.
79. Beck A, et al. Strategies and challenges for the next generation of therapeutic antibodies. Nat Rev Immunol. 2010;10:345.

80. Janetka JW, Jr RAG. Inhibitors of the growth-factor activating proteases matriptase, hepsin and HGFA: strategies for rational drug design and optimization. In: Extracellular targeting of cell signaling in c.ancer. Hoboken, NJ: Wiley; 2018.
81. Kirchhofer D, Eigenbrot C, Lazarus RA. Inhibitory antibodies of the proteases HGFA, matriptase and hepsin. In: Extracellular targeting of cell signaling in cancer. Hoboken, NJ: Wiley; 2018.
82. Sabari JK, et al. PD-L1 expression, tumor mutational burden, and response to immunotherapy in patients with MET exon 14 altered lung cancers. Ann Oncol. 2018;29(10):2085–91.

Targeting HER2 in Lung Cancer

Ajaz Bulbul, Alessandro Leal, and Hatim Husain

Abstract Human epidermal growth factor receptor 2 (*HER2*) amplification and mutations are oncogenic drivers in 2–5% of lung adenocarcinomas. *HER2* exon 20 in-frame mutations may be phenotypically related to the non-smoking Asian female population and mutually exclusive of other known lung mutations and *HER2* amplification. Although *HER2* amplification may be an important mechanism for acquired resistance to epidermal growth factor (EGFR) tyrosine kinase inhibitors (TKIs), the prognostic and predictive significance of the amplification event appears to be different in non-small cell lung cancer (NSCLC) compared to breast and gastric cancer. Single-agent HER2-targeted antibodies and dimerization inhibitor responses have been limited, however encouraging responses have been seen with TKIs targeting Pan-HER agents and antibody drug conjugates. Based on a small trial, the National Comprehensive Cancer Network (NCCN) recommends *HER2* exon 20 insertion mutants who have progressed on chemotherapy be considered for ado-trastuzumab emtansine. Further studies are needed in this population of patients. The type of *HER2* alterations (mutation/amplification) needs to be precisely defined, and the most compelling data for targeted approaches currently exists in select *HER2* mutation positive patients. Advances and approvals for next generation sequencing (NGS) technology have the potential to facilitate the identification of patients who may derive benefit for treatment options.

Keywords Human epidermal growth factor receptor 2 · Tyrosine kinase inhibitors · Trastuzumab · Lung cancer · Afatinib · Cetuximab

A. Bulbul · H. Husain (✉)
University of California San Diego, La Jolla, CA, USA
e-mail: hhusain@ucsd.edu

A. Leal
Johns Hopkins Sidney Kimmel Cancer Center, Baltimore, MD, USA

© Springer Nature Switzerland AG 2019
R. Salgia (ed.), *Targeted Therapies for Lung Cancer*, Current Cancer Research,
https://doi.org/10.1007/978-3-030-17832-1_6

Introduction

The human epidermal growth factor receptor 2 (HER2) (also known as erbB-2/neu) is a member of the erbB receptor tyrosine kinase family and is a major proliferative driver that activates downstream signaling through PI3K-AKT and MEK-ERK pathways [1]. (Fig. 1) *HER2* mutations and *HER2* amplifications have been reported in 2–3% and 2–5% of lung adenocarcinomas respectively [2–5]. The majority of patients with HER2-amplified lung cancers are male and former smokers, and patients with HER2 mutant lung cancers are usually women who are nonsmokers [6]. *HER2* mutations, specifically exon 20 in-frame insertions, have been described as an oncogenic driver alterations in a subset of non-small cell lung cancer with adenocarcinoma histology. While these insertions are small in-frame insertions in exon 20 (96%), point mutations in exon 20 have been observed in approximately 4% of cases. Generally, activating mutations in the tyrosine kinase domain of HER2 appear to be mutually exclusive with epidermal growth factor (EGFR) (exon 18–21), BRAF, ALK, PI3KCA, and KRAS mutations [2, 7, 8]. Mutations affecting the extracellular domain can result in constitutive dimerization [9]. Rare mutations in the transmembrane domain of HER2 may be seen in familial lung adenocarcinomas [10]. Herein, we will discuss the clinical characteristics of *HER2*-mutated or *HER2*-amplified NSCLC patients and the targeted therapies which have been explored in this space.

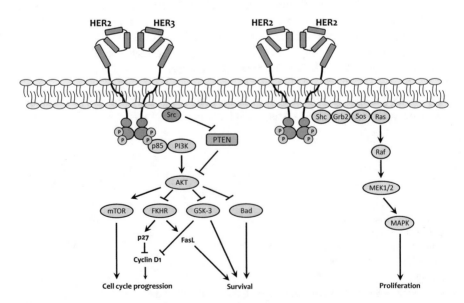

Fig. 1 HER2 downstream signaling through the PI3K and MAPK pathways

Clinical and Prognostic Implications

The oncogenic activation of HER2 can be caused by gene amplification or mutation resulting in molecular activation of the receptor or HER2 protein overexpression. The prognostic implications of these differences are not yet clear [8, 11]. HER2 has no known ligand, and it is activated by homo−/hetero-dimerization with other members of the erbB family. Under resting conditions, HER2 surface receptors are in a monomeric folded/closed inactive conformation [11]. Ligand binding to the extracellular domain leads to a conformational change to a dimerized/open state that exposes the receptor interface to drug targeting.

HER2 amplification has been found to have prognostic significance in breast cancer, gastric cancer, and gastric-esophageal junction (GEJ) adenocarcinomas. Historically, these subsets have had poor outcomes, and the addition of the anti-HER2 monoclonal antibody trastuzumab has led to significant improvement in clinical outcomes. The prognostic significance of HER2 in lung cancer has not been clear [1, 12]. *HER2* mutations did not have prognostic significance in a study of 504 Japanese lung cancer patients and involved 2.6% of the cases. When limiting testing to the subgroup of nonsmokers with adenocarcinoma without EGFR mutation, the frequency of *HER2* mutations increased to 14.1% (11/78).

Although not much is known about prognosis in this small subset of lung cancer, the incidence of brain metastases in patients with *HER2* mutant lung cancers appears to be lower than *EGFR* at diagnosis. CNS risk, however, worsens over the disease course. One third of patients with *HER2* mutant lung cancers develop brain metastases during treatment [13].

HER2 in NSCLC: Amplification Versus Mutations

Association between HER2 overexpression by immunohistochemistry (IHC), amplification by fluorescence in situ hybridization (FISH), or mutation is not entirely clear. Immunohistochemistry overexpression >2+ can be seen in approximately 16% of NSCLC, including adenocarcinomas and large cell carcinomas, while rare in squamous cell carcinomas (1%). IHC 3+ overexpression, however, is rare across all histologies and found in only 2–6% [4, 5]. The concordance between IHC intensity and FISH positivity was 4 of 7 patients and 2 of 76 patients, for 3+ IHC and 2+ IHC, respectively [7]. In a study of over 500 patients using a 23 gene hotspot amplification panel based on Ion AmpliSeq, at least one DNA mutation was detected in 374 patients (74.5%), and ERBB2 mutation was seen in 2% of cases in this cohort. Despite the paucity of data on *HER2* copy number assessment by NGS in lung cancer, a robust validation study conducted at MSKCC with 213 breast and 39 gastroesophageal cancers showed that NGS results for *HER2* amplification achieved 98.4% of overall concordance (248/252) with combined IHC/FISH [14]. A contemporary study called the SUMMIT trial evaluated *HER2/HER3* concordance of tumor testing local site NGS or RT-PCR testing versus central tumor

Table 1 Mutation location and response assessment to neratinib in the lung cohort of the SUMMIT trial

Mutation location	*Extracellular domain*	Kinase domain		Non-Hotspot
Mutation site	*S310*	Exon 20 ins	L755	Kinase domain
Response to Neratinib	+	+++	++	+

testing using hybridization-based exon capture and showed a concordance of 95% [15]. The distribution of identified mutations is listed in Table 1.

Tumor specimens from 175 patients with lung adenocarcinomas and no prior targeted therapy at Memorial Sloan Kettering and University of Colorado were studied and evaluated for the presence of *HER2* amplification, overexpression, and mutation. *HER2* amplification by FISH was identified in 3% of cases, and *HER2* mutation by NGS was detected in 3% with all aberrations in exon 20. None of the *HER2*-mutant tumors were amplified which is a finding consistent with The Cancer Genome Atlas (TCGA) data [16]. Negative IHC staining correlated with negative FISH results [6]. Recently, a subset of cases described have had both *HER2* amplification and mutation, and such overlap represents a small minority of cases [17, 18]. Among patients harboring *HER2* mutations, multivariate analysis showed that *HER2* amplification is an unfavorable prognostic factor, while those cases with HER2 phosphorylation identified may have a more favorable prognosis [18].

HER2 is known to be amplified in 12–13% of NSCLC that have acquired resistance to EGFR tyrosine kinase inhibitors [19]. Both in vitro and in vivo studies have shown that afatinib plus cetuximab may significantly reduce HER2 phosphorylation indicating a potential clinical use in *HER2*-amplified cancers [20]. *HER2* mutations have been evaluated in preclinical models and responses to the pan-HER inhibitor HKI-272, afatinib, and trastuzumab have been seen in these models [21, 22].

Few data exist describing details of the clinical course of patients with *HER2*-mutated NSCLC. Progression-free survival (PFS) for HER2 therapies was 5.1 months across cohorts. Median overall survival was 89 months and 23 months for early stage disease and metastatic patients, respectively [17].

Monoclonal Antibody Targeting HER2 Amplification in NSCLC

Single-agent activity of trastuzumab has been disappointing in HER2-amplified NSCLC. In 2005, a Phase II study was initiated to determine whether single-agent trastuzumab would affect outcomes in patients with Stage IIIB or Stage IV NSCLC expressing HER2 with 2+ or 3+ IHC expression of HER2. Trastuzumab at a dose of 4 mg/kg was given intravenously as loading followed by weekly doses of 2 mg/kg and did not exhibit significant clinical activity in this cancer and leukemia Group B (CALGB) study [23]. The failure to observe more than one response in the first 22 evaluable patients and the serious pulmonary toxicity observed in one patient led to the early closure of this CALGB trial. Single-agent responses in breast are higher at 25% with trastuzumab in those with IHC 2+/3+ metastatic breast cancer [24]. There was only one patient in that study with 3+ expression and such cases represent less than 2% of patients with NSCLC [23].

The combination of trastuzumab with chemotherapy appears to be more encouraging. Cisplatin and gemcitabine combined with trastuzumab was well tolerated with 38% partial response and a 62% 1-year survival rate (13/21). Additionally, 80% of patients with IHC 3+ disease on study treatment were alive after 6 months, compared with only 64% of the overall cohort. Given the small number of IHC 3+ (5%, 18/360), a larger study will be required to determine whether this combination is superior to chemotherapy alone [25].

In another phase II study, patients with HER2-positive tumors (2+ or 3+) were randomized to either single-agent trastuzumab or docetaxel. All patients received the trastuzumab/docetaxel combination in a sequential manner and had a partial response rate of 8%. In an ECOG phase II study, overall survival was similar to historical data using carboplatin and paclitaxel alone, while patients with 3+ HER2 expression had a higher median PFS of 3.3 months and a median overall survival of 10.1 months. The authors concluded that a phase III trial targeting HER2 should be limited to 3+ fluorescent in situ hybridization (FISH)-positive patients [26]. In a similar study, the response rate and time to progression in the chemotherapy only group was 41% and 7.2 months, respectively, compared to 36% and 6.3 months for patients receiving combination gemcitabine and cisplatin plus trastuzumab [27].

Both docetaxel and paclitaxel have been tested in a phase II setting with 23% response rate in the docetaxel plus trastuzumab group, and 26% in the paclitaxel plus trastuzumab cohort. HER2 positive patients had a 25% response rate compared to 24% in the HER2 negative group suggesting a limited value for this combination. Based on this data, HER2 expression status did not appear to affect outcomes [28].

In a retrospective cohort from Europe, an overall response rate of 50% and disease control rate (DCR) of 82% were seen with trastuzumab-based combinatorial therapies. The authors suggested a DCR of >90% for patients receiving trastuzumab-based combinations ($n = 15$) and 100% for patients receiving afatinib ($n = 3$) with the caveat of a limited sample size. Progression-free survival for HER2 therapies was 5.1 months with a median survival of 23 months in metastatic patients [17]. Pertuzumab, a first-in-class (HER2) dimerization inhibitor, approved in breast cancer binds at the receptor dimerization domain and inhibits HER2 signaling. Of 43 patients with NSCLC expressing HER2 treated with pertuzumab, no responses have been seen. Of the 22 patients who underwent FDG-PET as an exploratory pharmacodynamic endpoint, 6 patients (27.3%) had a metabolic response noted by a decrease in SUV avidity [29].

The overall disappointing clinical outcome results of *HER2* amplification in lung cancer indicate the importance of understanding how amplification may constitute a targetable oncogenic driver. The threshold of significance for HER2 overexpression and appropriate NGS cut-offs for gene amplification remain to be defined.

Tyrosine Kinase Inhibitors for *HER2* Mutations

Tyrosine kinase inhibitors have had more clinical efficacy; however, it is not known what is the optimal pan-HER TKI at this time to target *HER2* mutations. No responses were seen in 3 patients with *EGFR* mutations receiving lapatinib, and no mutations in *HER2* were found in a cohort of 75 patients receiving lapatinib. One of two patients with *HER2* amplification, however, had an unconfirmed response with a 51% decrease in tumor [30]. Two patients were treated with lapatinib, and all experienced disease progression [17]. Current clinical trials targeting HER2 mutated lung cancer are included in Table 2.

Promising data have been seen with irreversible TKIs targeting Pan-HER2/3 inhibitors such as afatinib and neratinib. In an exploratory phase II study of afatinib, 3/5 patients with *HER2*-mutated stage IV adenocarcinoma who received afatinib had an objective response [31]. In the updated analysis 5/7 of these *HER2*-mutated patients had stable disease [32].

Neratinib, an irreversible pan ErbB-receptor family inhibitor, was recently approved for maintenance use in HER2 overexpressing breast cancer and was evaluated in a phase I trial in combination with temsirolimus on the basis of preclinical data suggesting synergy. Responses were noted in patients with *HER2*-amplified breast cancer resistant to trastuzumab and in *HER2*-mutant NSCLC (partial responses in two of the six patients with *HER2*-mutant NSCLC) [33].

The SUMMIT trial (NCT01953926) is a basket trial evaluating the pan-HER tyrosine kinase inhibitor neratinib in 141 patients with 21 unique tumor types, mostly harboring *HER2* mutations. We now know that the efficacy of HER2 blockade in these HER2 mutant malignancies depends not just on the mutation but on the histologic type of tumor with greatest activity seen in breast and cervical cancers. Missense mutations were among the most common genomic alteration seen (74%). In-frame insertions were a distant second, presenting in 22% of patients involved.

In the 26 patients with lung cancer in the SUMMIT trial, *HER2* exon 20 insertions were the most prevalent, and only one objective response was seen in a patient with a L755S kinase domain missense mutation. Unfortunately, the lung cancer response rate did not meet the primary end-point for efficacy with only a 1% response rate and a 5.5-month median PFS [15].

Dacomitinib, another irreversible pan-HER TKI recently approved in first-line NSCLC based on the head-to-head comparison to gefitinib in the ARCHER 1050 trial, has been tested in HER2 mutant or HER2-amplified lung cancers and showed an overall 13% response rate in the 26 *HER2*-mutant patients. No response was seen in four patients with *HER2* amplification. In this study, 30 patients were included with *HER2* mutant lung cancer ($n = 26$, with 25 exon 20 insertions and 1 exon 20 missense mutation) or *HER2*-amplified lung cancers ($n = 4$). Three of 26 patients (12%) with tumors harboring *HER2* exon 20 mutations had a partial response lasting 3–14 months. No partial responses occurred in four patients with tumors with *HER2* amplifications. This has been the highest response so far noted in single-agent TKI treatment in *HER2* exon 20 insertions. Dacomitinib has recently

Table 2 Current clinical trials investigating anti-HER2 therapies in NCSLC

NCT number	Title	Interventions	Sponsor/Collaborators	Phases	Enrollment
NCT03318939	Phase 2 study of poziotinib in patients with NSCLC having EGFR or HER2 exon 20 insertion mutation	Drug: Poziotinib	Spectrum Pharmaceuticals, Inc.	Phase 2	314
NCT03505710	DS-8201a in human epidermal Growth factor receptor 2 (HER2)-expressing or -mutated non-small cell lung cancer	Drug: Trastuzumab deruxtecan (DS-82C1a)	Daiichi Sankyo, Inc.|Daiichi Sankyo Co., Ltd.	Phase 2	80
NCT03066206	Poziotinib in EGFR exon 20 mutant advanced non-small cell lung cancer (NSCLC) and HER2 exon 20 mutant NSCLC	Drug: Poziotinib	M.D. Anderson Cancer Center|Lung Cancer Research Foundation|Spectrum Pharmaceuticals, Inc	Phase 2	80
NCT02834936	A clinical study of pyrotinib in patients of advanced non-small cell lung cancer with HER2 mutation	Drug: pyrotinib	Jiangsu HengRui Medicine Co., Ltd.	Phase 2	55
NCT02716116	A trial of AP32788 in non-small cell lung cancer	Drug: AP32788	Ariad Pharmaceuticals|Takeda	Phase 1|Phase 2	250
NCT02500199	Phase I study of pyrotinib in patients with HER2-positive solid tumors	Drug: Pyrotinib	Hengrui Therapeutics, Inc.	Phase 1	50
NCT02314481	Deciphering antitumor response and resistance with intratumor heterogeneity	Drug: MPDL3280A|Drug: Vemurafenib|Drug: Alectinib|Drug: Trastuzumab emtansine	University College, London|Hoffmann-La Roche	Phase 2	119
NCT02912949	A study of MCLA-128 in patients with solid tumors	Drug: MCLA-128	Merus N.V.|Chiltern International Inc.|Covance|LGC Limited|Gustave Roussy, Cancer Campus, Grand Paris	Phase 1|Phase 2	130

(continued)

Table 2 (continued)

NCT number	Title	Interventions	Sponsor/Collaborators	Phases	Enrollment
NCT02117167	SAFIR02_lung efficacy of targeted drugs guided by genomic profiles in metastatic NSCLC patients	Drug: AZD2014|Drug: AZD4547|Drug: AZD5363|Drug: AZD8931|Drug: Selumetinib|Drug: Vandetanib|Drug: Standard maintenance for squamous NSCLC|Drug: Pemetrexed|Drug: MEDI4736	UNICANCER|IFCT|Fondation ARC|AstraZeneca	Phase 2	650
NCT03410927	A study of TAS0728 in patients with solid tumors With HER2 or HER3 abnormalities	Drug: TAS0728	Taiho Oncology, Inc.	Phase 1|Phase 2	204
NCT02892123	Trial of ZW25 in patients with advanced HER2-expressing cancers	Drug: ZW25, HER2 inhibitor|Combination Product: Paclitaxel|Combination Product: Capecitabine|Combination Product: Vinorelbine	Zymeworks Inc.	Phase 1	150
NCT03284723	PF-06804103 dose Escalation in HER2 positive solid tumors	Drug: PF-06804103	Pfizer	Phase 1	95

received FDA approval for EGFR-mutant lung cancer. A phase II study is currently evaluating the oral, quinazoline-based pan-HER inhibitor poziotinib in histologically or cytologically confirmed NSCLC with a documented *EGFR* or *HER2* exon 20 insertion mutation (NCT 03318939).

In another case, a pulse dosing strategy of afatinib at 280 mg weekly dose was noted to be reasonably well tolerated and induced antitumor activity in *HER2* -exon 20 insertion mutated lung adenocarcinomas. One of the 3 patients achieved a 5-month response, and stable disease was seen in another patient for approximately 11 months [34]. Additional clinical trials are needed to evaluate the clinical impact of pulse dosing.

Antibody Drug Conjugate

In a phase II basket trial performed at Memorial Sloan Kettering, 18 patients with *HER2* exon 20 insertions and point mutations in the kinase, transmembrane, and extracellular domains were treated with ado-trastuzumab emtansine intravenously at 3.6 mg/kg every 3 weeks until disease progression. Half of patients had received at least two prior therapies with *HER2*-based treatments. Objective partial response was observed in eight patients (44%) and stable disease in seven (39%). Interestingly, concurrent *HER2* amplification was seen in two patients, one having partial response and the other presenting with stable disease [35].

Practical Considerations

For patients with a *HER2*-exon 20 insertion mutation who have progressed on chemotherapy, clinical guidelines have incorporated HER2-targeted treatment into the next line of therapy and ado-trastuzumab emtansine has been included in the NCCN guidelines. As of this date, there is still no FDA approval for a targeted HER2 directed strategy in lung cancer. Pan-HER TKIs like afatinib or dacomitinib may be considered in *HER2*-mutant patients based on series and case reports; however, there has been limited activity for targeted therapy in HER overexpressed tumors. Additional approaches could combine active cytotoxic agents in lung cancer (e.g. gemcitabine, taxanes, vinorelbine) with trastuzumab as previously studied in earlier phase II trials in order to obtain synergistic effects [17, 35, 36]. Although combining trastuzumab and pertuzumab in breast cancer has led to additive effects, trastuzumab and/or pertuzumab have largely failed to show clinical benefit in lung cancer when administered as monotherapy or combined with chemotherapy [27]. More selective inhibitors against HER2 for activating mutations are likely a path forward and clinical trials of novel agents are underway.

Conclusion

As the cost of next generation sequencing continues to fall, broad-based molecular profiling will likely be a clinically important strategy to identify patients who may derive benefit from HER2-based therapies. *HER2* aberrations, whether mutation, amplification, or protein overexpression, need to be precisely defined as the most compelling data for targeted approaches suggest benefit for *HER2* mutations associated with gain of function. Patient selection to increase the positive predictive value of testing and additional biomarkers are needed in this clinical setting.

References

1. Spector NL, Blackwell KL. Understanding the mechanisms behind trastuzumab therapy for human epidermal growth factor receptor 2-positive breast cancer. J Clin Oncol. 2009;27(34):5838–47.
2. Arcila ME, Chaft JE, Nafa K, et al. Prevalence, clinicopathologic associations, and molecular spectrum of ERBB2 (HER2) tyrosine kinase mutations in lung adenocarcinomas. Clin Cancer Res. 2012;18(18):4910–8.
3. Network CGA. Comprehensive molecular characterization of human colon and rectal cancer. Nature. 2012;487(7407):330–7.
4. Heinmoller P, Gross C, Beyser K, et al. HER2 status in non-small cell lung cancer: results from patient screening for enrollment to a phase II study of herceptin. Clin Cancer Res. 2003;9(14):5238–43.
5. Hirsch FR, Varella-Garcia M, Franklin WA, et al. Evaluation of HER-2/neu gene amplification and protein expression in non-small cell lung carcinomas. Br J Cancer. 2002;86(9):1449–56.
6. Li BT, Ross DS, Aisner DL, et al. HER2 amplification and HER2 mutation are distinct molecular targets in lung cancers. J Thorac Oncol. 2016;11(3):414–9.
7. Stephens P, Hunter C, Bignell G, et al. Lung cancer: intragenic ERBB2 kinase mutations in tumours. Nature. 2004;431(7008):525–6.
8. Peters S, Zimmermann S. Targeted therapy in NSCLC driven by HER2 insertions. Transl Lung Cancer Res. 2014;3(2):84–8.
9. Greulich H, Kaplan B, Mertins P, et al. Functional analysis of receptor tyrosine kinase mutations in lung cancer identifies oncogenic extracellular domain mutations of ERBB2. Proc Natl Acad Sci U S A. 2012;109(36):14476–81.
10. Yamamoto H, Higasa K, Sakaguchi M, et al. Novel germline mutation in the transmembrane domain of HER2 in familial lung adenocarcinomas. J Natl Cancer Inst. 2014;106(1):djt338.
11. Ferguson KM, Berger MB, Mendrola JM, Cho HS, Leahy DJ, Lemmon MA. EGF activates its receptor by removing interactions that autoinhibit ectodomain dimerization. Mol Cell. 2003;11(2):507–17.
12. Bang YJ, Van Cutsem E, Feyereislova A, et al. Trastuzumab in combination with chemotherapy versus chemotherapy alone for treatment of HER2-positive advanced gastric or gastro-oesophageal junction cancer (ToGA): a phase 3, open-label, randomised controlled trial. Lancet. 2010;376(9742):687–97.
13. Kris MG, Offin MD, Feldman DL, et al. Frequency of brain metastases and outcomes in patients with HER2-, KRAS-, and EGFR-mutant lung cancers. J Clin Oncol. 2018;36(15_suppl):9081–9081.

14. Ross DS, Zehir A, Cheng DT, et al. Next-generation assessment of human epidermal growth factor receptor 2 (ERBB2) amplification status: clinical validation in the context of a hybrid capture-based, comprehensive solid tumor genomic profiling assay. J Mol Diagn. 2017;19(2):244–54.
15. Hyman DM, Piha-Paul SA, Won H, et al. HER kinase inhibition in patients with HER2- and HER3-mutant cancers. Nature. 2018;554(7691):189–94.
16. EA C, JD C, AN B, et al. Comprehensive molecular profiling of lung adenocarcinoma. Nature. 2014;511(7511):543–50.
17. Mazieres J, Peters S, Lepage B, et al. Lung cancer that harbors an HER2 mutation: epidemiologic characteristics and therapeutic perspectives. J Clin Oncol. 2013;31(16):1997–2003.
18. Suzuki M, Shiraishi K, Yoshida A, et al. HER2 gene mutations in non-small cell lung carcinomas: concurrence with Her2 gene amplification and Her2 protein expression and phosphorylation. Lung Cancer. 2015;87(1):14–22.
19. Yu HA, Arcila ME, Rekhtman N, et al. Analysis of tumor specimens at the time of acquired resistance to EGFR TKI therapy in 155 patients with EGFR mutant lung cancers. Clin Cancer Res. 2013;19(8):2240–7.
20. Takezawa K, Pirazzoli V, Arcila ME, et al. HER2 amplification: a potential mechanism of acquired resistance to EGFR inhibition in EGFR-mutant lung cancers that lack the second-site EGFRT790M mutation. Cancer Discov. 2012;2(10):922–33.
21. Shimamura T, Ji H, Minami Y, et al. Non-small-cell lung cancer and Ba/F3 transformed cells harboring the ERBB2 G776insV_G/C mutation are sensitive to the dual-specific epidermal growth factor receptor and ERBB2 inhibitor HKI-272. Cancer Res. 2006;66(13):6487–91.
22. Perera SA, Li D, Shimamura T, et al. HER2YVMA drives rapid development of adenosquamous lung tumors in mice that are sensitive to BIBW2992 and rapamycin combination therapy. Proc Natl Acad Sci U S A. 2009;106(2):474–9.
23. Clamon G, Herndon J, Kern J, et al. Lack of trastuzumab activity in nonsmall cell lung carcinoma with overexpression of erb-B2: 39810: a phase II trial of Cancer and Leukemia Group B. Cancer. 2005;103(8):1670–5.
24. Vogel CL, Cobleigh MA, Tripathy D, et al. Efficacy and safety of trastuzumab as a single agent in first-line treatment of HER2-overexpressing metastatic breast cancer. J Clin Oncol. 2002;20(3):719–26.
25. Zinner RG, Glisson BS, Fossella FV, et al. Trastuzumab in combination with cisplatin and gemcitabine in patients with Her2-overexpressing, untreated, advanced non-small cell lung cancer: report of a phase II trial and findings regarding optimal identification of patients with Her2-overexpressing disease. Lung Cancer. 2004;44(1):99–110.
26. Langer CJ, Stephenson P, Thor A, Vangel M, Johnson DH. Trastuzumab in the treatment of advanced non-small-cell lung cancer: is there a role? Focus on Eastern Cooperative Oncology Group study 2598. J Clin Oncol. 2004;22(7):1180–7.
27. Gatzemeier U, Groth G, Butts C, et al. Randomized phase II trial of gemcitabine-cisplatin with or without trastuzumab in HER2-positive non-small-cell lung cancer. Ann Oncol. 2004;15(1):19–27.
28. Krug LM, Miller VA, Patel J, et al. Randomized phase II study of weekly docetaxel plus trastuzumab versus weekly paclitaxel plus trastuzumab in patients with previously untreated advanced nonsmall cell lung carcinoma. Cancer. 2005;104(10):2149–55.
29. Herbst RS, Davies AM, Natale RB, et al. Efficacy and safety of single-agent pertuzumab, a human epidermal receptor dimerization inhibitor, in patients with non small cell lung cancer. Clin Cancer Res. 2007;13(20):6175–81.
30. Ross HJ, Blumenschein GR Jr, Aisner J, et al. Randomized phase II multicenter trial of two schedules of lapatinib as first- or second-line monotherapy in patients with advanced or metastatic non-small cell lung cancer. Clin Cancer Res. 2010;16(6):1938–49.
31. De Greve J, Teugels E, Geers C, et al. Clinical activity of afatinib (BIBW 2992) in patients with lung adenocarcinoma with mutations in the kinase domain of HER2/neu. Lung Cancer. 2012;76(1):123–7.

32. De Greve J, Moran T, Graas MP, et al. Phase II study of afatinib, an irreversible ErbB family blocker, in demographically and genotypically defined lung adenocarcinoma. Lung Cancer. 2015;88(1):63–9.
33. Gandhi L, Bahleda R, Tolaney SM, et al. Phase I study of neratinib in combination with temsirolimus in patients with human epidermal growth factor receptor 2-dependent and other solid tumors. J Clin Oncol. 2014;32(2):68–75.
34. Costa DB, Jorge SE, Moran JP, et al. Pulse afatinib for ERBB2 exon 20 insertion-mutated lung adenocarcinomas. J Thorac Oncol. 2016;11(6):918–23.
35. Li BT, Shen R, Buonocore D, et al. Ado-trastuzumab emtansine for patients with HER2-mutant lung cancers: results from a phase II basket trial. J Clin Oncol. 2018;36(24):2532–7.
36. Cappuzzo F, Bemis L, Varella-Garcia M. HER2 mutation and response to trastuzumab therapy in non-small-cell lung cancer. N Engl J Med. 2006;354(24):2619–21.

NTRK-Targeted Therapy in Lung Cancer

Xiaoliang Wu, Lin Zhu, and Patrick C. Ma

Abstract Gene rearrangements or fusions as a tumorigenic genomic driver event have been identified as a common recurrent occurrence in a variety of human malignancies. The neurotrophic tyrosine receptor kinase gene family contains *NTRK1*, *NTRK2*, and *NTRK3*, which encode the proteins tropomyosin receptor kinase A, B, and C (TRKA, TRKB, TRKC), respectively. TRKA, TRKB, and TRKC can be activated by the specific ligands, such as nerve growth factor (NGF), brain-derived neurotrophic factor (BDNF), and neurotrophin-3 (NT3). Interestingly, although *NTRK* gene fusions occur relatively rarely in human cancers overall, they have been found to be present broadly in many different tumor types, including both pediatric and adult malignancies. The recognition of *NTRK* fusions as driver genomic event in recent years have prompted impactful clinical therapeutic development which demonstrated the efficacy and safety of TRK inhibitors, with a recent approval of larotrectinib by the US Food and Drug Administration in a cancer-agnostic manner for *NTRK* fusion-positive cancers. Here, we reviewed the biology of *NTRK* gene fusions, antitumor activity of TRK inhibitors, clinical trials development, and challenges and future perspectives of *NTRK*-targeted therapies in human cancer with a special focus on lung cancer.

Keywords *NTRK* · Gene fusion · Tyrosine kinase inhibitor · Cancer · Biomarker · Targeted therapy · Lung cancer

X. Wu · L. Zhu · P. C. Ma (✉)
WVU Cancer Institute, Mary Babb Randolph Cancer Center, WVU Medicine,
West Virginia University, Morgantown, WV, USA
e-mail: pcma@hsc.wvu.edu

© Springer Nature Switzerland AG 2019
R. Salgia (ed.), *Targeted Therapies for Lung Cancer*, Current Cancer Research,
https://doi.org/10.1007/978-3-030-17832-1_7

Introduction

Chromosomal cancer gene rearrangements as a tumorigenic genomic event have initially been identified as a common recurrent occurrence in hematologic malignancies, e.g. *BCR/ABL* in chronic myelogenous leukemia (CML). Subsequently they become apparent also in solid tumor malignancies such as in prostate cancer (*TMPRSS2-ERG*) and sarcoma (t (11:22)(p24;q12)). In rennet years, it is more commonly recognized that cancer gene rearrangements, resulting in fusion oncogenes, are quite widespread in solid cancers including lung cancer. Furthermore, the discoveries and characterization of these activating cancer fusion genes have also fueled the development of multiple novel targeted therapeutics for clinical inhibition of the corresponding fusion oncoproteins. In lung cancer, targeted therapies against oncogenic fusion oncoproteins already include crizotinib, ceritinib, alectinib, brigatinib, and lorlatinib against *ALK* fusions; crizotinib against *ROS1* fusions, and cabozantinib against *RET* fusions. Recently, the neurotrophic tyrosine receptor kinase (*NTRK*) gene family has emerged as a novel class of oncogenic gene fusion that not only is relevant in lung cancer but also pivotal in the tumorigenesis of a wide array of human solid malignancies, pediatric, and adult tumors alike. More important, the development of targeted therapeutics against *NTRK* fusions has rapidly gained traction and recently received the Food and Drug Administration (FDA) approval of use in the United States, engendering a new era in precision genomics-guidance personalized cancer therapy.

The neurotrophic tyrosine receptor kinase gene family contains *NTRK1*, *NTRK2*, and *NTRK3*, and they encode the proteins tropomyosin receptor kinase A, B, and C (TRKA, TRKB, TRKC), respectively (Fig. 1). The *NTRK1* gene is located on chromosome 1q23.1, which was originally found as a fusion gene with tropomyosin in the 1980s and as one of the oncogenes in human cancer [45, 52, 60]. The TRKA protein is a 140 kDa glycoprotein, which is comprised of an extracellular ligand-binding domain, a transmembrane domain, and an intracellular tyrosine kinase domain [27]. TRKA dimerizes and undergoes autophosphorylation upon activation and then results in subsequent downstream activation of intracellular signaling pathways [27, 32].

The *NTRK2* gene is located on chromosome 9q21.33, encoding for a protein of 822 amino acid residues (TRKB). *NTRK2* was identified in 1991. TRKB has been shown to regulate a variety of cellular effects in human cell lines [37, 64]. *NTRK2* gene fusion involving are also becoming increasingly recognized in different cancers in recent years. Like TRKA, ligand binding to TRKB causes dimerization and autophosphorylation of its catalytic domain, resulting in the activation of multiple intracellular signaling pathways, including the RAS-MAPK, phospholipase-C gamma (PLCg), and PI3K pathways, which mediate its cellular effects [67].

The *NTRK3* gene is located on chromosome 15q25.3, encoding for a glycoprotein of 145 Kd (TRKC). A fusion between the *NTRK3* gene and an *ETV6* (ets-type

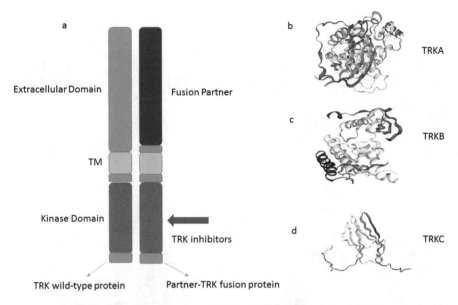

Fig. 1 Schematic diagrams showing structure of the TRK family proteins and fusion with partner genes. The neurotrophic tyrosine receptor kinases family contain *NTRK1*, *NTRK2*, and *NTRK3* genes, and they encode the proteins TRKA, TRKB, TRKC, respectively. (**a**) *Left*: TRKA, TRKB and TRKC structures contain extracellular domain, transmembrane region, and intracellular domain with a kinase domain. *Right*: a partner gene that contains a dimerization domain and the kinase domain of TRKA, TRKB, and TRKC. (**b**–**d**) the crystal structure of TRKA kinase with ligand, crystal structure of TRKB kinase domain, and NT3 binding domain of human TRKC, respectively. (Protein data bank. http://www.rcsb.org/)

transcription factor) was reported in congenital fibrosarcoma (CFS) in 1998. The fusion protein resulted in dysregulation of signaling pathways. TRKC promotes neuronal differentiation and survival. Mutations in TRKC resulting in an inactive protein have been identified as a cause for the Hirschsprung disease [30, 38, 41, 44, 49, 68, 70, 71, 76].

Physiological Roles and Signaling of TRK Receptors: Activation and Regulation (Fig. 2)

The *NTRK* family genes are particularly essential to neuronal development after embryogensis and play important roles in the development of the nervous system with differentiation, apoptosis, and survival [8, 31]. TRKA, TRKB, and TRKC can be activated by the specific ligands nerve growth factor (NGF), brain-derived neurotrophic factor (BDNF), and neurotrophin-3 (NT3), respectively. The TRKA, TRKB, and TRKC protein structure contains extracellular domain, transmembrane

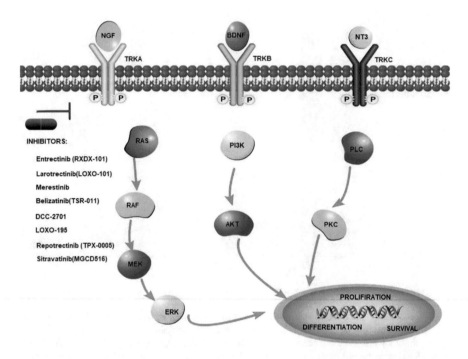

Fig. 2 TRK receptors signaling including three major pathways involved in cell differentiation and survival. NGF, BDNF, and NT-3 can bind to TRKA, TRKB, TRKC, respectively. Followed by activates three major different pathways including the RAS/RAF, PI3-K/AKT, PLCγ pathways, results in cell proliferation, differentiation, and survival. TRK inhibits, such as entrectinib, larotrectinib can inhibit of all of the three TRK receptors

region, and intracellular domain with a kinase domain. The extracellular domain is involved in specific ligand binding, followed by the oligomerization of the receptors and phosphorylation of specific tyrosine residues in the intracellular cytoplasmic kinase domain, ultimately leading to the activation of RAS/RAF, PI3-K/AKT, PLCγ signal pathways, and the regulation of cell proliferation, differentiation, and survival (Fig. 2) [48]. TRKA is the best known of the TRK family of proteins, and is activated by NGF. NGF can bind to TRKA, followed by activation of cell proliferation pathways, including the RAS/MAPK/ERK and the PLC/PI3-K pathways [42, 62]. Physiologically, TRKA is expressed in the nervous system, and it controls the differentiation of neurons [29]. The ligand BDNF can bind to TRKB which would result in dimerization and autophosphorylation of its catalytic domain, leading to activation of various downstream signaling pathways, including the RAS/RAF, PLCγ, and PI3-K/AKT pathways [67]. Douma et al. found that TRKB can act as a suppressor of anoikis of nonmalignant epithelial cells, resulting in the formation of large cellular aggregates [13]. The anti-EGFR monoclonal antibody cetuximab reduced both cell proliferation and the mRNA expression of BDNF and TRKB in human HT-29 CRC cells. BDNF/TRKB signaling might play a role in resistance to EGFR blockade [11]. Aberrant TRKB expression was implicated in central nervous system (CNS) pathology, and reduced TRKB protein was observed in Alzheimer's disease patients [1, 24, 58].

Neurotrophin-3 (NTF3, also known as NT-3) is the ligand for TRKC. Ligand binding leads to receptor dimerization, followed by autophosphorylation in the intracellular domain of the receptor, which then resulted in activation of down-stream signaling pathways including the RAS/RAF and PI3-K/AKT pathways to regulate cell survival and proliferation [2, 28, 41]. TRKC interacts with the c-SRC/JAK2 complex and can regulate JAK2/STAT3 to increases TWIST-1 and TWIST-2 levels [35].

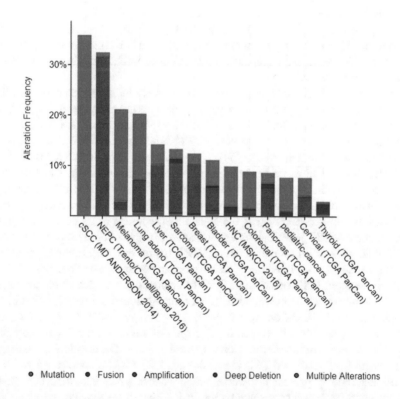

Fig. 3 *NTRK* genomic aberrations in human malignancies. *NTRK* genomic aberrations has been identified in a variety of malignancies. *NTRK* gene amplification: 31.6% of neuroendocrine prostate cancer (NEPC), 9.6% breast cancer, 9.4% liver cancer, 6.2% of lung adenocarcinoma, and 5.4% of pancreatic cancer. *NTRK* gene mutations: 35.9% of cutaneous squamous cell carcinoma (CSCC), 18.3% of melanoma, 13.1% lung adenocarcinoma, 2.2% breast cancer. *NTRK* gene fusions: 2.0% of thyroid cancer, 1.3% of head and neck cancer, 1.1% of pancreatic cancer, 1.0% of pediatric cancers, 0.8% of sarcoma, 0.5% of bladder cancer, 0.3% of colorectal cancer, 0.3% of cervical cancer, and 0.2% of lung adenocarcinoma

NTRK as Oncogenic "Drivers" in Human Cancers

NTRK genomic and TRK protein aberrations, including gene fusions, amplification, single nucleotide alterations, and protein overexpression, have been identified in many cancer types including NSCLC, breast cancer, colon cancer, and other cancers, with possible implications in tumorigenesis (Fig. 3). *NTRK* genomic amplification has been observed in a variety of malignancies. *NTRK* amplification has been reported in 31.6% of neuroendocrine prostate cancer (NEPC), 9.6% of breast cancer, 9.4% of liver cancer, 6.2% of lung adenocarcinoma, and 5.4% of pancreatic cancer (cBioPortal) [25]. A study by Aliccia et al. found that 4 of 10 (40%) breast cancer brain metastasis have *NTRK1* amplification [5]. Eggert et al. reported that children with Wilms' tumor expressing high levels of full-length *NTRKC2* mRNA (TRKB full) were associated with worse outcome [20]. *NTRK* gene mutations have been reported in 35.9% of cutaneous squamous cell carcinoma (CSCC), 18.3% of melanoma, 13.1% of lung adenocarcinoma, and 2.2% of breast cancer. However, the oncogenic nature and therapeutic implications of *NTRK* mutations have not been fully characterized yet.

Interestingly, *NTRK* fusions occur relatively rarely in human cancers overall but could be found present quite broadly across multiple types of congenital and acquired human malignancies, including both pediatric and adult forms. *NTRK* fusions are the best validated oncogenic aberration of *NTRK* family genes to this date, implicated in a wide array of human cancers [54]. The annual incidence of *NTRK* fusion-driven cancers in the United States has been estimated to be only in the range of 1500–5000 cases [33]. Nonetheless, the true frequency of *NTRK* fusions in human cancers arguably remains somewhat uncertain at the present time. One notable emerging theme in *NTRK* fusion-driven cancer is the apparent enrichment of its occurrence among rare tumors. *NTRK* gene fusions are infrequent in most cancer types, accounting for overall ~1% of all human cancers. *NTRK* fusion has been reported in 2.0% of thyroid cancer, 1.3% of head and neck cancer, 1.1% of pancreatic cancer, 1.0% of pediatric cancers, 0.8% of sarcoma, 0.5% of bladder cancer, 0.3% of colorectal cancer, 0.3% of cervical cancer, and 0.2% of lung adenocarcinoma (cBioPortal) [25] (Figs. 3 and 4). In *NTRK* oncogenic fusions, the 3′ region of *NTRK* gene (encoding the kinase domain) is joined with the 5′ region of a *NTRK* gene fusion partner via intrachromosomal or interchromosomal rearrangements. The novel hybrid oncogene has constitutively activated TRK kinase domain [33]. *NTRK* fusions are now known to be ubiquitously present in diverse human cancer types, including both pediatric and adult cancers. The resultant TRK fusion kinases become constitutively activated to dysregulate downstream cellular signaling, acting as an oncogenic addictive "driver." While *NTRK* fusion is rare in its incidence overall, accounting only up to ~1% of all solid cancers, it has been nonetheless implicated in up to 20 different cancer types. Many common cancer types harbor low frequencies of *NTRK* fusion occurrence (<5%), e.g. lung adenocarcinoma, large cell neuroendocrine cancer of the lung, colorectal cancer, pancreatic cancer, cholangiocarcinoma, breast cancer, sarcoma melanoma, and brain cancers. Yet, *NTRK* fusions can be found highly

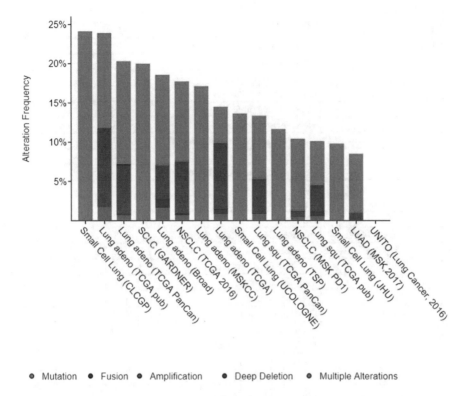

● Mutation ● Fusion ● Amplification ● Deep Deletion ● Multiple Alterations

Fig. 4 *NTRK* gene fusions in lung cancer. *NTRK* fusions have been reported in 0.2% (1/566 cases) lung adenocarcinoma from TCGA PanCancer

enriched in some rare cancer types (>75%), e.g. in infantile fibrosarcoma, mammary analog secretory carcinoma (MASC) of the salivary gland, and secretory breast cancer. *NTRK* fusions can be found in 5–25% in papillary thyroid cancer, congenital mesoblastic nephroma, Spitz tumor, and pontine glioma. Thus, *NTRK* fusion is considered a unique orphan molecular entity. While *NTRK* fusion is "rare overall, it can be also found occurring everywhere." This has rather enormous implications impacting cancer genomics-guided molecular-targeted therapy.

A large repertoire of multiple fusion partners has been identified in *NTRK1/ NTRK 2/NTRK3* fusion tumors to date (Table 1). Rudzinski et al. identified *NTRK* fusions in 19 of 79 pediatric mesenchymal tumors by NGS sequencing, including *ETV6-NTRK3, EML4-NTRK3, STRN-NTRK2,* and *TPM3-NTRK1, LMNA-NTRK1 (n = 2), TPR-NTRK1, SQSTM-NTRK1, MIR548F1-NTRK1* [56]. Another study by Taylor et al. investigated 7311 patients with a variety of hematologic malignancies and found 8 patients (0.1%) harboring *NTRK* fusions, including *LMNA-NTRK1, TFG-NTRK1, TPR-NTRK1, ETV6-NTRK3, ETV6-NTRK2, ETV6-NTRK3, UBE2R2-NTRK3,* and *HNRNPA2B1-NTRK3.* A 77-year-old man with chronic lymphocytic

Table 1 Different NTRK gene fusions and partners and corresponding tumor types

NTRK	Fusion partners	Tumor type	Refs.
NTRK1	ARHGEF2	Glioblastoma	[77]
	CHTOP	Glioblastoma	[77]
	MPRIP	Lung adenocarcinomas	[23]
	CD74	Lung adenocarcinomas	[69]
	LMNA	Pitzoid melanoma	[72]
		Hematologic malignancies	[66]
		Congenital infantile fibrosarcoma	[73]
		Colorectal cancer	[59]
		Pediatric mesenchymal tumor	[10]
		Soft tissue sarcoma	[12]
	NFASC	Glioblastoma multiforme	[34]
	BCAN	Gliomas	[26]
	RABGAP1L	Intrahepatic cholangiocarcinoma	[53]
	SQSTM1	Lung cancer	[23]
	TFG	Papillary thyroid carcinoma	[27]
	PPL	Thyroid carcinoma	[77]
	TP53	Spitzoid tumors	[72]
	TPM3	Colorectal cancer	[26]
		Glioblastoma	[26]
		Pediatric mesenchymal tumor	[10]
		Soft tissue sarcoma	[26]
		Cervical carcinoma	[26]
		Lung adenocarcinoma	[26]
		Papillary thyroid carcinoma	[27]
	TPR	Papillary thyroid carcinoma	[27]
		Hematologic malignancies	[66]
		Lung cancer	[23]
		Colorectal cancer	[9]
	MEF2D	Gliomas	[26]
	SCYL3	Colorectal cancer	[46]
	IRF2BP2	Lung cancer	[23]
NTRK2	AFAP1	Low-grade glioma	[65]
	AGBL4	Glioblastoma	[74]
	NACC2	Pilocytic astrocytoma	[50]
	PAN3	Head and neck squamous cell carcinoma	[65]
	QKI	Astrocytoma	[50]
	TRIM24	Non-small cell lung cancer	[65]
	VCL	Glioblastoma	[74]
	ETV6	Hematologic malignancies	[66]
	VCAN	Gliomas	[26]
	GKAP1	Gliomas	[26]
	KCTD8	Gliomas	[26]

(continued)

Table 1 (continued)

NTRK	Fusion partners	Tumor type	Refs.
	NOS1AP	Gliomas	[26]
	TBC1D2	Gliomas	[26]
	SQSTM1	Gliomas, lung adenocarcinoma	[26]
	BCR	Gliomas	[26]
	PRKAR2A	Gliomas	[26]
NTRK3	ETV6	Congenital fibrosarcoma	[38]
		Congenital mesoblastic nephroma	[55]
		Secretory breast carcinoma	[26]
		Acute myeloid leukemia	[63]
		Mammary analogue secretory carcinoma	[6]
		Gliomas	[26]
		AML	[21]
		GIST	[7]
		Lung adenocarcinoma	[26
		Thyroid carcinoma	[26]
	UBE2R2	Hematologic malignancies	[66]
	HNRNPA2B1	Hematologic malignancies	[66]
	VIM	Thyroid carcinoma	[26]
	SPECC1L	Uterine sarcoma	[26]
	SQSTM	Lung cancer	[23]

leukemia (CLL) harbored *ETV6-NTRK2* fusion. The patient received a TRK inhibitor larotrectinib and was found to experience a partial response by day 60 and a greater than 50% reduction over 10 weeks [66]. Gatalica et al. collected 11,502 cancer patients' tissue samples and analyzed for 53 gene fusions. *NTRK* fusions were confirmed in only 0/27% patients (31/11, 502). The most common fusions found included *ETV6-NTRK3, TPM3-NTRK1, TPM3-NTRK1, BCAN-NTRK1, VCAN-NARK2,* and *SQSTM1-NTRK2.* Gliomas had the highest number of *NTRK* fusions (14/982; 1.4%). Lung cancer patients had 0.09% (4/4073) with *NTRK* fusions (*NTRK1* fusion = 1, *NTRK2* fusion = 1, *NTRK3* fusion = 2) [26]. Using immunohistochemistry (IHC) to examine for TRKB expression in 58 small cell lung cancer (SCLC) patients, Shinichi Kimura et al. found 56.9% (33/58) to be positive [36]. A fusion between *ETV6* and the *NTRK3* gene was also found to be expressed in human secretory breast cancers (SBC) in 2004 [43].

NTRK fusions are also present in lung cancer as oncogenic aberration, leading to tumor cells transformation, proliferation, and survival. All three *NTRK1, NTRK2,* and *NTRK3* fusion types were found to be associated with poor outcome in lung cancers [51, 69].

Vaishnavi et al. found 3 of 91 lung cancer patients (3.3%) harboring *NTRK1* fusion, assayed by NGS or fluorescent in situ hybridization (FISH) [69]. Another study by Farago et al. investigated 4872 NSCLC tumors for the overall frequency of

NTRK fusions. They identified 11 total *NTRK* fusions (0.23%, 11/4872), including *SQSTM1-NTRK1, TPR-NTRK1, IRF2BP2-NTRK1, TPM3-NTRK1, MPRIP-NTRK1* (*n* = 7), and *ETV6-NTRK3, SQSTM1-NTRK3* (*n* = 4). Nine patients had adenocarcinoma, one patient had squamous cell carcinoma, and another one had neuroendocrine carcinoma. Interestingly, minimal or never smoking patient accounted for 73% (8 of 11) of the positive cases, 3/11 cases (27%) had a history of 30 pack-years or higher cigarette smoking [23].

Inhibition of TRK as Personalized Cancer-Targeted Therapy (Tables 2 and 3)

As the recognition of *NTRK* fusion as driver genomic event in human cancers grew recent years, the clinical development of *NTRK* cancer-targeted therapy has gained great momentum despite the overall rarity of the genomic aberration. We would review below the current clinical data available in the development of TRK kinase inhibition in human cancers, including both adult and pediatric studies.

Entrectinib (RXDX-101)

Entrectinibe, also known as RXDX-101 or NMS-E628, is an ATP-competitive small molecule inhibitor which inhibits TRKA/TRKB/TRKC, c-ros oncogene 1 (ROS1), and anaplastic lymphoma kinase (ALK). Entrectinib demonstrated potent antitumor effects in tumor cell lines and patient-derived xenograft (PDX) tumor models in preclinical studies. Furthermore, entrectinib can cross the blood–brain barrier (BBB) to impact primary brain tumors and brain metastases in patients with *NTRK1/NTRK2/NTRK3, ROS1*, and *ALK* fusion-driven cancers [3]. Drilon et al. investigated the antitumor activity and overall safety of entrectinib in a cohort of harboring *NTRK1/NTRK2/NTRK3, ROS1*, or *ALK* gene fusion patients with tumors. Two phase 1 clinical trials with entrectinib, ALKA-372-001 and STARTRK-1, for patients with advanced or metastatic solid tumors were conducted, including tumor types such as NSCLC, melanoma, breast, neuroblastoma, ovarian, pancreatic, and prostate. Initial tumor responses were demonstrated within cycles 1 or 2 (scans performed at 4 weeks or 8 weeks). The median duration of response for *ALK*- and *ROS1*-rearranged cancers was 7.4 months (95% CI: 3.7, not reached) and 17.4 months (95% CI: 12.7, not reached), respectively. And the durations of response were 2.6–15.1 months for the three patients with *NTRK* fusion cancers. The most serious treatment-related adverse events were fatigue/asthenia (grade 3, 4%), diarrhea (grade 3, 1%), and arthralgia (grade 3, 1%). The most common treatment-related adverse events were only grade 1 and 2 events. ALKA-372-001 was not found to have any dose-limiting toxicities (DLTs); whereas two DLTs were observed

Table 2 Different TRK inhibitors in corresponding tumor types

Drug	Targets	Phase	Cancer types	Sponsor	ClinicalTrials. gov identifier
Larotrectinib (LOXO-101)	NTRK1, NTRK2, or NTRK3 fusion	1	Advanced adult solid tumors	Loxo Oncology, Inc.	NCT02122913
		2	NTRK fusion-positive solid tumors		NCT02576431
			Cancers		NCT03025360
		1/2	Advanced pediatric solid or primary central nervous system tumors		NCT02637687
		2	Relapsed or refractory advanced solid tumors, non-Hodgkin lymphoma, or histiocytic disorders	National Cancer Institute (NCI)	NCT03213704
Entrectinib (RXDX-101)	NTRK 1/2/3 (Trk A/B/C), ROS1, or ALK fusion	2	Solid tumors	Hoffmann-La Roche	NCT02568267
		1/1b	Recurrent or refractory solid tumors and primary CNS tumors,		NCT02650401
		1	Locally advanced or metastatic cancer		NCT02097810
		2	BRAF/NRAS wild-type stage III-IV melanoma	University of California, San Francisco	NCT02587650
		N/A	Soft tissue sarcomas	Centre Leon Berard	NCT03375437
Cabozantinib	RET, ROS1, or NTRK fusion, or increased MET or AXL activity	2	Advanced non-small cell lung cancer	Memorial Sloan Kettering Cancer Center	NCT01639508
Merestinib	NTRK gene	2	Non-small cell lung cancer and solid tumors	Dana-Farber Cancer Institute	NCT02920996
Belizatinib (TSR-011)	ALK, TRKA, TRKB, and TRKC	1/2a	Advanced solid tumors and lymphomas	Tesaro, Inc.	NCT02048488

(continued)

Table 2 (continued)

Drug	Targets	Phase	Cancer types	Sponsor	ClinicalTrials. gov identifier
DS-6051b	ROS1 or NTRK gene	1	Advanced solid malignant tumors	Daiichi Sankyo Co., Ltd.	NCT02675491
		1	Solid tumors		NCT02279433
Sitravatinib (MGCD516)	Genetic alterations in MET, AXL, RET, TRK, DDR2, KDR, PDGFRA, KIT or CBL	1	Advanced cancer	Mirati Therapeutics Inc.	NCT02219711
		2	Urothelial carcinoma study		NCT03606174
		2	Non-small cell lung cancer		NCT02954991
PLX7486	Activating Trk (NTRK) point or NTRK fusion mutations	1	Advanced solid tumors	Plexxikon	NCT01804530
DCC-2701	TRK genomic alterations	1	Advanced solid tumors	Deciphera Pharmaceuticals LLC	NCT02228811
LOXO-195	NTRK fusion	1/2	Cancers	Loxo Oncology, Inc.	NCT03215511
Repotrectinib (TPX-0005)	ALK, ROS1, or NTRK rearrangements	1/2	Advanced solid tumors	TP Therapeutics, Inc.	NCT03093116

on the STARTRK-1 trial. Entrectinib was overall well tolerated, with predominantly grades 1/2 adverse events that were reversible with dose modification. Responses were observed in NSCLC, melanoma, colorectal cancer, and renal cell carcinoma, as early as 4 weeks, with treatment lasting as long as over 2 years. Notably, in three *NTRK1/2/3*-fusion advanced NSCLC (*SQSTM1-NTRK1*), mammary analog secretary carcinoma (MASC; *ETV6-NTRK3*), and colorectal cancer (*LMNA-NTRK1*), the overall response rate (ORR) was 100% (95% CI: 44, 100). The adverse effects of entrectnib were found to be acceptable and reversible, thus well-tolerated. It was concluded that entrectinib possesses promising antitumor effects for advanced cancer patients with acceptable tolerance and safety profile [14]. In the study by Sartore-Bianchi et al., a metastatic colorectal cancer (CRC) patient with *LMNA-NTRK1* fusion was treated with entrectinib 1,600 mg/m² orally once daily for 4 consecutive days per week and for 3 consecutive weeks every 28 days. Tumor measurement decreased from 6.8 and 8.2 cm in longest diameter to 4.7 and 4.3 cm in hepatic segments 6 and 5, respectively [59]. Farago AF et al. used anchored multiplex polymerase chain reaction (AMP) to screen 1378 NSCLC; one stage IV lung adenocrcinoma with *SQSTM1-NTRK1* fusion patient was treated with entrectinib. CT scans indicated partial response (PR) and complete response (CR) of all brain metastases [22]. Drilon et al. reported a mammary analogue secretory carcinoma

Table 3 TRK inhibitors under ongoing clinical trials

ClinicalTrials.gov identifier	Content	Sponsor	First posted
NCT02122913	Oral TRK inhibitor LOXO-101 for treatment of advanced adult solid tumors	Loxo Oncology, Inc.	4/25/14
NCT02576431	Study of LOXO-101 (larotrectinib) in subjects with NTRK fusion-positive solid tumors	Loxo Oncology, Inc.	10/15/15
NCT02637687	Oral TRK inhibitor LOXO-101 (larotrectinib) for treatment of advanced pediatric solid or primary central nervous system tumors	Loxo Oncology, Inc.	12/22/15
NCT03215511	Phase 1/2 study of LOXO-195 in patients with previously treated NTRK fusion cancers	Loxo Oncology, Inc	7/12/17
NCT02568267	Basket study of entrectinib (RXDX-101) for the treatment of patients with solid tumors harboring NTRK 1/2/3 (Trk A/B/C), ROS1, or ALK gene rearrangements (fusions) (STARTRK-2)	Hoffmann-La Roche	10/5/15
NCT02650401	Study of RXDX-101 in children with recurrent or refractory solid tumors and primary CNS tumors, with or without TRK, ROS1, or ALK fusions	Hoffmann-La Roche	1/8/16
NCT03375437	RNASARC: molecular screening program of soft tissue sarcomas with complex genomic profile to detect NTRK1/2/3, ROS1 or ALK gene fusions	Centre Leon Berard	12/18/17
NCT01639508	Cabozantinib in patients with RET fusion-positive advanced non-small cell lung cancer and those with other genotypes: ROS1 or NTRK fusions or increased MET or AXL activity	Memorial Sloan Kettering Cancer Center	7/12/12
NCT02920996	Merestinib as a treatment for solid tumors that have an alteration in the NTRK gene	Dana-Farber Cancer Institute	9/30/16
NCT02587650	Entrectinib in treating BRAF/NRAS wild-type stage III-IV melanoma with NTRK1, NTRK2, NTRK3, or ROS1 fusion	University of California, San Francisco	10/27/15
NCT02219711	Phase 1/1b study of MGCD516 in patients with advanced cancer	Mirati Therapeutics Inc.	8/19/14
NCT03556228	Oral TrkA inhibitor VMD-928 for treatment of advanced adult solid tumors or lymphoma	VM Oncology, LLC	6/14/18
NCT03093116	TPX-0005 in patients with advanced solid tumors harboring ALK, ROS1, or NTRK1–3 rearrangements	TP Therapeutics, Inc.	3/28/17
NCT03213704	Larotrectinib in treating patients with relapsed or refractory advanced Solid Tumors, non-Hodgkin lymphoma, or histiocytic disorders with NTRK fusions	National Cancer Institute (NCI)	7/11/17

(MASC) patient harboring *ETV6-NTRK3* fusion, and treated by entrectinib, that experienced a dramatic and durable response achieved. However, acquired resistance was identified eventually, with a novel *NTRK3*-G623R mutation [15]. Sigal et al. found the first reported metastatic well-differentiated neuroendocrine cancer with *ETV6-NTRK3* fusion in a patient, was identified and treated with entrectinib, resulting in improvement of the patient's clinical condition [61]. In a study by Mariangela Russo et al., a patient with metastatic colorectal cancer harboring *LMNA–NTRK1* fusion was treated with entrectinib, who displayed a remarkable response; and the patient eventually experienced acquired drug resistance. The investigators collected and analyzed circulating tumor DNA (ctDNA) and tumor tissue biopsies during treatment, and found two acquired resistant point mutations in *NTRK1*, p.G595R and p.G667C [57].

Larotrectinib (LOXO-101)

Larotrectinib, also known as LOXO-101 and ARRY-470, is a small molecule that was designed to block the ATP-binding site of the TRKA, TRKB, and TRKC, serving as a highly specific and potent inhibitor of all of the three tropomyosin kinase receptors [12, 19, 40]. Recently a pooled analysis of three multicenter open-label single-arm treatment clinical studies with larotrectinib (NCT02122913, NCT02637687, and NCT02576431) was reported [14]. These three studies are (1) a phase 1 study involving adults with advanced solid tumors (LOXO-TRK-14001; $n = 8$), (2) a pediatric phase 1–2 study (SCOUT; $n = 12$), and (3) a phase 2 "basket" study involving adolescents/adults (NAVIGATE; $n = 35$). The results of the pooled-analysis of the first 55 consecutive patients enrolled in these studies have been published [14], forming the basis of the FDA approval. The enrolled subjects' ages ranged from 4 months to 76 years. There were a total of 17 diverse cancer types included. Majority of patients had *NTRK1*, and *NTRK3* fusions. *NTRK* fusions were identified by next-gene sequencing (NGS) or fluorescence in situ hybridization. The TRK fusion tumor types included mammary analogue secretory carcinoma (MASC) of the salivary gland ($n = 12$), infantile fibrosarcoma ($n = 7$), thyroid tumor ($n = 5$), lung tumor ($n = 4$), melanoma ($n = 4$), colon tumor ($n = 4$), gastrointestinal stromal tumor ($n = 3$), and other cancers ($n = 16$) (Fig. 5). *NTRK1*, *NTRK2*, *NTRK3* infusions were found in 25 patients (45.4%), 1 patient (2%), and 29 patients (53%), respectively. One patient had central nervous system metastases, while the rest did not. The overall response rate (ORR) was 75% (95% CI, 61–85) according to independent review including 7 patients (13%) with complete response (CR) and 34 patients (62%) with partial response (PR). Seven patients (13%) had stable disease (SD), 5 patients (9%) had progressive disease (PD), and 2 patients (4%) could not be evaluated owing to early withdrawal. ORR was 80% (95% CI, 67–90) according to investigator assessment. The median time to response was 1.8 months (range,

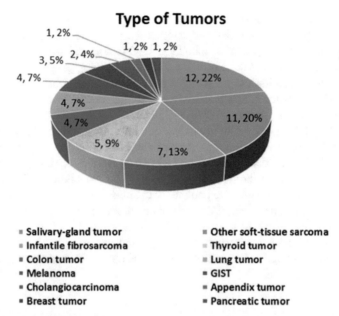

Fig. 5 Diverse of cancer types included in larotrectinib clinical studies. In the 3 multicenter open-label clinical studies (NCT02122913, NCT02637687, and NCT02576431) which enrolled 55 patients in the pooled analysis leading to the FDA approval of larotrectinib, there were 17 unique tumor types included that harbored TRK fusions, including mammary analogue secretory carcinoma of the salivary gland ($n = 12$), infantile fibrosarcoma ($n = 7$), thyroid tumor ($n = 5$), lung tumor ($n = 4$), melanoma ($n = 4$), colon tumor ($n = 4$), gastrointestinal stromal tumor ($n = 3$), and other cancers ($n = 16$)

0.9–6.4). The median progression-free survival (PFS) and duration of response had not been reached after a median follow-up duration of 9.9 months, 8.3 months, respectively. Seventy-one percent (71%) of responses were ongoing, and 55% of all patients remained progression-free at 1 year. The longest response patient had was the first patient who was still receiving therapy at 27 months. Eighty-six percent (86%; 38/44) of the patients with a response were continuing treatment or had undergone surgery. The majority of adverse events (AEs) (93%, 964 of 1038 events) were of grade 1 or 2. Regardless of attribution, few AEs were of grade 3 or 4, and the most common ones were anemia (11%), weight gain (7%), elevated alanine aminotransferase or aspartate aminotransferase level (7%), and decrease in neutrophil count (7%). No grade 4 or 5 events related to the treatment were reported by the investigators and no treatment-related grade 3 adverse events occurred in more than 5% of the patients. No patients came off treatment with larotrectinib due to drug-related adverse events response.

Six patients (11%) were found to have primary resistance to larotrectinib. One patient who had been treated with entrectinib, followed by was identified to express a *NTRK3*-G623R mutation in the ATP-binding site of the kinase domain before the administration of larotrectinib [15]. The *NTRK1*-G595R and *NTRK3*-G623R mutation are termed "solvent-front" mutations, as it can reduce the inhibitory potency of larotrectinib. Central pan-TRK IHC testing did not confirm positive TRK fusion expression in three of these patients, implying potential false positive *NTRK* fusion test results or that the TRK fusion proteins were not expressed despite the genomic alterations. Ten patients were found to experience acquired drug resistance mutations, including *NTRK1*-G595R, *NTRK3*-G623R, *NTRK1*-F589 L, *NTRK1*-G667S, or *NTRK3*-G696A to larotrectinib. Acquired drug resistance was defined as disease progression during treatment after objective response or stable disease at least 6 months. The US Food and Drug Administration (FDA) granted accelerated approval to larotrectinib (Vitrakvi®) on November 26th, 2018, as a treatment for adult and pediatric patients with solid tumors that have *NTRK* gene fusions without a known acquired resistance mutation, are metastatic or where surgical resection is likely to result in severe morbidity, and have no satisfactory alternative treatments or that have progressed following treatment on. In the approval statement by FDA, a complete response rate of 22% and partial response rate of 53% were cited.

Merestinib

Merestinib, also known as LY2801653, is a small molecule that has been shown in vitro to be a reversible type II ATP-competitive inhibitor of MET. Preclinical testing also has shown merestinib to inhibit several other receptor tyrosine oncokinases including MST1R, FLT3, AXL, MERTK, TEK, ROS1, and NTRK1/2/3 [39]. An ongoing, open-label, phase 2 study of merestinib is being conducted in patients with advanced cancer harboring an *NTRK1/2/3* fusion or advanced NSCLC with MET exon 14 mutation (NCT02920996) [75].

TSR-011

Belizatinib, also known as TSR-011, is an oral inhibitor of ALK and TRK. In 2014, TSR-011 began a phase 1/2 open-label, dose-escalation trial in patients with advanced solid tumors harboring TRK or ALK activity, including NSCLC ($n = 10$), pancreatic ($n = 3$), ovarian ($n = 2$), salivary gland ($n = 2$) and papillary thyroid, bladder ($n = 1$), carcinoid ($n = 1$), cholangiocarcinoma ($n = 1$), colon ($n = 1$), and leiomyosarcoma ($n = 1$). All patients have been enrolled at oral daily doses between 30 and 480 mg. TSR-011 was found to be well tolerated. (NCT02048488) [4].

DS-6051b

DS-6051b is an oral inhibitor of the *NTRK* and *ROS1*. A first-in-human study to evaluate the safety, tolerability, and pharmacokinetics in cancer patients and identify a recommended phase 2 dose (RP2D) is ongoing (NCT02279433).

Sitravatinib (MGCD516)

Sitravatinib, known as MGCD516, is a multikinase (*MET, RET, AXL, NTRK1*, or *NTRK3* genes) inhibitor used in a phase 1/1b clinical trial (NCT02219711) for patients with advanced cancers (NCT02219711). Another phase 2 study evaluates the clinical activity of combined sitravatinib and the PD-1 immune checkpoint inhibitor nivolumab in patients with advanced or metastatic urothelial carcinoma, and NSCLC (NCT03606174, NCT02954991).

Repotrectinib (TPX-0005)

Repotrectinib, also known as TPX-0005, is a multikinase (ROS1, ALK, and TRKA/B/C) inhibitor that is tested in an ongoing first-in-human phase 1/2 trail (NCT03093116). Repotrectinib has advantage with central nervous system (CNS) penetration, aimed to target both wide-type (WT) and solvent-front mutations (SFM) kinases and other resistance mutations including ROS1-G2032R and ROS1-D2033N, TRKA-G595R, TRKB-G639R, TRKC-G623R, and ALK-G1202R. There was a patient with mammary analogue secretory carcinoma (MASC) lung metastases harboring *ETV6–NTRK3* rearrangement, who was previously enrolled into a clinical trial under entrectinib treatment, with a partial response for 6 months, followed by doxorubicin treatment upon progression, and then later with combined entrectinib and trametinib treatment for 2 months with progressive disease. Rebiopsy studies revealed that the tumor developed a new *NTRK3*-G623E resistance mutation. He was then enrolled in the clinical study under repotrectinib treatment (40 mg per day); and within the first few days, a rapid and dramatic response to repotrectinib was observed [17].

LOXO-195

LOXO-195 is an orally available, highly potent, and selective TRK kinase inhibitor designed to overcome drug resistance mediated by acquired mutations. Although responses to TRK inhibition can be dramatic and durable; however, eventually emergence of acquired resistance is found to be inevitable. A multicenter, open-label phase 1/2 trial in patients with TRK fusion cancers who have progressed while receiving another TRK inhibitor or are intolerant to another TRK inhibitor (NCT03215511) using LOXO-196 was conducted. In the study, there was a colorectal cancer patient with *LMNA-NTRK1* who achieved a rapid partial response to larotrectinib, followed by progressed after 6 months with acquired TRKA-G595R resistance mutation. Another pediatric patient in the study had infantile fibrosarcoma expressing *ETV6-NTRK3* fusion was treated by larotrectinib, with resultant tumor regression as partial response, followed by progression with acquired TRKC-G623R mutation after 8 months. These two patients were treated with LOXO-195 under FDA-allowed single patient protocols. Both of these two patients experienced a rapid clinical response after LOXO-195 treatment [16].

New Paradigm: "Cancer-Agnostic" Targeted Therapy and Molecular Diagnostics

The approval of larotrectinib as a "cancer-agnostic" *NTRK*-targeting therapy impacts considerably the development of personalized cancer genomics-guided molecular-targeted therapy. It is hailed as a novel paradigm-changing drug approval of larotrectinib, as treatment for *NTRK* fusion-positive solid tumors. The clinical efficacy, duration of responses, and the safety profile of larotrectinib are all considered to be rather remarkable. Larotrectinib's approval particularly highlights the relevance and significance of molecular-genomic classification, which is nowadays indispensable in addition to anatomic or histologic cancer classification. Moreover, it is also remarkable that the observed responses in the larotrectinib registration clinical studies were found "agnostic" to age, sex, anatomic or histologic cancer types, and molecular fusion partners of *NTRK*.

Nowadays, the recognition of the highly "actionable" nature of *NTRK* fusions along with the availability of the FDA-approved targeted drug larotrectinib marks another small and yet highly significant fraction of the modern lung cancer genomic pie, besides the other actionable aberrations such as *EGFR* mutations; *ALK, ROS1, RET* fusions; *MET* amplification; and *MET* exon 14 skipping mutations. In order to effectively and efficiently arrive at potentially targetable aberrations in lung cancer, it would be advisable nowadays for the adoption of an unbiased and comprehensive tumor molecular profiling, preferably with NSG-based platform, as state-of-the-art personalized genomics-guided cancer therapy standard-of-care. It is also clear that regulatory adaptation is needed to keep pace with the evolution and progress of human cancer genomics and genomics-guided personalized therapeutics. Individual companion diagnostics accompanying targeted therapeutics regulatory approval would likely become obsolete and replaced with more broad-based NGS tumor tissues or liquid biopsy platforms of molecular profiling.

With the advent of genomic profiling and recent approval of larotrectinib for *NTRK* fusion-targeting personalized therapy, a number of practical considerations emerge as relevant to modern-day oncologists clinical practices. As the trend of migration of molecular tumor testing from individual genotype tests into more broad-based multiplexed gene panels or comprehensive NGS-based genomics profiling, oncologists and pathologists alike are confronted with many critical issues of optimal tissue prioritization for testing and choices for tumor profiling platforms. With respect to optimal *NTRK* fusion testing at this time, one should recognize that there are several method options available in principle. However, the IHC and FISH platforms are considered to be in research and phase presently. On the other hand, the NGS platform is available with several commercially accessible vendors with the genomics profiling platform encompassing the *NTRK* fusions (Table 4).

Table 4 NGS Test Platforms for Detecting of *NTRK* Fusions

Company	Assay	Genes
OHSU Knight Diagnostic Laboratories	GeneTrails® Solid Tumor Fusion Gene Panel	Including NTRK1, NTRK2, and NTRK3
Caris Life Sciences, Irving, TX	MI Profile™	Including NTRK1, NTRK2, and NTRK3
Sirona Dx, Lake Oswego, OR	Oncomine™ Focus Assay	Including 23 genes for fusions
PathGroup, Brentwood, TN	SmartGenomics™ NGS Solid Tumor	126 genes for fusions
OmniSeq, Buffalo, NY	OmniSeq ComprehensiveSM	Including NTRK1, NTRK2, and NTRK3
NeoGenomics Laboratories, Fort Myers, FL	NGS ALK, NTRK, RET, ROS1 Fusion Profile	Including NTRK1 and NTRK3
Tempus, Chicago, IL	xO Onco-seq	Including NTRK1, NTRK2, and NTRK3
Cancer Genetics, Rutherford, NJ	Solid Tumor FOCUS: Oncomine™ NGS Panel	Fusion analysis optional
Foundation Medicine, Cambridge, MA	FoundationOne® Heme	Including NTRK1, NTRK2, and NTRK3
Foundation Medicine, Cambridge, MA	FoundationOne®	Including NTRK1, NTRK2 and ETV6-NTRK3

However, it is important to point out that not all commercial NGS panels have fusion testing included. Similarly, not all *NTRK* genes are always included in the commercial profiling panel platforms. For instance, the FoundationOne assay (Foundation Medicine) for solid tumors incorporates *NTRK1*, *NTRK2* fusions, but only *ETV6-NTRK3* fusion in its current platform. Caris Molecular Intelligence (Caris Life Sciences) profiling platform included in the fusion detection panel all of *NTRK1*, *NTRK2*, and *NTRK3* fusions. On the other hand, in the liquid biopsy profiling arena, the Guardant360 assay (Guardant Health) has a six-gene panel of fusion detection in the assay platform, which included only *NTRK1* besides *ALK*, *FGFR2*, *FGFR3*, *RET*, and *ROS1* fusions. Thus it is imperative that the treating oncologists understand which genes and genomic alterations are included in the molecular-genomic profiling assay they are ordering. Also equally important, one needs to understand the assay methodologies and limitations inherent within the profiling platform per se.

Another consideration one needs to decide for *NTRK* fusion patient identification is whether there are key clinical or pathologic parameters that one can reliably utilized as basis for selective *NTRK* gene fusion testing. Nonetheless, while there are certain rare tumor types that evidently have the essential pathognomonic occurrence of *NTRK* fusions such as in MASC tumors, MSI-high malignancies, and certain pediatric cancers, e.g., infantile fibrosarcoma, no clinical or pathologic features of the tumors can be justifiably adopted as screening criteria for selective *NTRK* fusion testing in lung or other solid cancers. One only needs to recall the landmark IPASS study (Iressa Pan-Asia Survival Study) which elegantly brought forth the consensus principle of molecular profiling in lieu of clinicopathologic profiling as the essential *EGFR* mutation-driven lung cancer first-line therapy principle of decision-making [47]. It is the molecular-genomic aberration that drives the therapeutic response, and not the correlative clinicopathologic features or characteristics.

Future Perspectives

While the use of *NTRK* fusion-targeted therapeutics with potent activities against the oncogenic fusion TRKA, TRKB, and TRKC kinases can result in significant clinical benefit in lung cancer as well as other diverse malignancies harboring the fusions, acquired drug resistance invariably develops. Identification of acquired resistance mechanisms and the development of new drugs for acquired resistance mechanisms are still necessary to further optimize the impact of personalized *NTRK* targeting cancer therapy. Clinical studies in development of second-generation TRK inhibitors to target and overcome first-generation TRK inhibitors resistance are already actively in progress.

Another area of development would likely be the development of more CNS-active TRK inhibitors. As in the case of *EGFR* mutant and *ALK* fusion lung cancer therapies, the CNS as a tumor sanctuary to evade systemic targeted therapeutic inhibition represent a paramount clinical problem. With the advent of CNS-active new-generation TKI such as osimertinib and alectinib, respectively, against *EGFR*-mutant and *ALK* fusion-positive diseases, one is almost certain to predict that the same principle of extending the clinical benefits of targeted therapies can be applicable to *NTRK* fusion personalized therapeutics. It remains to be seen whether other forms of *NTRK* genomic and molecular aberrations such as amplification, mutations, overexpression can also be adopted as "actionable" targets as in the case of oncogenic fusions. Undoubtedly more basic and translational research in these areas would be urgently necessary to address these issues.

Last, the rapidly emerging and expanding roles of single agent and combination cancer immunotherapies in human cancer treatments raise many important questions that are yet to be fully resolved. Whether there can be a rational role of immune checkpoint PD-1/PD-L1 blockade in *NTRK* fusion-positive human malignancies remains to be tested. Whether immunotherapy, be it immune checkpoint of other combination immune-oncology regimens, can impact further clinical benefits in *NTRK* fusion-targeted therapy is an attractive question that requires answers sooner rather than later. One could envision potential role of concurrent or maintenance use of I-O therapy with *NTRK*-targeted inhibitors. Furthermore, there may be a role of similar I-O combination regimens with or without anti-angiogenesis therapy in salvage therapy of acquired *NTRK*-inhibitor resistance. Certainly, we definitely need to have robust preclinical models and well-designed clinical studies to properly test out these interesting hypothesis.

Conflicts of Interest Advisory Board/Committee: AstraZeneca, Cymeta, Takeda, Caris Life Sciences

Speakers Bureau: Merck, Takeda, AstraZeneca, Bristol Myers-Squibb, Bayer

Research Funding (to Institution): AstraZeneca, Bristol Myers-Squibb, AbbVie, Loxo, CBT Pharmaceuticals, Pfizer, Cymeta Biopharmaceuticals, Incyte, Medimmune, Tesaro, XCovery, Spectrum, EpicentRx

References

1. Allen SJ, Wilcock GK, Dawbarn D. Profound and selective loss of catalytic TrkB immunoreactivity in Alzheimer's disease. Biochem Biophys Res Commun. 1999;264:648–51. https://doi.org/10.1006/bbrc.1999.1561.
2. Amatu A, Sartore-Bianchi A, Siena S. NTRK gene fusions as novel targets of cancer therapy across multiple tumour types. ESMO Open. 2016;1:e000023. https://doi.org/10.1136/esmoopen-2015-000023.
3. Ardini E, Menichincheri M, Banfi P, et al. Entrectinib, a pan-TRK, ROS1, and ALK inhibitor with activity in multiple molecularly defined cancer indications. Mol Cancer Ther. 2016;15:628–39. https://doi.org/10.1158/1535-7163.MCT-15-0758.
4. Arkenau HT, Sachdev JC, Mita MM, et al. Phase (Ph) 1/2a study of TSR-011, a potent inhibitor of ALK and TRK, in advanced solid tumors including crizotinib-resistant ALK posi-

tive non-small cell lung cancer. J Clin Oncol. 2015;33:8063–8063. https://doi.org/10.1200/jco.2015.33.15_suppl.8063.

5. Bollig-Fischer A, Michelhaugh SK, Wijesinghe P, et al. Cytogenomic profiling of breast cancer brain metastases reveals potential for repurposing targeted therapeutics. Oncotarget. 2015;6:14614–24. https://doi.org/10.18632/oncotarget.3786.

6. Boon E, Valstar MH, van der Graaf WTA, Bloemena E, Willems SM, Meeuwis CA, Slootweg PJ, Smit LA, Merkx MAW, Takes RP, Kaanders JHAM, Groenen PJTA, Flucke UE, van Herpen CML. Clinicopathological characteristics and outcome of 31 patients with ETV6-NTRK3 fusion geneconfirmed (mammary analogue) secretory carcinoma of salivary glands. Oral Oncol. 2018;82:29–33.

7. Brenca M, Rossi S, Polano M, Gasparotto D, Zanatta L, Racanelli D, Valori L, Lamon S, Dei Tos AP, Maestro R. Transcriptome sequencing identifies ETV6-NTRK3 as a gene fusion involved in GIST. J Pathol. 2016;238(4):543–9.

8. Brodeur GM, Minturn JE, Ho R, et al. Trk receptor expression and inhibition in neuroblastomas. Clin Cancer Res. 2009;15:3244–50. https://doi.org/10.1158/1078-0432.CCR-08-1815.

9. Créancier L, Vandenberghe I, Gomes B, Dejean C, Blanchet JC, Meilleroux J, Guimbaud R, Selves J, Kruczynski A. Chromosomal rearrangements involving the NTRK1 gene in colorectal carcinoma. Cancer Lett. 2015;365(1):107–11.

10. Davis JL, Lockwood CM, Albert CM, Tsuchiya K, Hawkins DS, Rudzinski ER. Infantile NTRK-associated Mesenchymal Tumors. Pediatr Dev Pathol. 2018;21(1):68–78.

11. De Farias CB, Heinen TE, Dos Santos RP, et al. BDNF/TrkB signaling protects HT-29 human colon cancer cells from EGFR inhibition. Biochem Biophys Res Commun. 2012;425:328–32. https://doi.org/10.1016/j.bbrc.2012.07.091.

12. Doebele RC, Davis LE, Vaishnavi A, et al. An oncogenic NTRK fusion in a patient with soft-tissue sarcoma with response to the tropomyosin-related kinase inhibitor LOXO-101. Cancer Discov. 2015;5:1049–57. https://doi.org/10.1158/2159-8290.CD-15-0443.

13. Douma S, Van Laar T, Zevenhoven J, et al. Suppression of anoikis and induction of metastasis by the neurotrophic receptor TrkB. Nature. 2004;430:1034–9. https://doi.org/10.1038/nature02765.

14. Drilon A, Laetsch TW, Kummar S, et al. Efficacy of larotrectinib in TRK fusion-positive cancers in adults and children. N Engl J Med. 2018a;378:731–9. https://doi.org/10.1056/NEJMoa1714448.

15. Drilon A, Li G, Dogan S, et al. What hides behind the MASC: clinical response and acquired resistance to entrectinib after ETV6-NTRK3 identification in a mammary analogue secretory carcinoma (MASC). Ann Oncol. 2016;27:920–6. https://doi.org/10.1093/annonc/mdw042.

16. Drilon A, Nagasubramanian R, Blake JF, et al. A next-generation TRK kinase inhibitor overcomes acquired resistance to prior TRK kinase inhibition in patients with TRK fusion-positive solid tumors. Cancer Discov. 2017a;7:963–72. https://doi.org/10.1158/2159-8290.CD-17-0507.

17. Drilon A, Ou SH, Cho BC, et al. Repotrectinib (TPX-0005) is a next-generation ROS1/TRK/ALK inhibitor that potently inhibits ROS1/TRK/ALK solvent-front mutations. Cancer Discov. 2018b;8:1227–36. https://doi.org/10.1158/2159-8290.CD-18-0484.

18. Drilon A, Siena S, Ou SH, et al. Safety and antitumor activity of the multitargeted pan-TRK, ROS1, and ALK inhibitor entrectinib: combined results from two phase I trials (ALKA-372-001 and STARTRK-1). Cancer Discov. 2017b;7:400–9. https://doi.org/10.1158/2159-8290.CD-16-1237.

19. DuBois SG, Laetsch TW, Federman N, et al. The use of neoadjuvant larotrectinib in the management of children with locally advanced TRK fusion sarcomas. Cancer. 2018;124:4241–7. https://doi.org/10.1002/cncr.31701.

20. Eggert A, Grotzer MA, Ikegaki N, et al. Expression of the neurotrophin receptor TrkB is associated with unfavorable outcome in Wilms' tumor. J Clin Oncol. 2001;19:689–96. https://doi.org/10.1200/JCO.2001.19.3.689.

21. Eguchi M, Eguchi-Ishimae M, Tojo A, Morishita K, Suzuki K, Sato Y, Kudoh S, Tanaka K, Setoyama M, Nagamura F, Asano S, Kamada N. Fusion of ETV6 to neurotrophin-3 receptor TRKC in acute myeloid leukemia with t(12;15)(p13;q25). Blood. 1999;93(4):1355–63.

22. Farago AF, Le LP, Zheng Z, et al. Durable clinical response to entrectinib in NTRK1-rearranged non-small cell lung cancer. J Thorac Oncol. 2015;10:1670–4. https://doi.org/10.1097/01. JTO.0000473485.38553.f0.

23. Farago AF, Taylor MS, Doebele RC et al Clinicopathologic features of non-small-cell lung cancer harboring an NTRK gene fusion. JCO Precis Oncol. 2018;2018. https://doi.org/10.1200/ PO.18.00037.

24. Ferrer I, Marín C, Rey MJ, et al. BDNF and full-length and truncated TrkB expression in Alzheimer disease. Implications in therapeutic strategies. J Neuropathol Exp Neurol. 1999;58:729–39.

25. Gao J, Aksoy BA, Dogrusoz U, et al. Integrative analysis of complex cancer genomics and clinical profiles using the cBioPortal. Sci Signal. 2013;6:pl1. https://doi.org/10.1126/ scisignal.2004088.

26. Gatalica Z, Xiu J, Swensen J, et al. Molecular characterization of cancers with NTRK gene fusions. Mod Pathol. 2019;32:147–53. https://doi.org/10.1038/s41379-018-0118-3.

27. Greco A, Miranda C, Pierotti MA. Rearrangements of NTRK1 gene in papillary thyroid carcinoma. Mol Cell Endocrinol. 2010;321:44–9. https://doi.org/10.1016/j.mce.2009.10.009.

28. Gromnitza S, Lepa C, Weide T, et al. Tropomyosin-related kinase C (TrkC) enhances podocyte migration by ERK-mediated WAVE2 activation. FASEB J. 2018;32:1665–76. https://doi. org/10.1096/fj.201700703R.

29. Indo Y. Neurobiology of pain, interoception and emotional response: lessons from nerve growth factor-dependent neurons. Eur J Neurosci. 2014;39:375–91. https://doi.org/10.1111/ ejn.12448.

30. Ivanov SV, Panaccione A, Brown B, et al. TrkC signaling is activated in adenoid cystic carcinoma and requires NT-3 to stimulate invasive behavior. Oncogene. 2013;32:3698–710. https:// doi.org/10.1038/onc.2012.377.

31. Kaplan DR, Martin-Zanca D, Parada LF. Tyrosine phosphorylation and tyrosine kinase activity of the trk proto-oncogene product induced by NGF. Nature. 1991;350:158–60. https://doi. org/10.1038/350158a0.

32. Kaplan DR, Miller FD. Neurotrophin signal transduction in the nervous system. Curr Opin Neurobiol. 2000;10:381–91.

33. Kheder ES, Hong DS. Emerging targeted therapy for tumors with NTRK fusion proteins. Clin Cancer Res. 2018;24:5807–14. https://doi.org/10.1158/1078-0432.CCR-18-1156.

34. Kim J, Lee Y, Cho HJ, Lee YE, An J, Cho GH, Ko YH, Joo KM, Nam DH. NTRK1 fusion in glioblastoma multiforme. PLoS One. 2014;9(3):e91940.

35. Kim MS, Jeong J, Seo J, et al. Dysregulated JAK2 expression by TrkC promotes metastasis potential, and EMT program of metastatic breast cancer. Sci Rep. 2016;6:33899. https://doi. org/10.1038/srep33899.

36. Kimura S, Harada T, Ijichi K, et al. Expression of brain-derived neurotrophic factor and its receptor TrkB is associated with poor prognosis and a malignant phenotype in small cell lung cancer. Lung Cancer. 2018;120:98–107. https://doi.org/10.1016/j.lungcan.2018.04.005.

37. Klein R, Nanduri V, Jing S, et al. The trkB tyrosine protein kinase is a receptor for brain-derived neurotrophic factor and neurotrophin-3. Cell. 1991;66:395–403.

38. Knezevich SR, McFadden DE, Tao W, et al. A novel ETV6-NTRK3 gene fusion in congenital fibrosarcoma. Nat Genet. 1998;18:184–7. https://doi.org/10.1038/ng0298-184.

39. Konicek BW, Capen AR, Credille KM, et al. Merestinib (LY2801653) inhibits neurotrophic receptor kinase (NTRK) and suppresses growth of NTRK fusion bearing tumors. Oncotarget. 2018;9:13796–806. https://doi.org/10.18632/oncotarget.24488.

40. Laetsch TW, DuBois SG, Mascarenhas L, et al. Larotrectinib for paediatric solid tumours harbouring NTRK gene fusions: phase 1 results from a multicentre, open-label, phase 1/2 study. Lancet Oncol. 2018;19:705–14. https://doi.org/10.1016/S1470-2045(18)30119-0.

41. Lamballe F, Klein R, Barbacid M. trkC, a new member of the trk family of tyrosine protein kinases, is a receptor for neurotrophin-3. Cell. 1991;66:967–79.

42. Lange AM, Lo HW. Inhibiting TRK proteins in clinical cancer therapy. Cancers (Basel). 2018;10. https://doi.org/10.3390/cancers10040105.

43. Makretsov N, He M, Hayes M, et al. A fluorescence in situ hybridization study of ETV6-NTRK3 fusion gene in secretory breast carcinoma. Genes Chromosomes Cancer. 2004;40:152–7. https://doi.org/10.1002/gcc.20028.
44. Mardy S, Miura Y, Endo F, et al. Congenital insensitivity to pain with anhidrosis: novel mutations in the TRKA (NTRK1) gene encoding a high-affinity receptor for nerve growth factor. Am J Hum Genet. 1999;64:1570–9. https://doi.org/10.1086/302422.
45. Martin-Zanca D, Hughes SH, Barbacid M. A human oncogene formed by the fusion of truncated tropomyosin and protein tyrosine kinase sequences. Nature. 1986;319:743–8. https://doi.org/10.1038/319743a0.
46. Milione M, Ardini E, Christiansen J, Valtorta E, Veronese S, Bosotti R, Pellegrinelli A, Testi A, Pietrantonio F, Fucà G, Wei G, Murphy D, Siena S, Isacchi A, De Braud F. Identification and characterization of a novel *SCYL3-NTRK1* rearrangement in a colorectal cancer patient. Oncotarget. 2017;8(33):55353–60.
47. Mok TS, Wu YL, Thongprasert S, et al. Gefitinib or carboplatin–paclitaxel in pulmonary adenocarcinoma. N Engl J Med. 2009;361:947–57.
48. Nakagawara A. Trk receptor tyrosine kinases: a bridge between cancer and neural development. Cancer Lett. 2001;169:107–14.
49. Nakagawara A, Liu XG, Ikegaki N, et al. Cloning and chromosomal localization of the human TRK-B tyrosine kinase receptor gene (NTRK2). Genomics. 1995;25:538–46.
50. Ni J, Xie S, Ramkissoon SH, Luu V, Sun Y, Bandopadhayay P, Beroukhim R, Roberts TM, Stiles CD, Segal RA, Ligon KL, Hahn WC, Zhao JJ. Tyrosine receptor kinase B is a drug target in astrocytomas. Neuro Oncol. 2017;19(1):22–30.
51. Okamura K, Harada T, Wang S, et al. Expression of TrkB and BDNF is associated with poor prognosis in non-small cell lung cancer. Lung Cancer. 2012;78:100–6. https://doi.org/10.1016/j.lungcan.2012.07.011.
52. Pulciani S, Santos E, Lauver AV, et al. Oncogenes in solid human tumours. Nature. 1982;300:539–42.
53. Ross JS, Wang K, Gay L, Al-Rohil R, Rand JV, Jones DM, Lee HJ, Sheehan CE, Otto GA, Palmer G, Yelensky R, Lipson D, Morosini D, Hawryluk M, Catenacci DV, Miller VA, Churi C, Ali S, Stephens PJ. New routes to targeted therapy of intrahepatic cholangiocarcinomas revealed by next-generationsequencing. Oncologist. 2014;19(3):235–42.
54. Rubin JB, Segal RA. Growth, survival and migration: the Trk to cancer. Cancer Treat Res. 2003;115:1–18.
55. Rubin BP, Chen CJ, Morgan TW, Xiao S, Grier HE, Kozakewich HP, Perez-Atayde AR, Fletcher JA. Congenital mesoblastic nephroma t(12;15) is associated with ETV6-NTRK3 gene fusion: cytogenetic and molecular relationship to congenital (infantile) fibrosarcoma. Am J Pathol. 1998;153(5):1451–8.
56. Rudzinski ER, Lockwood CM, Stohr BA, et al. Pan-Trk immunohistochemistry identifies NTRK rearrangements in pediatric mesenchymal tumors. Am J Surg Pathol. 2018;42:927–35. https://doi.org/10.1097/PAS.0000000000001062.
57. Russo M, Misale S, Wei G, et al. Acquired resistance to the TRK inhibitor entrectinib in colorectal cancer. Cancer Discov. 2016;6:36–44. https://doi.org/10.1158/2159-8290.CD-15-0940.
58. Salehi A, Verhaagen J, Dijkhuizen PA, et al. Co-localization of high-affinity neurotrophin receptors in nucleus basalis of Meynert neurons and their differential reduction in Alzheimer's disease. Neuroscience. 1996;75:373–87.
59. Sartore-Bianchi A, Ardini E, Bosotti R et al. Sensitivity to entrectinib associated with a novel LMNA-NTRK1 gene fusion in metastatic colorectal cancer. J Natl Cancer Inst. 2016;108. https://doi.org/10.1093/jnci/djv306.
60. Shaw AT, Hsu PP, Awad MM, et al. Tyrosine kinase gene rearrangements in epithelial malignancies. Nat Rev Cancer. 2013;13:772–87. https://doi.org/10.1038/nrc3612.
61. Sigal D, Tartar M, Xavier M, et al. Activity of entrectinib in a patient with the first reported NTRK fusion in neuroendocrine cancer. J Natl Compr Cancer Netw. 2017;15:1317–22. https://doi.org/10.6004/jnccn.2017.7029.

62. Singer HS, Hansen B, Martinie D, et al. Mitogenesis in glioblastoma multiforme cell lines: a role for NGF and its TrkA receptors. J Neuro-Oncol. 1999;45:1–8.

63. Smith KM, Fagan PC, Pomari E, Germano G, Frasson C, Walsh C, Silverman I, Bonvini P, Li G. Antitumor activity of entrectinib, a Pan-TRK, ROS1, and ALK inhibitor, in *ETV6-NTRK3*-Positive acute myeloid leukemia. Mol Cancer Ther. 2018;17(2):455–63.

64. Squinto SP, Stitt TN, Aldrich TH, et al. trkB encodes a functional receptor for brain-derived neurotrophic factor and neurotrophin-3 but not nerve growth factor. Cell. 1991;65:885–93.

65. Stransky N, Cerami E, Schalm S, Kim JL, Lengauer C. The landscape of kinase fusions in cancer. Nat Commun. 2014;5:4846.

66. Taylor J, Pavlick D, Yoshimi A, et al. Oncogenic TRK fusions are amenable to inhibition in hematologic malignancies. J Clin Invest. 2018;128:3819–25. https://doi.org/10.1172/JCI120787.

67. Thiele CJ, Li Z, McKee AE. On Trk--the TrkB signal transduction pathway is an increasingly important target in cancer biology. Clin Cancer Res. 2009;15:5962–7. https://doi.org/10.1158/1078-0432.CCR-08-0651.

68. Tognon C, Garnett M, etal KE. The chimeric protein tyrosine kinase ETV6-NTRK3 requires both Ras-Erk1/2 and PI3-kinase-Akt signaling for fibroblast transformation. Cancer Res. 2001;61:8909–16.

69. Vaishnavi A, Capelletti M, Le AT, et al. Oncogenic and drug-sensitive NTRK1 rearrangements in lung cancer. Nat Med. 2013;19:1469–72. https://doi.org/10.1038/nm.3352.

70. Valent A, Danglot G, Bernheim A. Mapping of the tyrosine kinase receptors trkA (NTRK1), trkB (NTRK2) and trkC(NTRK3) to human chromosomes 1q22, 9q22 and 15q25 by fluorescence in situ hybridization. Eur J Hum Genet. 1997;5:102–4.

71. Weier HU, Rhein AP, Shadravan F, et al. Rapid physical mapping of the human trk protooncogene (NTRK1) to human chromosome 1q21-q22 by P1 clone selection, fluorescence in situ hybridization (FISH), and computer-assisted microscopy. Genomics. 1995;26:390–3.

72. Wiesner T, He J, Yelensky R, Esteve-Puig R, Botton T, Yeh I, Lipson D, Otto G, Brennan K, Murali R, Garrido M, Miller VA, Ross JS, Berger MF, Sparatta A, Palmedo G, Cerroni L, Busam KJ, Kutzner H, Cronin MT, Stephens PJ, Bastian BC. Kinase fusions are frequent in Spitz tumours and spitzoid melanomas. Nat Commun. 2014;5:3116.

73. Wong V, Pavlick D, Brennan T, Yelensky R, Crawford J, Ross JS, Miller VA, Malicki D, Stephens PJ, Ali SM, Ahn H. Evaluation of a congenital infantile fibrosarcoma by comprehensive genomic profiling revealsan LMNA-NTRK1 gene fusion responsive to crizotinib. J Natl Cancer Inst. 2015;108:1. pii: djv307.

74. Wu G, Diaz AK, Paugh BS, Rankin SL, Ju B, Li Y, Zhu X, Qu C, Chen X, Zhang J, Easton J, Edmonson M, Ma X, Lu C, Nagahawatte P, Hedlund E, Rusch M, Pounds S, Lin T, Onar-Thomas A, Huether R, Kriwacki R, Parker M, Gupta P, Becksfort J, Wei L, Mulder HL, Boggs K, Vadodaria B, Yergeau D, Russell JC, Ochoa K, Fulton RS, Fulton LL, Jones C, Boop FA, Broniscer A, Wetmore C, Gajjar A, Ding L, Mardis ER, Wilson RK, Taylor MR, Downing JR, Ellison DW, Zhang J, Baker SJ. The genomic landscape of diffuse intrinsic pontine glioma and pediatric non-brainstem high-grade glioma. Nat Genet. 2014;46(5):444–50.

75. Yan SB, Um SL, Peek VL, et al. MET-targeting antibody (emibetuzumab) and kinase inhibitor (merestinib) as single agent or in combination in a cancer model bearing MET exon 14 skipping. Investig New Drugs. 2018;36:536–44. https://doi.org/10.1007/s10637-017-0545-x.

76. Yeo GS, Hung CC, Rochford J, et al. A de novo mutation affecting human TrkB associated with severe obesity and developmental delay. Nat Neurosci. 2004;7:1187–9. https://doi.org/10.1038/nn1336.

77. Zheng Z, Liebers M, Zhelyazkova B, Cao Y, Panditi D, Lynch KD, Chen J, Robinson HE, Shim HS, Chmielecki J, Pao W, Engelman JA, Iafrate AJ, Le LP. Anchored multiplex PCR for targeted next-generation sequencing. Nat Med. 2014;20(12):1479–84.

Novel Therapies for Small Cell Lung Cancer

Marianna Koczywas and Idoroenyi Amanam

Abstract Small cell lung cancer (SCLC) is an aggressive illness with an overall poor prognosis. A large number of therapeutics have been utilized in the past without much success. Cisplatin (or carboplatin) and etoposide are the hallmarks of the therapy. A large number of current novel therapeutics are targeting the immune system, and based on the recent results, nivolumab and atezolizumab have been approved in certain settings. Targeting with antibody conjugates and bispecifics are coming to fruition. Also, downstream targeting with transcription inhibitors such as EZH2 inhibitors, aurora kinase inhibitors, mitochondrial inhibitors of BCL-2, DLL3/DLL4, and stem cell signaling are currently being tested in the clinics. With novel therapies and immune therapies, there is hope that the bleak overall survival for SCLC will be improved considerably.

Keywords Small cell lung cancer · Cisplatin · Crizotinib · Immunotherapy · Anti-angiogenesis

Introduction

Small cell lung cancer (SCLC) is a poorly differentiated neuroendocrine tumor that is highly associated with smoking. Histologically, small cell lung cancer consists of small round, oval, and spindle-shaped cells with scant cytoplasm, ill-defined borders, finely granular nuclear chromatin, prominent nuclear molding, and high mitotic rate and absent on inconspicuous nucleoli. It is an aggressive malignancy with different clinical, pathological, and molecular features from non-small cell lung cancer with frequently advanced stage at presentation and poor prognosis [1]. SCLC constitutes approximately 13% of all diagnosed lung cancers in the United

M. Koczywas (✉) · I. Amanam
Department of Medical Oncology and Experimental Therapeutics,
City of Hope National Medical Center, Duarte, CA, USA
e-mail: mkoczywas@coh.org

© Springer Nature Switzerland AG 2019
R. Salgia (ed.), *Targeted Therapies for Lung Cancer*, Current Cancer Research,
https://doi.org/10.1007/978-3-030-17832-1_8

163

States and approximately 35,000 new cases are diagnosed annually. This is a significant decline from 20% to 25% 20 years ago mostly as a result of reduced smoking. For more than three decades, combination chemotherapy served as the primary treatment, with the platinum and etoposide combination being the gold standard. However, majority of patients have short-lived benefit from the frontline treatment with poor outcome [2, 3]. More recently, immunotherapy is coming to fruition in SCLC. There are limited options for second line treatment with topotecan being the only chemotherapy agent approved in this setting [4, 5]. Therefore, novel therapies are urgently needed. SCLC is almost always smoking induced and has a high frequency of genetic alterations, including alterations of tumor suppressor genes, and copy number gains and other somatic mutations in transcription factors, enzymes involved in chromatin modification, and receptor tyrosine kinases and their downstream signaling component [6, 7]. One of the hallmarks of SCLC is high frequency of mutations in *TP53* and *RB1*. Given the luck of therapeutic options, research focused on a better understanding of genomic changes may lead to development of new effective therapies [8, 9].

Immunotherapy

Autoimmune paraneoplastic syndromes are frequently observed in patients diagnosed with SCLC indicating that the disease may be primed to generate T-cell responses, which in some cases leads to improved survival [10, 11]. Recent SCLC tumor genome analyses have shown large number of acquired mutations that generated many neoantigens, which favor immunotherapy [6, 9, 12]. One would expect that recently developed antagonistic antibodies targeting the inhibitory immune-checkpoint proteins cytotoxic T-lymphocyte-associated protein 4 (CTLA-4), programmed cell death protein 1 (PD −1), or its ligand PD-L1, will result in activity in SCLC and provide new treatment options for patients [13]. These agents showed activity across multiple tumor types [14–18]. Ipilimumab, a fully human monoclonal antibody, binds to CTLA-4 expressed by T cells and blocks the interaction of this receptor with its ligands CD80 and CD86 on antigen-presenting cells, promoting T-cell activation and anticancer immune response [19]. Reck et al. investigated the activity of ipilimumab in combination with paclitaxel and carboplatin versus paclitaxel and carboplatin alone in patients with previously untreated extensive stage SCLC [20]. In that phase II trial, 130 patients were randomized 1:1:1 to receive paclitaxel (175 mg/m^2)/carboplatin AUC 6) with either placebo (control) or ipilimumab 10 mg/kg in two alternate regimens, concurrent ipilimumab (ipilimumab plus paclitaxel/carboplatin followed by placebo plus paclitaxel/carboplatin) and phased ipilimumab (placebo plus paclitaxel/carboplatin followed by ipilimumab plus paclitaxel/carboplatin). Treatment was administered every 3 weeks for a maximum of 18 weeks (induction), followed by maintenance ipilimumab or placebo every 12 weeks. The patients were not stratified by tumor PD-L1 expression and the immune-related response criteria (irRC) were used to assess response to therapy. Phase ipilimumab, but not concurrent ipilimumab, improved irPFS versus control, (HR 0.64, $p = 0.03$). However, no significant improvement in progression-free survival (PFS) (HR $= 0.93$; $p = 0.37$) or OS (HR $= 0.75$; $p = 0.13$) was observed. In a similar setting, in phase III clinical trial, 1132 patients were randomly assigned at as ratio 1:1 to receive chemotherapy with etoposide and platinum (either cisplatin or carboplatin) plus ipilimumab 10 mg/kg or placebo every 3 weeks for a total of four doses each in phased induction schedule (chemotherapy in cycles 1–4; ipilimumab or placebo beginning in cycle 3 up to cycle 6), followed by ipilimumab or placebo maintenance every 12 weeks [21]. Median overall survival (OS) was 11.0 months for chemotherapy plus ipilimumab versus 10.9 months for chemotherapy plus placebo (HR $= 0.94$, $p = 0.3775$). Median PFS was 4.6 months for the experimental arm versus 4.4 months. Ipilimumab was associated with higher rate and severity of some toxicities, including diarrhea, rash, and colitis, and higher rate of treatment-related discontinuation (18% vs 2% with chemotherapy plus placebo). Five treatment-related deaths occurred with chemotherapy plus ipilimumab and two with chemotherapy and placebo. Preclinical data from malignant melanoma research suggests that combining CTLA-4 and PD-1 exhibits synergy in enhancing activation of tumor-specific T cells and antitumor activity through complementary mechanism [22]. CheckMate 032, a multicenter, open-label, phase I/II trial of nivolumab alone and nivolumab plus ipilimumab in patient with recurrent extensive stage SCLC, has been reported in 2016 [13]. The investigators enrolled and treated 216 patients: 98 with nivolumab 3 mg/kg, 3 with nivolumab 1 mg/kg plus ipilimumab 1 mg/kg, 61 with nivolumab 1 mg/kg plus ipilimumab 3 mg/kg, and 54 with nivolumab 3 mg/kg plus ipilimumab 1 mg/kg. The overall response rates (ORRs) were 10% in nivolumab arm and 19–33% in the combination arms. The 1-year survival was 33% and 35–43%, respectively. Toxicities were similar to prior studies, higher as expected in the combination arms. Based on these results, the combination regimen was incorporated in the NCCN guidelines. Subsequently, on August 16, 2018, FDA granted nivolumab accelerated approval for the treatment of patients with SCLC who progressed after platinum-based therapy and at least one other line of therapy [23]. The results from the phase IB KEYNOTE assessing the safety and efficacy of single agent pembrolizumab were published in 2016 [24]. Among 24 patients with PD-L1 expressing pretreated SCLC, one patient had complete response, and 7 patients had partial response, with ORR of 33%. The safety of pembrolizumab was consistent with known safety profile. The role of check point inhibitors was explored in the maintenance setting. In phase II trial, Gadgeel et al. investigated pembrolizumab in patients with extensive stage SCLC with response or stable disease after induction of chemotherapy (4–6 cycles of platinum and etoposide) [25]. Maintenance pembrolizumab did not appear to improve median PFS compared with historical data. However, the 1-year PFS rate of 1% and OS rate of 37% suggest that a subset of patients did benefit from pembrolizumab. Clinical activity, safety, and predictive biomarkers result from phase Ia atezolizumab trial in extensive stage SCLC, leading to the IMpower133 trial, which evaluated the efficacy and safety of adding atezolizumab or placebo to first-line treatment with carboplatin and etoposide for four cycles (induction phase) followed by maintenance phase with either atezolizumab or placebo (according to the previous random assignment) [26]. At a median follow up of 13.9 months, the median OS was 12.3 months in the atezolizumab arm and 10.3 months in the placebo group (HR = 0.70, p = 0.007). The median PFS was 5.2 months and 4.3 months, respectively (HR = 0.77, p = 0.02). The safety profile of atezolizumab plus carboplatin and etoposide was consistent with previously reported safety profile of the individual agents, and this has been approved by the FDA. In contrast to a prior report, exploratory subgroup analyses showed no clear suggestion that blood-based tumor mutation burden (TMB) levels at either cutoff (10 or 16 mutations per megabase) were predictive of benefit with atezolizumab in this population. However, this trial suggests that combining checkpoint inhibitor with cytotoxic therapy during induction followed by maintenance with checkpoint inhibitor may be a better approach than chemotherapy alone followed by maintenance checkpoint inhibitor in patients with newly diagnosed extensive stage small cell lung cancer [25, 26].

In addition to extensively studied checkpoint inhibitors, vaccine and immunotoxin therapies have been investigated in clinical trials [27]. An immunotoxin targeting the neoantigen HuD (a neuronal RNA-binding protein that is expressed in 100% of SCLC tumor cells) has been tested in preclinical and animal studies [28]. Krug et al. studied vaccination with NP-polySA-KLH in patients with SCLC who completed initial treatment and had no evidence of disease. Polysialic acid (polySA) is a polymer side chain bound to the neural cell adhesion molecule that is extensively expressed on the surface of SCLC cells. Vaccination produced robust antibody response [29]. Another investigational vaccination approach was targeting the *p53* gene, which is mutated in majority of SCLC patients. Transduction of dendritic cells with adenovirus expressing p53 produced a T-cell response in 57.1% of ED-SCLC patients with high rate of objective clinical responses to subsequent chemotherapy (61.9%) that immediately followed vaccination [29]. Ganglioside GD3, cell surface glycosphingolipid antigen, is expressed on the surface of most SCLC tumors, with limited expression in normal tissues, making it an appropriate antigenic target for active immunization to eliminate microscopic disease and improve survival. However, clinical trials with preBec2/BCG as adjuvant vaccination in responding patient with limited stage SCLC showed no improvement in the survival, PFS, or quality of life [30, 31]. CD47 is a cell surface molecule that promotes immune evasion by engaging signal-regulatory protein alpha, which serves as an inhibitory receptor on macrophages, with high level of expression on the surface of SCLC. Preclinical data from human cell lines and xenografts suggests that blocking CD47 strongly promotes the phagocytosis of SCLC cells by macrophages and inhibits tumor growth by T-cell-mediated processes [32]. Phase I trial with Hu5F9-G4, a CD47 targeting antibody in patients with AML and solid tumors, is ongoing (NCT02216409). Patients with SCLC have often been found to have functional deficiency in a variety of immunocytes; therefore cellular immunotherapy (CIT) with ex vivo activated and expanded immunocytes may be feasible and effective. Several immunotherapies to induce cytotoxic T lymphocyte (CTL) have been tried with limited success due to the complexity of the immune escape in this malignancy. Ding et al. investigated the safety and efficacy of autologous natural killer, gamma delta ($\gamma\delta$) T, and cytokine-induced killer (CIK) cells as maintenance therapy in patients with extensive stage SCLC, who responded to initial chemotherapy [33]. CIT maintenance therapy prolonged overall survival with minimal side effects in the experimental arm as compared to control (13.2 months vs. 8.2 months). Natural killer (NK) cells can kill a broad array of tumor cells in a nonmajor histocompatibility complex (MHC)-restricted manner. A phase II clinical trial is currently evaluating maintenance therapy with autologous adaptive transfer of NK cells after response from first-line treatment, comparing with conventional observation group (NCT03410368).

Antibody-Drug Conjugates (ADCs)

Antibody-drug conjugates (ADCs) are a type of human or humanized monoclonal antibody conjugated with cytotoxic drugs directed to antigens differentially overexpressed in tumor cells [34]. Development of these drugs represents a paradigm shift in chemotherapy. Rovalpituzumab tesirine (Rova-T) is an antibody-drug conjugate that recognizes delta-like protein 3 (DLL3), a NOTCH ligand, which is expressed on the surface of approximately 80% of SCLC cells but absent on normal cells. Phase I clinical trial was conducted in patients who progressed after one or more previous regimen. Among 60 assessable patients, 11 (18%) had a confirmed objective response, including 10 (38%) of 26 patients confirmed to have high DLL3 expression (expression in 50% or more of tumor cells) [35]. Dose-limiting toxicity included grade 4 thrombocytopenia, grade 4 liver function abnormalities. Other toxicities of concern were pleural effusion, increased lipase level. AMG 757 is a half-life extended bispecific T-cell engager (Bite®) targeting DLL3 currently undergoing safety and tolerability evaluation in phase I trial in the refractory and first-line consolidation setting in patient with SCLC (NCT03319940). Trop-2 is a glycoprotein expressed in many epithelial cancers (including SCLC) and shown to be an attractive and selective target for antibody-based therapy. Sacituzumab govitecan is a novel antibody-drug conjugate comprising 7-ethyl-10-hydroxy-camptothecin (active metabolite of irinotecan) conjugated to an anti-Trop-2 humanized antibody. In phase I/II clinical trial in previously treated extensive stage SCLC, overall response to sacituzumab govitecan was 14%, the median duration of response 5.7 months and median OS 7.5 months. Grade 3 plus drug-related toxicities included neutropenia (34%), anemia (6%) and diarrhea (9%) [36]. CD56, a cell surface marker highly expressed in majority of SCLC, is a promising therapeutic target. Recently, a novel CD56 targeting antibody-drug conjugate, IMGN901 (lorvotuzumab mertansine), designed for tumor-selective delivery of the cytotoxic maytansinoid DM1 and characterized by high affinity, internalization, and tumor specificity, was evaluated in CD56-expressing solid tumors. A dose- expansion phase accrued patients with SCLC. Responses included one complete response (CR), one clinical CR, and one unconfirmed partial response (PR) in MCC and one unconfirmed PR in SCLC. Stable disease was seen for 25% of all evaluable patients who received doses ≥ 60 mg/m^2 [37].

Transcription Inhibitors

Lurbinectedin (PM01183, L) is a novel anticancer drug that inhibits activated transcription, induces DNA double-strand breaks generating apoptosis, and modulates tumor microenvironment. In a phase II basket trial of patients with advanced solid tumors, lurbinectedin has shown promising activity in a cohort of patients with SCLC. Sixty six patients with previously treated disease received intravenous lurbinectedin 3.2 mg/m^2 every 3 weeks. An objective response was observed in 24 (39.3%) of 61 evaluable patients [38]. ATLANTIS: Global, randomized phase III study of lurbinectedin with doxorubicin vs. CAV or topotecan in patients after failure of first-line platinum doublets, reached its accrual goal in July of 2018, and the results are expected at the end on 2019 [39]. In August of 2018, the FDA has granted lurbinectedin (PM1183), an orphan drug designation for the treatment of patients with SCLC.

Antiangiogenic Agents

A large body of literature suggests that angiogenesis plays a fundamental role in determining the growth rate, invasiveness, and development of metastasis in SCLC [40]. It is well known that the formation of structurally and functionally abnormal neovessels from the existing blood vessels mediates resistance to chemotherapy [41]. Low serum vascular endothelial growth factor (VEGF) concentration is a significant and independent prognostic factor in patients with SCLC; however, it was found not to be useful in predicting response to chemotherapy [42]. A meta-analysis of 7 randomized controlled phase II and phase III trials with angiogenesis inhibitors, with 1322 patients enrolled (669 received angiogenesis inhibitors: bevacizumab, thalidomide, vandetanib, sunitinib, and endostatin), showed that adding angiogenesis inhibitors to chemotherapy did not improve PFS, OS, ORR, 1-year survival rate, 2-year survival rate or 1-year PFS rate for SCLC. However, subgroup analysis revealed that bevacizumab enhanced PFS. All 7 trials used antiangiogenesis agents as maintenance and first-line therapies were platinum-based chemotherapy [43].

Cancer Stem Cell-Targeted Therapy

SCLC responds extremely well to first-line therapy; however, all patients with extensive stage and majority with limited stage will relapse within a short period of time with disease relatively resistant to second-line therapies. Cancer stem cells (CSCs) have been studied as a potential cause of the heterogeneity, drug resistance, recurrence, and metastasis of several types of tumors. Some characteristics of SCLC, such as aggressiveness, suggest that this kind of tumor could be enriched in CSCs, and drug resistance in SCLC could be attributable to the existence of a CSC subpopulation in SCLC [44–46]. There has been significant research interest focusing on the signaling pathways, which are critical for stem cell development and self-renewal: the Hedgehog, Notch and Wnt. A number of agents blocking the Hedgehog pathway have been investigated in SCLC, including bromodomain, visomodegib, GDC-0449 (NCT00887159), LDE225 (NCT 01579929) [47–49]. Belani et al. evaluated, in phase II randomized study of 103 patients, concurrent and maintenance visomodegib with cisplatin and etoposide in the first-line extensive stage SCLC and reported no significant differences in response rate, progression free survival, or overall survival between the arms [49]. The Notch signaling pathway has also been shown to regulate normal stem cells and neoplastic transformation when deregulated. In the phase Ib/II "PINNACLE" trial, ant-Notch 2/3 (Tarextumab) was tested in combination with etoposide in first-line extensive stage SCLC. Combination treatment was well tolerated and encouraging anti-tumor activity has been observed [50]. Monoclonal antibodies targeting Wnt-1 and Wnt-2 (aberrations of the Wnt pathway) are being developed: SM08502 (NCT03355066) [51].

PARP Inhibitor

Dysregulation of transcription and response to DNA damage has been identified as a hallmark of malignancy. The most common mutations identified are inactivation of the tumor suppressors *TP53* and *RB1* [6]. However, unfortunately, to date, there has not been success at inhibiting these targets. A unique approach that is currently under investigation involves poly-ADP ribose polymerase (PARP). PARP is a critical component to DNA damage repair [52] and has been shown to be overexpressed in SCLC [53].

In each cell, DNA is damaged by a variety of different mechanisms and can lead to single- and double-stranded breaks which require repair to ensure cell survival. One of the pathways involved in DNA repair involved includes PARP. PARP1 is a nuclear globular protein that contains three functional domains. The N-terminus DNA binding domain containing several zinc finger motifs, a central automodification domain and a C-terminus catalytic domain that has the protein's enzymatic activity and substrate binding sites for nicotinamide adenine dinucleotide (NAD) which powers the protein. The catalytic (cat) domain contains a WGR motif which serves to activate the enzymatic activity of the cat region in addition to conserved histidine and tyrosine residues which are necessary for NAD+ binding.

A PARP inhibitor will compete with NAD+ at this substrate binding site. In the absence of an inhibitor, PARP will be recruited to a single-stranded break site and initiates poly-ADP ribosylation of histones and chromatin remodeling enzymes leading to recruitment of PARP-dependent DNA damage repair proteins. At presence of PARP inhibitor, PARP is still recruited to single-stranded DNA breaks but can't recruit DNA repair proteins because catalytic activity is inhibited. PARP will stay attached to DNA, and the stalling at the replication fork leads to a double-stranded break and eventually leading to cell death.

Current standard of care for limited and extensive stage SCLC include DNA-damaging agents (radiotherapy and chemotherapy) and thus make utilization of PARP inhibitors an ideal treatment modality. PARP inhibitors have been evaluated in the frontline setting in combination with standard chemotherapy due to success in cell lines and animal models [53–55]. Byers et al. showed that there was an equal decrease in viability of cell lines when exposed to standard chemotherapy (cisplatin and etoposide) or a PARP inhibitor. When chemotherapy was combined with a PARP inhibitor, there was synergistic effect in inhibition of cell viability [53].

A phase II study ECOG-ACRIN 2511 by Owonikoko et al. evaluated veliparib added to cisplatin and etoposide in extensive stage small cell lung cancer. Veliparib is a potent inhibitor of PARP-1 and PARP-2 that has been shown to have good oral bioavailability, crosses the blood-brain barrier, and potentiates other cytotoxic agents including platinum and radiation [56]. Patient received four cycles of cisplatin and etoposide with or without veliparib. The median PFS was 6.1 months for patients who received veliparib compared to 5.5 months for those that didn't (HR: 0.75; $p = 0.06$). The median OS was 10.3 months and 8.9 months (HR: 0.83; $p = 0.17$) with ORR 72% compared to 66% ($p = 0.57$) in veliparib and placebo, respectively. This study showed that PARP inhibition can be used with good activity in the frontline setting [57] for extensive stage disease.

Maintenance after frontline treatment is also of interest and has been shown to be successful in other tumors. In ovarian cancer, maintenance with PARP inhibition showed a PFS benefit with a 70% lower risk of progression [58]. STOMP, a phase II study evaluating patients with extensive stage SCLC who responded to first-line chemotherapy and received either olaparib or placebo, attempted to evaluate if maintenance PARP inhibition would yield any benefit in this population. Olaparib, a first-generation PARP inhibitor approved for use in ovarian and breast cancer, is currently being evaluated in a variety of tumors. STOMP did not show any statistical improvement in PFS compared to placebo (2.6 vs 3.6 month; HR 0.87; $p = 0.29$) nor did OS [59]. These results were disappointing, considering the success of PARP in advanced ovarian cancer maintenance setting. Niraparib, another PARP-1 and PARP-2 inhibitor, is currently enrolling patients in a phase III study evaluating maintenance after response with chemotherapy in extensive disease SCLC (NCT03516084).

The median survival of extensive stage SCLC ranges between 9.4 and 12.8 months [60, 61] with recurrence occurring within 5 to 6 months. PARP inhibition has been tested in the relapsed setting, with veliparib combined with temozolomide. This phase II study evaluated 104 relapsed SCLC patients treated with temozolomide with or without veliparib. Though ORR (39% vs 14%; $p = 0.16$) was improved with PARP inhibition there was no significant improvement in survival (mOS 8.2 months vs 7.0 months; $p = 0.50$). An exploratory marker using SLFN11, a biomarker of PARP inhibitor sensitivity, showed promising results. Those tumors harboring SLFN11 positivity had significant survival benefit (PFS 5.7 vs 3.6 months; $p = 0.009$; OS 12.2 vs 7.5 months; $p = 0.014$) with PARP inhibition [62].

A newer more potent PARP inhibitor, talazoparib, with more efficient PARP-trapping capability than older PARP inhibitors has been shown to have activity as a single agent in small cell lung cancer patients [63]. In preclinical models, it was shown that temzolomide potentiates talazoparib leading to synergistic lethality, and there is a phase II study planned that will evaluate this combination (NCT03672773). A combination of interest identified in talazoparib's preclinical models was an inhibition of PARP and PI3K pathways. PI3K is activated in SCLC cell lines treated with talazoparib and activation was blocked by PI3K inhibition [64]. Talazoparib is an exciting new PARP inhibitor currently under investigation with, as of October 2018, 20 active clinical trials evaluating activity in a variety of solid neoplasms and combination therapies including small cell lung cancer (https://clinicaltrials.gov/ct2/results?term=BMN+673&Search=Apply&recrs=a&age_v=&gndr=&type=&rslt=).

EZH2 Inhibitor

The tumor suppressor RB1 is inactivated in over 90% of SCLC cases [8]. This disruption of RB1/E2 promoter binding factor (E2F) is postulated to be a major factor in pathogenesis of SCLC. EZH2, a factor in this pathway, is found to be upregulated in SCLC [53]. EZH2 is a histone methyltransferase and its activation leads to alteration in cell cycle regulation, proliferation, and cancer progression [65]. High expression and mutation of EZH2 are in a variety of malignancies and usually portend for a poor prognosis [66].

EZH2 has been shown to repress the cell cycle inhibitor p21 and other pro-apoptotic factors, thereby promoting cell cycling in SCLC cells [67]. In various SCLC cell lines, suppression of EZH2 leads to reduction of cells in S, G2/M phase with increased p21 expression [67]. EZH2 was also shown to prevent apoptosis by inhibition of TGF-β via histone methyltransferase methylation of lysine 27 in histone H3 (H3K27me3) [68]. In addition, it has been shown that in platinum-resistant cancer cells, protein and mRNA expression EZH2 is upregulated and by silencing EZH2 overcomes drug resistance [69], making EZH2 a target of interest in SCLC.

Various EZH2 inhibitors have been investigated in preclinical and clinical studies. 3-Deazaadenosine A (DZnep) is a nonspecific EZH2 inhibitor that inhibits EZH2 via SAH-hydrolase inhibition. DZnep has been shown in animals to be effective [70]. Tazemetostat, an oral EZH2 inhibitor that decreases the levels of H3K27me3, has shown promise. It was the first-in-class drug to complete a phase I study with favorable safety and antitumor activity [71]. The FDA placed a partial clinical hold on any additional Tazemetostat studies due a pediatric patient developing a secondary malignancy. GSK2816126 is a SAM-competitive inhibitor of EZH2, and its phase I study was terminated due to insufficient evidence of clinical activity. There are many other EZH2 inhibitors with preclinical data awaiting clinical evaluation [66].

Aurora Like Kinase Inhibitor

Aurora kinases are a group of serine/threonine kinases, consisting of Aurora A, Aurora B, and Aurora C, and are essential in cell division and regulators of mitosis [72]. These three kinases are involved with chromosomal segregation, deletions, or deficiency of Aurora kinases, leading to cell instability and eventual cell death [73, 74]. Overexpression or amplification of Aurora kinases have been detected in multiple malignancies and usually predict for a poorer prognosis [75].

MYC amplification is a frequent event in SCLC, occurring in SCLC up to 50% of the time. In conjunction with *TP53* and *RB1* loss, it makes a SCLC a highly aggressive and lethal malignancy. *MYC* has been associated with resistance to treatment, progression, and overall a poorer outcome [76].

Concurrent overexpression/activation of MYC and Aurora kinases are found often in malignancies. Aurora kinases can transcriptionally upregulate expression of c-MYC [77], and on the other hand, c-MYC can bind to the promoter of AURKA and increase the expression of AURKA [78]. AURKA also protects N-MYC from degradation [79]. c-MYC also upregulates cyclin-dependent kinases, leading to increased proliferation [80].

In animal models, SCLC driven by high expression of MYC showed high response to chemotherapy but rapid relapse following treatment [81], thus making MYC a target of interest in this disease, but so far has proved a difficult target. Aurora kinase inhibition may prove to be a novel and attractive approach considering AURKA's relationship to MYC.

MLN8237 (Alisertib) has so far shown the most promise in SCLC as it has been specifically studied in this disease. A phase II study evaluated 60 patients with small cell lung cancer receiving MLN8237 as a single agent with 21% having an objective response rate. The overall PFS was 2.1 months; those with a chemotherapy-sensitive relapse had a longer PFS (2.6 months) compared to those with refractory or chemotherapy-resistant disease (1.7 months). The median duration of response was 4.1 months, with 33% of patients having stable disease and 4% having stable disease >6 months [82].

MLN8237 is being evaluated in combination with paclitaxel in SCLC patient who progressed after initial chemotherapy. Preliminary results were favorable with patients who received the combination compared to those who received paclitaxel alone. The median PFS 101 days compared to 66 days in the chemotherapy alone arm (HR 0.72; $p = 0.038$) with responses observed in 22% of patients who received the combination. Though these results are favorable, there were higher rates of adverse events with combination [83].

BCL-2

Evasion from apoptosis is one of the many foundations of carcinogenesis and one of the mechanisms of eventual drug resistance. It was discovered that elevated expression of the antiapoptotic protein Bcl-2 is highly expressed in SCLC [84].

BCL-2 has been characterized in SCLC via immunohistochemistry, microarray detection of mRNA, genomic sequencing and proteomic profiling with levels up to 84% [85–88].

In preclinical models, BCL-2 binds and sequesters BH3-only proapoptotic proteins BID or BIM and prevents them from interacting with the pore-forming effectors that lead to apoptosis and cell death. Understanding of the mechanism of BCL-2 proteins has led to two approaches to inhibiting this pathway, either by direct inhibition of BCL-2 or using BH-3 mimetics.

ABT-263, a BH3 mimetic, demonstrated antitumor activity in laboratory models of SCLC but unfortunately has not led to repeated success in the clinic [89–93]. Phase II trials of ABT-263 have not demonstrated success. Out of 26 patients, only 1 showed a response to treatment with ABT-263 [94].

Venetoclax, an effective BCL-2 inhibitor which has been effective clinically in treating a variety of hematologic malignancies, has also been investigated. Preclinical data appears promising as venetoclax, dosed at 100 mg/kg/qd, induced tumor regression in mouse models, and further investigation is required [95].

DLL4

The Notch pathway has been identified as one of the most commonly activated pathways in cancer [96, 97]. This signaling cascade is crucial for cell growth, differentiation, and survival [98]. Notch signaling has been identified as possibly having an impact in survival [99] in those who have a diagnosis of cancer and thus makes this a pathway of interest.

The Notch pathway is activated when a Notch receptor binds to a ligand. The mammalian Notch family contains five ligands, delta-like ligand 1 (DLL1), delta-like ligand 3 (DLL3), delta-like ligand 4 (DLL4), Jagged-1 (JAG1), and Jagged-2 (JAG2), and four receptors, Notches 1–4. For the purpose of this review, we will focus on DLL4, which has been studied in SCLC and implicated in activating NF-$\kappa\beta$ leading to enhanced VEGF secretion and promotion of metastases [100].

During tumorigenesis, induction of DLL4 expression by VEGF in endothelial cells of the tumor leads to improved angiogenesis. Interruption of DLL4-Notch signaling led to suppression of tumor growth via nonproductive angiogenesis and hypoxia of tumors [101]. High levels of DLL4 are expressed in cancer stem cells in preclinical models using SCLC cell lines. In human tumor xenografts, targeting DLL4-Notch with anti-DLL4 monoclonal antibodies as a single agent or in combination with cisplatin/etoposide or topotecan resulted in reduction of cancer stem cells [102].

Demcizumab, a humanized IgG monoclonal antibody, directed against DLL4 was successful in showing single-agent activity in its phase I study with overall disease control rate of 40% and some of the best responses identified in patients with lung malignancies [103]. A phase II study looking at demcizumab in NSCLC in combination with standard frontline therapy did not meet its primary endpoint, and the drug developer halted further development of this agent.

MEDI0639, another humanized monoclonal antibody targeting DLL4-signaling, was also evaluated in the clinic. A phase I study evaluating 9 SCLC patients who received single agent MEDI0639 showed efficacy in reduction in number of cancer stem cells after treatment [104]. Another phase I study evaluating this monoclonal antibody, which included 4 SCLC patients, showed encouraging antitumor activity [105]. Unfortunately, as in the case of demcizumab, the drug developer stopped all development on MEDI0639. There are other viable targets in the Notch signaling pathway that are currently under investigation.

Conclusion

In the era of personalized medicine in oncology, treatment of SCLC remains challenging, with limited therapeutic options. Many of the agents with promising activity in the preclinical or phase I trials failed in phase II/III clinical trials. It is difficult to replicate the success stories seen with targeted personalized treatment in other solid tumors. However, over the last few years, there has been a worldwide renewed interest in studying SCLC, including comprehensive molecular mapping, development of patient-derived xenografts, discoveries of new potentially targetable pathways, and a multitude of clinical trials focusing on new therapeutic agents. As we make progress in our understanding of the biology of SCLC, we hope to be able to identify new targets and develop personalized treatment that will provide long-term benefit to our patient diagnosed with SCLC.

References

1. Govindan R, et al. Changing epidemiology of small-cell lung cancer in the United States over the last 30 years: analysis of the surveillance, epidemiologic, and end results database. J Clin Oncol. 2006;24(28):4539–44.
2. Sabari JK, et al. Unravelling the biology of SCLC: implications for therapy. Nat Rev Clin Oncol. 2017;14(9):549–61.
3. Lara PN Jr, et al. Phase III trial of irinotecan/cisplatin compared with etoposide/cisplatin in extensive-stage small-cell lung cancer: clinical and pharmacogenomic results from SWOG S0124. J Clin Oncol. 2009;27(15):2530–5.
4. Faria AL, et al. Topotecan in second-line treatment of small-cell lung cancer--how it works in our daily clinical practice? Curr Drug Saf. 2010;5(2):114–7.
5. von Pawel J. The role of topotecan in treating small cell lung cancer: second-line treatment. Lung Cancer. 2003;41(Suppl 4):S3–8.
6. George J, et al. Comprehensive genomic profiles of small cell lung cancer. Nature. 2015;524(7563):47–53.
7. Wistuba AFG II, Minna JD. Molecular genetics of small cell lung carcinoma. Semin Oncol. 2001;28(2 Suppl 4):3–13.
8. Peifer M, et al. Integrative genome analyses identify key somatic driver mutations of small-cell lung cancer. Nat Genet. 2012;44(10):1104–10.
9. Rudin CM, et al. Comprehensive genomic analysis identifies SOX2 as a frequently amplified gene in small-cell lung cancer. Nature Genetics. 2012;44(10):1111.

10. Darnell RB, Posner JB. Paraneoplastic syndromes involving the nervous system. N Engl J Med. 2003;349(16):1543–54.
11. Graus F, et al. Anti-Hu antibodies in patients with small-cell lung cancer: association with complete response to therapy and improved survival. J Clin Oncol. 1997;15(8):2866–72.
12. Rizvi NA, et al. Cancer immunology. Mutational landscape determines sensitivity to PD-1 blockade in non-small cell lung cancer. Science. 2015;348(6230):124–8.
13. Antonia SJ, et al. Nivolumab alone and nivolumab plus ipilimumab in recurrent small-cell lung cancer (CheckMate 032): a multicentre, open-label, phase 1/2 trial. Lancet Oncol. 2016;17(7):883–95.
14. Reck M, Heigener D, Reinmuth N. Immunotherapy for small-cell lung cancer: emerging evidence. Future Oncol. 2016;12(7):931–43.
15. Gettinger S, et al. Nivolumab Monotherapy for First-Line Treatment of Advanced Non-Small-Cell Lung Cancer. J Clin Oncol. 2016;34(25):2980–7.
16. Garon EB. Current Perspectives in Immunotherapy for Non-Small Cell Lung Cancer. Semin Oncol. 2015;42(Suppl 2):S11–8.
17. Brahmer JR, et al. Safety and activity of anti-PD-L1 antibody in patients with advanced cancer. N Engl J Med. 2012;366(26):2455–65.
18. Topalian SL, et al. Safety, activity, and immune correlates of anti-PD-1 antibody in cancer. N Engl J Med. 2012;366(26):2443–54.
19. Hoos A, et al. Improved Endpoints for Cancer Immunotherapy Trials. JNCI: J Natl Cancer Inst. 2010;102(18):1388–97.
20. Reck M, et al. Ipilimumab in combination with paclitaxel and carboplatin as first-line therapy in extensive-disease-small-cell lung cancer: results from a randomized, double-blind, multicenter phase 2 trial. Ann Oncol. 2013;24(1):75–83.
21. Reck M, et al. Phase III randomized trial of ipilimumab plus etoposide and platinum versus placebo plus etoposide and platinum in extensive-stage small-cell lung cancer. J Clin Oncol. 2016;34(31):3740–8.
22. Curran MA, et al. PD-1 and CTLA-4 combination blockade expands infiltrating T cells and reduces regulatory T and myeloid cells within B16 melanoma tumors. Proc Natl Acad Sci USA. 2010;107(9):4275–80.
23. Ready N, et al. Third-line nivolumab monotherapy in recurrent small cell lung cancer: checkmate 032. J Thorac Oncol. 2019;14(2):237–244.
24. Ott PA, et al. Pembrolizumab in patients with extensive-stage small-cell lung cancer: results from the phase ib KEYNOTE-028 study. J Clin Oncol. 2017;35(34):3823–9.
25. Gadgeel SM, et al. Phase II study of maintenance pembrolizumab in patients with extensive-stage small cell lung cancer (SCLC). J Thorac Oncol. 2018;13(9):1393–9.
26. Horn L, et al. First-line atezolizumab plus chemotherapy in extensive-stage small-cell lung cancer. N Engl J Med 2018;379:2220–2229.
27. Freeman-Keller M, Goldman J, Gray J. Vaccine immunotherapy in lung cancer: clinical experience and future directions. Pharmacol Ther. 2015;153:1–9.
28. Ehrlich D, et al. Intratumoral anti-HuD immunotoxin therapy for small cell lung cancer and neuroblastoma. J Hematol Oncol. 2014;7:91.
29. Krug LM, et al. Immunization with N-propionyl polysialic acid-KLH conjugate in patients with small cell lung cancer is safe and induces IgM antibodies reactive with SCLC cells and bactericidal against group B meningococci. Cancer Immunol Immunother. 2012;61(1):9–18.
30. Giaccone G, et al. Phase III study of adjuvant vaccination with Bec2/bacille Calmette-Guerin in responding patients with limited-disease small-cell lung cancer (European Organisation for Research and Treatment of Cancer 08971-08971B; Silva Study). J Clin Oncol. 2005;23(28):6854–64.
31. Bottomley A, et al. Symptom and quality of life results of an international randomised phase III study of adjuvant vaccination with Bec2/BCG in responding patients with limited disease small-cell lung cancer. Eur J Cancer. 2008;44(15):2178–84.
32. Weiskopf K, et al. CD47-blocking immunotherapies stimulate macrophage-mediated destruction of small-cell lung cancer. J Clin Invest. 2016;126(7):2610–20.

33. Ding X, et al. Cellular immunotherapy as maintenance therapy prolongs the survival of the patients with small cell lung cancer. J Transl Med. 2015;13:158.
34. Bouchard H, Viskov C, Garcia-Echeverria C. Antibody-drug conjugates-A new wave of cancer drugs. Bioorg Med Chem Lett. 2014;24(23):5357–63.
35. Rudin CM, et al. Rovalpituzumab tesirine, a DLL3-targeted antibody-drug conjugate, in recurrent small-cell lung cancer: a first-in-human, first-in-class, open-label, phase 1 study. Lancet Oncol. 2017;18(1):42–51.
36. Gray JE, et al. Phase 2 study of sacituzumab govitecan (IMMU-132), an anti-Trop-2/SN-38 antibody-drug conjugate (ADC), in patients with pretreated metastatic small-cell lung cancer (mSCLC). Cancer Res. 2017;23(19):5711–5719.
37. Shah MH, et al. Phase I study of IMGN901, a CD56-targeting antibody-drug conjugate, in patients with CD56-positive solid tumors. Invest New Drugs. 2016;34(3):290–9.
38. Perez JMT, et al. Efficacy and safety of lurbinectedin (PM1183) in small cell lung cancer (SCLC): results from a phase 2 study. J Clin Oncol. 2018;36(15). Abstract 8570.
39. Farago AF, et al. ATLANTIS: global, randomized phase III study of lurbinectedin (L) with doxorubicin (DOX) vs. CAV or topotecan (T) in small-cell lung cancer after platinum therapy. J Clin Oncol. 2018;36(15). Abstract TPS8587.
40. Lucchi M, et al. Small cell lung carcinoma (SCLC): the angiogenic phenomenon. Eur J Cardiothorac Surg. 2002;21(6):1105–10.
41. Salven P, et al. High pre-treatment serum level of vascular endothelial growth factor (VEGF) is associated with poor outcome in small-cell lung cancer. Int J Cancer. 1998;79(2):144–6.
42. Ustuner Z, et al. Prognostic and predictive value of vascular endothelial growth factor and its soluble receptors, VEGFR-1 and VEGFR-2 levels in the sera of small cell lung cancer patients. Med Oncol. 2008;25(4):394–9.
43. Li Q, et al. Angiogenesis inhibitors for the treatment of small cell lung cancer (SCLC) A meta-analysis of 7 randomized controlled trials. Medicine. 2017;96(13). e6412.
44. Codony-Servat J, Verlicchi A, Rosell R. Cancer stem cells in small cell lung cancer. Transl Lung Cancer Res. 2016;5(1):16–25.
45. Pore M, et al. Cancer stem cells, epithelial to mesenchymal markers, and circulating tumor cells in small cell lung cancer. Clin Lung Cancer. 2016;17(6):535–42.
46. Koren A, Motaln H, Cufer T. Lung cancer stem cells: a biological and clinical perspective. Cell Oncol (Dordr). 2013;36(4):265–75.
47. Kaur G, et al. Bromodomain and hedgehog pathway targets in small cell lung cancer. Cancer Lett. 2016;371(2):225–39.
48. Abe Y, Tanaka N. The Hedgehog signaling networks in lung cancer: the mechanisms and roles in tumor progression and implications for cancer therapy. Biomed Res Int. 2016.
49. Belani CP, et al. Vismodegib or cixutumumab in combination with standard chemotherapy for patients with extensive-stage small cell lung cancer: a trial of the ECOG-ACRIN Cancer Research Group (E1508). Cancer. 2016;122(15):2371–8.
50. Pietanza MC, et al. Final results of phase Ib of tarextumab (TRXT, OMP-59R5, anti-Notch2/3) in combination with etoposide and platinum (EP) in patients (pts) with untreated extensive-stage small-cell lung cancer (ED-SCLC). J Clin Oncol. 2015;33(15). Abstract 7508.
51. Pan F, et al. Inhibitory effects of XAV939 on the proliferation of small-cell lung cancer H446 cells and Wnt/beta-catenin signaling pathway in vitro. Oncol Lett. 2018;16(2):1953–8.
52. Rouleau M, et al. PARP inhibition: PARP1 and beyond. Nature reviews. Cancer. 2010;10(4):293–301.
53. Byers LA, et al. Proteomic profiling identifies dysregulated pathways in small cell lung cancer and novel therapeutic targets including PARP1. Cancer Discov. 2012;2(9):798–811.
54. Cardnell RJ, et al. Proteomic markers of DNA repair and PI3K pathway activation predict response to the PARP inhibitor BMN 673 in small cell lung cancer. Clin Cancer Res. 2013;19(22):6322–6328.
55. Spigel D, et al. 1472P Phase II Study Of Carboplatin/Etoposide Plus LY2510924, A CXCR4 peptide antagonist, versus carboplatin/etoposide in patients with extensive-stage small cell lung canceR (SCLC). Ann Oncol. 2014;25(suppl_4):iv514.

56. Donawho CK, et al. ABT-888, an orally active poly(ADP-Ribose) polymerase inhibitor that potentiates DNA-damaging agents in preclinical tumor models. Clin Cancer Res. 2007;13(9):2728–37.
57. Owonikoko, T.K., et al., Randomized trial of cisplatin and etoposide in combination with veliparib or placebo for extensive stage small cell lung cancer: ECOG-ACRIN 2511 study. J Clin Oncol. 2017;37:222–229.
58. Moore K, et al. Maintenance olaparib in patients with newly diagnosed advanced ovarian cancer. New England J Med. 2018;379:2495.
59. Woll P, et al. P1. 07–015 STOMP: a UK national cancer research network randomised, double blind, multicentre phase II trial of olaparib as maintenance therapy in SCLC: topic: drug treatment alone and in combination with radiotherapy. J Thoracic Oncol. 2017;12(1):S704–5.
60. Noda K, et al. Irinotecan plus cisplatin compared with etoposide plus cisplatin for extensive small-cell lung cancer. N Engl J Med. 2002;346(2):85–91.
61. El Maalouf G, et al. Could we expect to improve survival in small cell lung cancer? Lung Cancer. 2007;57(Suppl 2):S30–4.
62. Pietanza MC, et al. Randomized, double-blind, phase II study of temozolomide in combination with either veliparib or placebo in patients with relapsed-sensitive or refractory small-cell lung cancer. J Clin Oncol. 2018;36(23):2386–94.
63. Wainberg, Z.A., et al., Safety and antitumor activity of the PARP inhibitor BMN673 in a phase 1 trial recruiting metastatic small-cell lung cancer (SCLC) and germline BRCA-mutation carrier cancer patients. Am Soc Clin Oncol. 2014.
64. Feng Y, et al. 242 BMN 673 as single agent and in combination with temozolomide or PI3K pathway inhibitors in small cell lung cancer and gastric cancer models. Eur J Cancer. 2014;50:81.
65. Gall Troselj K, Novak Kujundzic R, Ugarkovic D. Polycomb repressive complex's evolutionary conserved function: the role of EZH2 status and cellular background. Clin Epigenetics. 2016;8:55.
66. Yan K-S, et al. EZH2 in cancer progression and potential application in cancer therapy: a friend or foe? Int J Mol Sci. 2017;18(6):1172.
67. Hubaux R, et al. EZH2 promotes E2F-driven SCLC tumorigenesis through modulation of apoptosis and cell-cycle regulation. J Thorac Oncol. 2013;8(8):1102–6.
68. Murai F, et al. EZH2 promotes progression of small cell lung cancer by suppressing the TGF-β-Smad-ASCL1 pathway. Cell Discovery. 2015;1:15026.
69. Zhou W, et al. siRNA silencing EZH2 reverses cisplatin-resistance of human non-small cell lung and gastric cancer cells. Asian Pac J Cancer Prev. 2015;16(6):2425–30.
70. Mayr C, et al. 3-deazaneplanocin a may directly target putative cancer stem cells in biliary tract cancer. Anticancer Res. 2015;35(9):4697–705.
71. Italiano A, et al. Tazemetostat, an EZH2 inhibitor, in relapsed or refractory B-cell non-Hodgkin lymphoma and advanced solid tumours: a first-in-human, open-label, phase 1 study. Lancet Oncol. 2018;19(5):649–59.
72. Nigg EA. Mitotic kinases as regulators of cell division and its checkpoints. Nat Rev Mol Cell Biol. 2001;2(1):21–32.
73. Lu LY, et al. Aurora A is essential for early embryonic development and tumor suppression. J Biol Chem. 2008;283(46):31785–90.
74. Torchia EC, et al. Aurora kinase-A deficiency during skin development impairs cell division and stratification. J Invest Dermatol. 2013;133(1):78–86.
75. Tang A, et al. Aurora kinases: novel therapy targets in cancers. Oncotarget. 2017;8(14):23937–54.
76. Sos ML, et al. A framework for identification of actionable cancer genome dependencies in small cell lung cancer. Proc Natl Acad Sci USA. 2012;109(42):17034–9.
77. Lu L, et al. Aurora kinase A mediates c-Myc's oncogenic effects in hepatocellular carcinoma. Mol Carcinog. 2015;54(11):1467–79.
78. den Hollander J, et al. Aurora kinases A and B are up-regulated by Myc and are essential for maintenance of the malignant state. Blood. 2010;116(9):1498–505.
79. Brockmann M, et al. Small molecule inhibitors of aurora-a induce proteasomal degradation of N-myc in childhood neuroblastoma. Cancer Cell. 2013;24(1):75–89.

80. Keller UB, et al. Myc targets Cks1 to provoke the suppression of p27Kip1, proliferation and lymphomagenesis. Embo j. 2007;26(10):2562–74.
81. Mollaoglu G, et al. MYC drives progression of small cell lung cancer to a variant neuroendocrine subtype with vulnerability to aurora kinase inhibition. Cancer cell. 2017;31(2):270–85.
82. Melichar B, et al. Safety and activity of alisertib, an investigational aurora kinase A inhibitor, in patients with breast cancer, small-cell lung cancer, non-small-cell lung cancer, head and neck squamous-cell carcinoma, and gastro-oesophageal adenocarcinoma: a five-arm phase 2 study. Lancet Oncol. 2015;16(4):395–405.
83. Owonikoko T, et al. Randomized phase 2 study of investigational aurora A kinase (AAK) inhibitor alisertib (MLN8237)+ paclitaxel (P) vs placebo+ P as second line therapy for small-cell lung cancer (SCLC). Ann Oncol. 2016;27(6):493–496.
84. van Meerbeeck JP, Fennell DA, De Ruysscher DK. Small-cell lung cancer. Lancet. 2011;378(9804):1741–55.
85. Kaiser U, et al. Expression of bcl-2—protein in small cell lung cancer. Lung Cancer. 1996;15(1):31–40.
86. Lawson M, et al. Bcl-2 and β 1-integrin predict survival in a tissue microarray of small cell lung cancer. Br J Cancer. 2010;103(11):1710.
87. Hodgkinson CL, et al. Tumorigenicity and genetic profiling of circulating tumor cells in small-cell lung cancer. Nature Med. 2014;20(8):897.
88. Byers LA, et al. Proteomic profiling identifies dysregulated pathways in small cell lung cancer and novel therapeutic targets including PARP1. Cancer Discov. 2012;2(9):798–811.
89. Tse C, et al. ABT-263: a potent and orally bioavailable Bcl-2 family inhibitor. Cancer Res. 2008;68(9):3421–8.
90. Shoemaker AR, et al. Activity of the Bcl-2 family inhibitor ABT-263 in a panel of small cell lung cancer xenograft models. Clin Cancer Res. 2008;14(11):3268–77.
91. Hann CL, et al. Therapeutic efficacy of ABT-737, a selective inhibitor of BCL-2, in small cell lung cancer. Cancer Res. 2008;68(7):2321–8.
92. Sartorius UA, Krammer PH. Upregulation of bcl-2 is involved in the mediation of chemotherapy resistance in human small cell lung cancer cell lines. Int J Cancer. 2002;97(5):584–92.
93. Gandhi L, et al. Phase I study of Navitoclax (ABT-263), a novel Bcl-2 family inhibitor, in patients with small-cell lung cancer and other solid tumors. J Clin Oncol. 2011;29(7):909.
94. Rudin CM, et al. Phase II study of single-agent navitoclax (ABT-263) and biomarker correlates in patients with relapsed small cell lung cancer. Clin Cancer Res. 2012;18(11):3163–3169.
95. Lochmann TL, et al. Venetoclax is effective in small-cell lung cancers with high BCL-2 expression. Clin Cancer Res. 2018;24(2):360–9.
96. D'Angelo RC, et al. Notch reporter activity in breast cancer cell lines identifies a subset of cells with stem cell activity. Mol Cancer Ther. 2015;14(3):779–786.
97. Yuan X, Ma W. Mapped B-spline basis functions for shape design and isogeometric analysis over an arbitrary parameterization. Comput Methods Appl Mech Eng. 2014;269:87–107.
98. Ranganathan P, Weaver KL, Capobianco AJ. Notch signalling in solid tumours: a little bit of everything but not all the time. Nat Rev Cancer. 2011;11:338.
99. Donnem T, et al. Prognostic impact of Notch ligands and receptors in nonsmall cell lung cancer. Cancer. 2010;116(24):5676–85.
100. Yuan X, et al. Notch signaling: an emerging therapeutic target for cancer treatment. Cancer Lett. 2015;369(1):20–7.
101. Yamanda S, et al. Role of ephrinB2 in nonproductive angiogenesis induced by Delta-like 4 blockade. Blood. 2009;113(15):3631–9.
102. Strout P, et al. Abstract A49: anti-DLL4 antibodies inhibit cancer stem cells in small cell lung cancer. Mol Cancer Ther. 2013;12(11 Suppl):A49.
103. Smith DC, et al. A phase I dose escalation and expansion study of the anticancer stem cell agent demcizumab (Anti-DLL4) in patients with previously treated solid tumors. Clin Cancer Res. 2014;20(24):6295–303.
104. Bao H, et al. Evaluation of anti-cancer stem cell activity of the anti-DLL4 antibody MEDI0639 in a phase I clinical trial of SCLC. Am Soc Clin Oncol. 2016:e20093.
105. Falchook GS, et al. Phase I study of MEDI0639 in patients with advanced solid tumors. Am Soc Clin Oncol. 2015:3024.

Complexities of the Lung Tumor Microenvironment

Colt A. Egelston and Peter P. Lee

Abstract Successful development of the next wave of immunotherapies for lung cancer will require a deeper understanding of the tumor microenvironment (TME). Tumors are composed of heterogeneous cancer cells, stromal cells, and immune cells. Various subsets of tumor-infiltrating immune cells have been shown to have prominent protumor or anti-tumor effects, and correlate either positively or negatively with patient survival and response to therapy. Nonimmune tumor components, including fibroblasts, extracellular matrix, and various metabolites, also play increasingly recognized roles in shaping the TME. Furthermore, chronic inflammation often associated with lung cancer has been shown to transform the lung TME, highlighting the complex interplay between immune and nonimmune components of tumors. In this chapter, we review recent findings on the composition of the lung TME and how these functionally varied components modulate tumor progression and response to therapy.

Keywords Tumor microenvironment · Lung cancer · Nonimmune stromal cells · Immuno-oncology · Immunoediting

Introduction

Our current view of tumors has greatly expanded from simply a mass of homogeneous cancer cells to a complex ecosystem consisting of heterogeneous cancer cells, stromal cells, and immune cells—collectively termed the tumor microenvironment (TME). Mounting evidence demonstrate that patient outcome, in lung cancer and other cancers, is significantly impacted by the immune contexture of the tumor as a reflection of host immune surveillance. Furthermore, immune cell infiltration and function within tumors is now increasingly appreciated to be shaped not only by cancer cells but also by nonimmune stromal cells, extracellular matrix (ECM), and

C. A. Egelston · P. P. Lee (✉)
Department of Immuno-Oncology, Beckman Research Institute, City of Hope,
Duarte, CA, USA
e-mail: plee@coh.org

© Springer Nature Switzerland AG 2019   179
R. Salgia (ed.), *Targeted Therapies for Lung Cancer*, Current Cancer Research,
https://doi.org/10.1007/978-3-030-17832-1_9

metabolic activity. Recent advances in cancer immunotherapy have demonstrated significant clinical successes, especially in patients with preexisting, antitumor-immune activity. A paradigm shift in cancer treatment has occurred, with immune modulating agents becoming the foundation rather than regimens that solely target cancer cells or cancer cell pathways. Here, we will discuss the various immune (adaptive and innate), nonimmune, and extracellular components that make up the tumor microenvironment. The complex interweaving of these components has been shown to have a profound impact on patient response to therapy and clinical outcome.

The presence of immune cells within tumors is now widely accepted as associated with beneficial outcome in a multitude of cancer types, including lung cancer [21, 28]. However, immune infiltration of different tumors can vary widely, with a mix of protumor and antitumor immune cell subsets that reflects the yin-yang nature of the mature immune system [66]. For instance, while CD8+ T cell infiltration into tumors is prognostically favorable, infiltration of FOXP3+ CD4+ regulatory T cells is unfavorable [32]. Numerous studies such as these have reinforced the central idea that infiltration of the TME by specific immune cell types, rather than immune cells in general, is critical for prognostic and therapeutic benefit for cancer patients. Thus, while immune cell subsets can be broadly categorized as either innate (dendritic cells, macrophages, neutrophils, mast cells, basophils, natural killer cells) or adaptive (T cells, B cells), immuno-oncology research must carefully consider the protumor or anti-tumor facets of each of these elements (Fig. 1).

Immune Features of the TME

Early studies in murine models demonstrated that lack of functional immune cells allowed for more rapid outgrowth of both induced and spontaneous tumors [77]. Interactions between immune cells and cancer cells go beyond simple immune surveillance, as under immune pressure the more immunogenic subclones of cancer cells are removed by immune cells, allowing for outgrowth of other less immunogenic subclones of cancer cells. This paradoxical phenomenon, now commonly termed "immunoediting," encompasses elimination of cancer cells by immune cells, equilibrium between cancer cell growth and immune control of cancer cells, and escape of cancer cell subclones from recognition by immune cells leading to clinically observable manifestations of cancer [51].

CD8+ cytotoxic T cells are central to immune recognition and elimination of cancer cells. Tumor-reactive CD8+ T cells that are able to specifically recognize and kill cancer cells have been identified in both small cell lung cancer (SCLC) and non-small cell lung cancer (NSCLC) [94]. In the clinic, adoptive cellular therapy of autologous tumor infiltrating lymphocytes (TILs) in combination with the cytokine IL-2 led to increased overall survival and reduced time to relapse among Stage III NSCLC patients [70]. Expression of human leukocyte antigen (HLA) class I molecules, which mediate antigen peptide presentation to CD8+ T cell receptors, has been shown to have a critical role in immune surveillance of lung cancer.

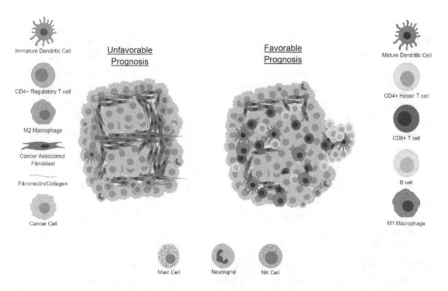

Fig. 1 Tumor microenvironment composition correlates with patient outcomes. The presences or absences of certain immune and nonimmune cell subsets have been associated with patient prognosis, either unfavorable or favorable. Immature dendritic cells, CD4+ regulatory T cells, M2 macrophages, and cancer associated fibroblasts have all negatively associated with relapse-free outcome. On the other hand, the presence of mature dendritic cells, CD4+ helper T cells, CD8+ T cells, B cells, and M1 macrophages have associated positively with relapse-free outcome. The role of other immune subsets, such as mast cells, neutrophils, and NK cells is less clear in the tumor microenvironment of lung cancer tumors

Downregulation of HLA class I expression in NSCLC tumors was found to contain lower densities of CD8+ T cells and associate with poor prognosis [49]. Lung cancer cells with loss of HLA class I molecules have indeed exhibited the ability to escape from CD8+ T cell-mediated killing, highlighting CD8+ T cell recognition of tumor antigen as critical for immune-mediated control of cancer cell growth [83]. As a result, an explosion of preclinical and clinical studies to evaluate the mechanisms of immune cell recognition of cancer cells has occurred over the past two decades.

Early searches for the antigens of lung tumor-specific T cells focused on those overexpressed by cancer cells relative to normal lung epithelial cells [45]. These antigens included melanoma associated antigen A3 (MAGE-A3), mucin-1 (MUC-1), and epidermal growth factor (EGF). Clinical trials involving vaccination attempts to elicit antitumor immunity via these antigens have yielded mixed or negative results, although efforts to improve efficacy and identify biomarkers of response continue [13, 74, 92].

More recent work in identifying CD8+ T cell targets within the TME have focused on mutation derived neoantigens [76]. This shift in focus to neoantigens from overexpressed self-antigens was motivated by the discovery that tumor-reactive T cells in patients responsive to immune checkpoint blockade (ICB) therapy are often specific for neoantigens [37]. In lung cancer, the level of neoantigen burden has been linked to overall survival in patients and is predictive of response to ICB therapy [60, 72]. Furthermore, neoantigen specificity by CD8+ T cells has also been described in checkpoint blockade responsive lung cancer patients [4]. Unsurprisingly then, recent studies have conclusively found that lung cancer patients with a history of smoking have higher tumor mutational burdens and importantly a higher overall response rate to checkpoint blockade therapies [20, 53]. Currently the evolution of neoantigen expression and reactivity by CD8+ T cells in the context of immunotherapy pressure is being studied to understand resistance and relapse in these settings. In a return to interest for vaccines, neoantigen vaccines have demonstrated efficacy in cancer patients and are currently in preclinical testing for lung cancer [39, 67].

A recently described subset of CD8+ T cells termed resident memory T cells (TRM) has been shown to be of particular importance in immune control of cancer cells [24]. TRM expression of the integrin CD103 allows for their attachment to epithelial (cancer) cells via binding to E-cadherin. Among other molecular features of TRM, this allows for retention of TRM within epithelial cell-rich tissues [27]. This retention contrasts TRMs from other memory T cells that recirculate amongst the blood to lymphoid tissue; instead, TRMs are poised at peripheral sites for immediate responses to antigen encounter [59]. CD8+ TRM have been linked to prognostic survival and to mediate cytolytic killing of autologous cancer cells in NSCLC patients [22]. Importantly, the association between CD8+ TRM presence in the TME with NSCLC patient survival has been found to be independent of the overall density CD8+ T cells, highlighting CD8+ TRM as a cornerstone of antitumor immunity within the TME [30]. Recent preclinical efforts to establish CD8+ TRM at mucosal sites using cancer vaccines have demonstrated efficacy, suggesting a new wave of vaccine-based approaches eliciting tumor-specific TRM may soon yield results in the clinic [62].

Despite the presence of tumor-reactive CD8+ T cells within the TME, cancer cell growth often outraces the immune system capacity for control, resulting in the chronic presence of tumor antigens [90]. Repeated exposure of tumor-specific CD8+ T cells to their cognate antigens, in combination with exposure to various TME inflammatory cues, often results in induction of T cell dysfunction. This dysfunction can be described as a general loss of polyfunctional capacity to exert various effector functions, such as effector cytokine secretion, cytotoxic capacity, and proliferation—in a process termed T cell exhaustion [95]. Tumor antigen-induced T cell exhaustion has been described in progressing lung tumors, which includes accumulated CD8+ T cell dysfunction and expression of inhibitory checkpoint molecules, such as PD-1, LAG-3, and TIM-3 [38, 89]. An understanding of the characteristics of exhausted T cells and the ability of these checkpoint molecules to suppress T cells has led to development of numerous checkpoint blockade monoclonal antibody therapies. Antibodies targeting PD-1 and its ligand PD-L1 have demonstrated the ability to restore functional T cell receptor signaling in T cells, which is normally deactivated via PD-1:PD-L1 engagement [3, 17, 26].

While reduced T cell functionality within the TME may reflect failure to control tumor growth, recent work also point to the presence of exhausted T cells as indicative of an immune response to tumor antigen. Indeed, the presence of PD-1$^+$ CD8$^+$ T cells predicts response to PD-1 targeting checkpoint blockade monoclonal antibody therapy [88]. Additionally, expression of the ligand for PD-1, PD-L1 is thought to reflect interferon gamma secretion and effector activity by CD8$^+$ T cells within the TME. Interestingly, PD-L1 expression is predictive of response to PD-1 blockade in NSCLC, but not SCLC, suggesting differences between the two in some aspects of CD8$^+$ T cell tumor reactivity [8, 10]. Further research is needed to understand what TME features and T cell qualities predict response to checkpoint blockade and how checkpoint blockade therapies can reinvigorate these exhausted CD8$^+$ T cell responses to cancer cells.

Importantly, CD8$^+$ T cells do not function independently of other immune subsets within the TME. CD4$^+$ T helper cells, which have a critical role in providing cytokine support for CD8$^+$ T cells, have an important role as well. Studies have shown that NSCLC tumors infiltrated with high levels of CD8$^+$ T cells, but low levels of CD4$^+$ T cells still lack favorable prognostic outcome [43]. Instead, concurrent infiltration of both CD8$^+$ T cells and CD4$^+$ T cells allows for potent antitumor activity. In contrast to the beneficial effects of CD4$^+$ T helper cells, regulatory CD4$^+$ T cells have been shown to exert protumor effects within the TME, and lung tumors with higher levels of regulatory CD4$^+$ T cells have been shown to have poor outcome in patients [50, 86].

Natural killer (NK) cells are known to kill HLA-deficient/mismatched target cells. However, despite the frequent loss of HLA molecules on lung cancer cells, NK cells are rarely found within NSCLC tumors [14]. Nonetheless, levels of NK cells within the TME have been associated with positive prognosis in lung cancer patients, although larger confirmatory studies are needed [46]. In contrast, presence of other innate immune subtypes within the lung TME has lacked prognostic significance. Tumor infiltration of neutrophils has been shown to correlate with markers of circulating inflammatory mediators such as C-reactive protein but has no clear association with prognosis [15]. Mast cells, important mediators of inflammatory factors such as histamine, have been shown to correlate with vasculature formation and cancer cell proliferation, but also have not been tied to prognostic outcome [48, 85, 91].

Antigen presenting cells (APCs) have also been shown to have an important role to support T cell function within the lung TME. Recent work demonstrated the critical role of dendritic cells in promoting CD8$^+$ T cell function within tumors [84]. However, dendritic cells analyzed from lung tumors have been shown to lack maturation markers or full antigen presentation capacity [69]. Clear evidence for the local role of dendritic cells within the lung TME was also shown by demonstrating a positive correlation between mature dendritic cell levels and levels of CD8$^+$ effector cells within the NSCLC TME [34].

The role of B cells in cancer is less clear. In addition to producing antibodies, B cells also have antigen presentation functions and can produce various cytokines. Presence of activated B cells within NSCLC tumors correlates with increased level of interferon-γ producing CD4$^+$ T cells, while less activated B cells correlated with increased levels of regulatory CD4+ T cells [12]. Overall, the density of B cells within the TME correlates with overall survival in NSCLC patients [2]. Tumor-infiltrating B cells tend to form tertiary lymphoid structures (TLSs) in the periphery of tumors; TLSs are often seen as aggregates of B cells, T cells, and mature dendritic cells in proximity to high endothelial venules. Likely a site for antigen exchange, presentation, and T cell proliferation, TLSs themselves are prognostically favorable in NSCLC patients [21, 33].

While macrophages are potent APCs, they may have both protumor and antitumor roles within the TME. Tumor associated macrophages (TAMs) may be subclassified according to their pro-inflammatory (M1) or anti-inflammatory (M2) functions [57]. M1 macrophages produce IL-1β, TNF-α, IL-6, and IL-12, while M2 macrophages produce potent T cell inhibitors IL-10 and arginase. NSCLC tumors with elevated levels of M1 macrophages had increased survival as compared to those with elevated levels of M2 macrophages [57]. Recent work characterizing lung TAMs in great detail has also suggested that the cellular origin of macrophages, whether embryonic resident macrophages or migratory monocyte, may be linked to their protumor or antitumor potential, respectively [56]. In support of this, alveolar macrophages have been demonstrated to precondition a "metastatic niche" within the lung, for other tumor types via TGFβ mediate suppression of dendritic cell and T cell function [18, 79].

Nonimmune Features of the TME

The importance of stroma-cancer and stroma-immune interactions within the TME is now becoming more appreciated. NSCLC patients with stroma-rich tumors (>50% stroma) have decreased overall survival as compared with stroma-poor (<50% stroma) tumors [96]. Fibrous-rich tissue features, such as large fibroblasts and thick collagen deposits, within lung tumors have been associated with unfavorable outcome in treatment-naïve cancer patients [87]. Fibroblasts found within the TME are termed cancer associated fibroblasts (CAFs) and are noted for their expression of α-smooth muscle actin, fibroblast specific protein-1, and fibroblast activating protein [5]. How CAFs arise from normal tissues in response to cancer remains unclear. Preclinical research pointed to activation of quiescent normal tissue fibroblasts, epithelial to mesenchymal transition (EMT), recruitment of progenitors from bone marrow, and also endothelial to mesenchymal transition as potential mechanisms [97]. Acquisition of CAF features are most likely elicited by cancer cell production of transforming growth factor-β (TGF-β), platelet-derived growth factor (PDGF), epidermal growth factor (EGF), and fibroblast growth factor (FGF) [98]. Adding to this complexity, recent studies using single cell sequencing technology have shown that the lung cancer TME may contain over 50 subtypes of stromal cells, ranging from endothelial to mesenchymal to fibroblasts, stressing the need for further studies to understand the complex stromal ecosystem of the TME [52].

Cancer cells in near proximity to CAFs displayed features of increased metastatic potential, such as loss of E-cadherin and increased expression of matrix metalloproteinases. CAF secreted IL-6 and TGF-β propagate EMT of neighboring cancer cells and resistance to chemotherapy induced cytotoxicity [1, 80]. CAF production of tryptophan 2,3-dioxygenase (TDO2), which converts tryptophan to kynurenine, has also demonstrated the ability to promote EMT transition and metastatic features [44]. Similarly, CAF secreted cytokines have been shown to promote CD4+ T cell conversion to regulatory T cells, thereby dampening the immune response within the TME [50]. As a result, CAF mediate increased metastatic potential of neighboring cancer cells and spread of disseminated disease [93].

Given the importance of CD8+ T cell elimination of cancer cells for control of disease and metastatic spread, the effects of the TME on CD8+ T cell infiltration into cancer nests has been an area of major translational research interest. Analysis of immune infiltration via immunohistochemistry approaches revealed that spatial location, rather than simply overall density, is important in lung cancer patient survival. Tumors are composed geographically of epithelial cell-derived "cancer nests" with intervening stromal areas composed of fibroblasts, mesenchymal stem cells, and various immune cells. CD8+ T cell and macrophage infiltration into the cancer nests of NSCLC patient tumors has been associated with favorable prognosis [48]. Undoubtedly, therefore, spatial relationships between cancer cells, immune cells, and nonimmune cells are heterogeneously diverse within and between patient tumors (Fig. 2). Understanding these relationships continues to be a major avenue

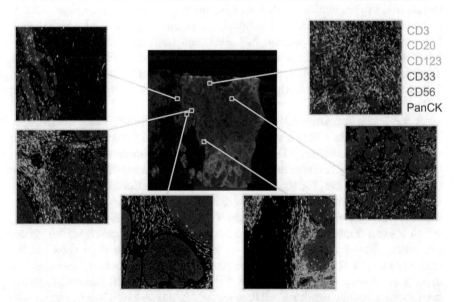

Fig. 2 Patient tumors have heterogeneous cell composition and spatial relationships. Multiplex immunohistochemistry allows for visualization of numerous cell types in relationship to each other in the tumor microenvironment. Various immune subsets can be identified by canonical markers (CD3, CD20, CD123, CD33, CD56) and examined for their relationship to epithelial cancer cells (panCytokeratin; panCK). (Lee Lab: Multiplex immunofluorescence images of a human tumor)

of research with the goal of identifying mechanisms and signatures of patient responses to therapy and prognostic outcomes.

Lack of T cell infiltration into cancer nests, despite general T cell infiltration into the tumor, has been termed "T cell exclusion" [47]. Different facets of the TME have been shown to contribute to the promotion of T cell exclusion. Fibroblast derived ECM, such as fibronectin and collagen, has been shown to have a critical effect on T cell motility within the TME and T cell capacity to infiltrate cancer nests. Thus, cancer nests with dense fibrous stroma surroundings exhibit limited T cell infiltration, whereas looser fibrous contents surrounding vascularization allows for T cell trafficking in and out of blood vessels [75]. CAF secreted chemokines, such as CXCL12, have also been shown to contribute to T cell exclusion from cancer nests [25]. In addition to ECM effects on T cell motility, macrophages within the stroma have been shown to mediate T cell exclusion from cancer nests via long-lasting T cell interactions [68]. Recently, TGF-β signaling in CAFs has been described as central to the stroma and ECM features promoting T cell exclusion and is currently a major target of therapeutic intervention for numerous cancer types [58].

Beyond ECM-driven exclusion of T cell infiltration into cancer nests, TME-derived metabolites have been shown to dampen T cell proliferation and inhibit T cell function. Indoleamine 2,3-dioxygenase (IDO), which may be secreted by a number of immune or nonimmune cells, has been shown to elicit increased IL-6 productions via the IDO metabolite kynurenic acid [82]. Cyclooxygenase-2 (COX-2), often overexpressed by lung cancer epithelial cells, and its derivative metabolite, prostaglandin E_2 (PGE2), have been shown to promote regulatory T cell formation in the TME [78]. Arginase, a potent suppressor of immune cell function via arginine depletion, has also been described to be produced by tumor cells themselves in a murine model as result of PGE2 signaling [73]. Together, metabolic regulation of the TME by COX2, IDO, arginase, and other enzymes creates a protumorigenic environment hostile to antitumor immune cell effector function.

Energy metabolism features of the TME are now increasingly being studied. The lung cancer TME has been shown to be heterogeneously composed of different metabolically active regions [41]. Increased uptake and consumption of glucose by cancer cells actively utilizing aerobic glycolysis is a common feature of numerous tumor types [40]. This process, also termed the Warburg effect, is a response to the increased energy demands of proliferative cancer cells and their hypoxic environment. Increased consumption of glucose, fatty acids, and amino acids by cancer cells leads to a competitive metabolic TME that may also alter immune cell function and phenotypes. T cell effector function within the TME has been shown to be critically dependent on glucose consumption, while T cell memory formation is dependent on fatty acid oxidation [16, 61]. Additionally, lipid accumulation has been shown to inhibit dendritic cell function, and hypoxia-driven hypoxia-inducible factor-1α signaling has been shown to upregulate PD-L1, together creating an immunosuppressive TME [42, 63].

Chronic Inflammation and the Lung Tumor Microenvironment

Chronic inflammation is strongly linked to the development and progression of cancer [35]. In its function of respiratory gas exchange, the lung tissue microenvironment is left susceptible to airborne sources of inflammation and irritants. Pulmonary disease in general has been attributed to inhaled environmental factors such as allergens, particulate matters, and toxic gases [11]. Inhalation of carcinogens, such as tobacco smoke, air pollution, arsenic, radon, or asbestos, is a major driver of lung cancer development [29]. While these carcinogens have clear roles in the induction of mutations in epithelial cells and resulting malignancy transformation, they have also been observed to mediate lung microenvironment remodeling and chronic inflammation [65]. Clearly, lung inflammation and lung cancer are intertwined, as patients with a history of chronic obstructive pulmonary disorder have a significantly higher risk for lung cancer development [81].

Lung cancer has long been associated with fibrosis of the lung and characteristic scarring similar to those observed with history of chronic inflammation [7]. Cigarette smoke has been demonstrated to hinder lung fibroblast proliferation, via p53 pathway induced senescence [64]. As a result, lung tissue exposed to chronic smoking and the associated epithelial damage has limited ability to repair tissue injuries and develop chronic inflammatory features. Additionally, smoking induces changes in secretory products of fibroblasts, including elevated levels of matrix metalloproteinases and IL-6, that allow for promotion of epithelial cell malignancy, growth, and possible EMT [19, 55]. In a murine model, cigarette smoke has been shown to induce recruitment of inflammatory immune cells to the lung microenvironment, likely contributing to a premalignant state conducive to cancer cell transformation [9].

Mechanistic studies have gone on to demonstrate that particulate matter and cigarette smoke elicit toll-like receptor signaling and pro-inflammatory responses in lung epithelial cells [6]. Asbestos and silica have specifically been demonstrated to elicit IL-1β production by macrophages via NALP3 inflammasome signaling [23]. Together, IL-1β and toll-like receptor sensing of particulate matter have been demonstrated to be critical to inflammation and fibrosis in the pulmonary tract [31]. Further evidence of the effects of inhalation of toxins on the lung TME, a comparison of the immune composition of lung tumors from patients with or without a history of smoking demonstrated increased levels of activated mast cells and activated CD4$^+$ T cells in the smoking history cohort [54]. These immune alterations were linked to altered chemokine network expression and likely to inflammation-induced perturbations of the lung microenvironment.

A greater understanding of the role of chronic inflammation through environmental toxins on lung cancer development has led to potential sites of therapeutic intervention. Anti-inflammatory agents, such as COX-2 inhibitors, have achieved mixed results in the prevention or treatment of lung cancer [36]. However, IL-1β targeting monoclonal antibody therapy (canakinumab) has demonstrated impressive reduced incidence of lung cancer in a large cohort of patients with atherosclerotic disease [71]. Canakinumab treatment was also associated with decreased levels of circulating CRP and IL-6, indicating successful reduction of systemic inflammation. Intriguingly, this trial demonstrated slightly increased benefit of the anti-inflammatory therapy in current smokers. Together, these results highlight the role of inflammation in lung cancer progression and demonstrate the potential of anti-inflammatory inhibitors in cancer prevention and therapy.

Conclusion

Over the past decade, a dramatically new perspective of the lung TME has emerged. Rather than a mass of homogeneous cancer cells, each tumor represents a unique complex ecosystem consisting of heterogeneous cancer cells, stromal cells, and immune cells. The complex interplay between these diverse cell types determines clinical outcome and response to therapy. As such, cancer treatments must progress beyond surgery, radiation, and chemotherapy to a multimodal therapeutic approach that takes into account the complexities of the TME. While emergence of the immune checkpoint blockade era has provided new technologies to stimulate T cell proliferation and reinvigoration from exhaustion, combinatorial approaches to synergize with checkpoint blockade are currently a major area of research. Reduction of suppressive macrophages, enhancement of dendritic cell function, and modulation of ECM and stromal barriers are some examples of potential targets to increase therapeutic efficacy and durable responses in patients. To achieve these goals, recent advances in single cell sequencing, high-dimensional flow cytometry, and multiplex immunohistochemistry will allow for an unprecedented view of the TME before and after therapeutic intervention—hopefully leading soon to unprecedented therapeutic success in the clinic for lung cancer patients.

References

1. Abulaiti A, Shintani Y, Funaki S, Nakagiri T, Inoue M, Sawabata N, Minami M, Okumura M. Interaction between non-small-cell lung cancer cells and fibroblasts via enhancement of TGF-beta signaling by IL-6. Lung Cancer. 2013;82:204–13.
2. Al-Shibli KI, Donnem T, Al-Saad S, Persson M, Bremnes RM, Busund LT. Prognostic effect of epithelial and stromal lymphocyte infiltration in non-small cell lung cancer. Clin Cancer Res. 2008;14:5220–7.
3. Alsaab HO, Sau S, Alzhrani R, Tatiparti K, Bhise K, Kashaw SK, Iyer AK. PD-1 and PD-L1 checkpoint signaling inhibition for cancer immunotherapy: mechanism, combinations, and clinical outcome. Front Pharmacol. 2017;8:561.
4. Anagnostou V, Smith KN, Forde PM, Niknafs N, Bhattacharya R, White J, Zhang T, Adleff V, Phallen J, Wali N, et al. Evolution of neoantigen landscape during immune checkpoint blockade in non-small cell lung cancer. Cancer Discov. 2017;7:264–76.
5. Augsten M. Cancer-associated fibroblasts as another polarized cell type of the tumor microenvironment. Front Oncol. 2014;4:62.

6. Bauer RN, Diaz-Sanchez D, Jaspers I. Effects of air pollutants on innate immunity: the role of Toll-like receptors and nucleotide-binding oligomerization domain-like receptors. J Allergy Clin Immunol. 2012;129:14–24; quiz 25–16.

7. Bobba RK, Holly JS, Loy T, Perry MC. Scar carcinoma of the lung: a historical perspective. Clin Lung Cancer. 2011;12:148–54.

8. Borghaei H, Paz-Ares L, Horn L, Spigel DR, Steins M, Ready NE, Chow LQ, Vokes EE, Felip E, Holgado E, et al. Nivolumab versus docetaxel in advanced nonsquamous non-small-cell lung cancer. N Engl J Med. 2015;373:1627–39.

9. Bracke KR, D'Hulst AI, Maes T, Moerloose KB, Demedts IK, Lebecque S, Joos GF, Brusselle GG. Cigarette smoke-induced pulmonary inflammation and emphysema are attenuated in CCR6-deficient mice. J Immunol. 2006;177:4350–9.

10. Brahmer J, Reckamp KL, Baas P, Crino L, Eberhardt WE, Poddubskaya E, Antonia S, Pluzanski A, Vokes EE, Holgado E, et al. Nivolumab versus docetaxel in advanced squamous-cell non-small-cell lung cancer. N Engl J Med. 2015;373:123–35.

11. Brain JD. The respiratory tract and the environment. Environ Health Perspect. 1977;20:113–26.

12. Bruno TC, Ebner PJ, Moore BL, Squalls OG, Waugh KA, Eruslanov EB, Singhal S, Mitchell JD, Franklin WA, Merrick DT, et al. Antigen-presenting intratumoral B cells affect CD4(+) TIL phenotypes in non-small cell lung cancer patients. Cancer Immunol Res. 2017;5:898–907.

13. Butts C, Socinski MA, Mitchell PL, Thatcher N, Havel L, Krzakowski M, Nawrocki S, Ciuleanu TE, Bosquee L, Trigo JM, et al. Tecemotide (L-BLP25) versus placebo after chemo-radiotherapy for stage III non-small-cell lung cancer (START): a randomised, double-blind, phase 3 trial. Lancet Oncol. 2014;15:59–68.

14. Carrega P, Ferlazzo G. Natural killers are made not born: how to exploit NK cells in lung malignancies. Front Immunol. 2017;8:277.

15. Carus A, Ladekarl M, Hager H, Pilegaard H, Nielsen PS, Donskov F. Tumor-associated neutrophils and macrophages in non-small cell lung cancer: no immediate impact on patient outcome. Lung Cancer. 2013;81:130–7.

16. Chang CH, Qiu J, O'Sullivan D, Buck MD, Noguchi T, Curtis JD, Chen Q, Gindin M, Gubin MM, van der Windt GJ, et al. Metabolic competition in the tumor microenvironment is a driver of cancer progression. Cell. 2015;162:1229–41.

17. Chemnitz JM, Parry RV, Nichols KE, June CH, Riley JL. SHP-1 and SHP-2 associate with immunoreceptor tyrosine-based switch motif of programmed death 1 upon primary human T cell stimulation, but only receptor ligation prevents T cell activation. J Immunol. 2004;173:945–54.

18. Chen XW, Yu TJ, Zhang J, Li Y, Chen HL, Yang GF, Yu W, Liu YZ, Liu XX, Duan CF, et al. CYP4A in tumor-associated macrophages promotes pre-metastatic niche formation and metastasis. Oncogene. 2017;36:5045–57.

19. Coppe JP, Boysen M, Sun CH, Wong BJ, Kang MK, Park NH, Desprez PY, Campisi J, Krtolica A. A role for fibroblasts in mediating the effects of tobacco-induced epithelial cell growth and invasion. Mol Cancer Res MCR. 2008;6:1085–98.

20. Desrichard A, Kuo F, Chowell D, Lee KW, Riaz N, Wong RJ, Chan TA, Morris LGT. Tobacco smoking-associated alterations in the immune microenvironment of squamous cell carcinomas. J Natl Cancer Inst. 2018;110:1386–92.

21. Dieu-Nosjean MC, Antoine M, Danel C, Heudes D, Wislez M, Poulot V, Rabbe N, Laurans L, Tartour E, de Chaisemartin L, et al. Long-term survival for patients with non-small-cell lung cancer with intratumoral lymphoid structures. J Clin Oncol. 2008;26:4410–7.

22. Djenidi F, Adam J, Goubar A, Durgeau A, Meurice G, de Montpreville V, Validire P, Besse B, Mami-Chouaib F. CD8+CD103+ tumor-infiltrating lymphocytes are tumor-specific tissue-resident memory T cells and a prognostic factor for survival in lung cancer patients. J Immunol. 2015;194:3475–86.

23. Dostert C, Petrilli V, Van Bruggen R, Steele C, Mossman BT, Tschopp J. Innate immune activation through Nalp3 inflammasome sensing of asbestos and silica. Science. 2008;320:674–7.

24. Dumauthioz N, Labiano S, Romero P. Tumor resident memory T cells: new players in immune surveillance and therapy. Front Immunol. 2018;9:2076.
25. Feig C, Jones JO, Kraman M, Wells RJ, Deonarine A, Chan DS, Connell CM, Roberts EW, Zhao Q, Caballero OL, et al. Targeting CXCL12 from FAP-expressing carcinoma-associated fibroblasts synergizes with anti-PD-L1 immunotherapy in pancreatic cancer. Proc Natl Acad Sci U S A. 2013;110:20212–7.
26. Francisco LM, Salinas VH, Brown KE, Vanguri VK, Freeman GJ, Kuchroo VK, Sharpe AH. PD-L1 regulates the development, maintenance, and function of induced regulatory T cells. J Exp Med. 2009;206:3015–29.
27. Franciszkiewicz K, Le Floc'h A, Jalil A, Vigant F, Robert T, Vergnon I, Mackiewicz A, Benihoud K, Validire P, Chouaib S, et al. Intratumoral induction of CD103 triggers tumor-specific CTL function and CCR5-dependent T-cell retention. Cancer Res. 2009;69:6249–55.
28. Fridman WH, Pages F, Sautes-Fridman C, Galon J. The immune contexture in human tumours: impact on clinical outcome. Nat Rev Cancer. 2012;12:298–306.
29. Fucic A, Gamulin M, Ferencic Z, Rokotov DS, Katic J, Bartonova A, Lovasic IB, Merlo DF. Lung cancer and environmental chemical exposure: a review of our current state of knowledge with reference to the role of hormones and hormone receptors as an increased risk factor for developing lung cancer in man. Toxicol Pathol. 2010;38:849–55.
30. Ganesan AP, Clarke J, Wood O, Garrido-Martin EM, Chee SJ, Mellows T, Samaniego-Castruita D, Singh D, Seumois G, Alzetani A, et al. Tissue-resident memory features are linked to the magnitude of cytotoxic T cell responses in human lung cancer. Nat Immunol. 2017;18:940–50.
31. Gasse P, Mary C, Guenon I, Noulin N, Charron S, Schnyder-Candrian S, Schnyder B, Akira S, Quesniaux VF, Lagente V, et al. IL-1R1/MyD88 signaling and the inflammasome are essential in pulmonary inflammation and fibrosis in mice. J Clin Invest. 2007;117:3786–99.
32. Geng Y, Shao Y, He W, Hu W, Xu Y, Chen J, Wu C, Jiang J. Prognostic role of tumor-infiltrating lymphocytes in lung cancer: a meta-analysis. Cell Physiol Biochem. 2015;37:1560–71.
33. Germain C, Gnjatic S, Tamzalit F, Knockaert S, Remark R, Goc J, Lepelley A, Becht E, Katsahian S, Bizouard G, et al. Presence of B cells in tertiary lymphoid structures is associated with a protective immunity in patients with lung cancer. Am J Respir Crit Care Med. 2014;189:832–44.
34. Goc J, Germain C, Vo-Bourgais TK, Lupo A, Klein C, Knockaert S, de Chaisemartin L, Ouakrim H, Becht E, Alifano M, et al. Dendritic cells in tumor-associated tertiary lymphoid structures signal a Th1 cytotoxic immune contexture and license the positive prognostic value of infiltrating CD8+ T cells. Cancer Res. 2014;74:705–15.
35. Grivennikov SI, Greten FR, Karin M. Immunity, inflammation, and cancer. Cell. 2010;140:883–99.
36. Groen HJ, Sietsma H, Vincent A, Hochstenbag MM, van Putten JW, van den Berg A, Dalesio O, Biesma B, Smit HJ, Termeer A, et al. Randomized, placebo-controlled phase III study of docetaxel plus carboplatin with celecoxib and cyclooxygenase-2 expression as a biomarker for patients with advanced non-small-cell lung cancer: the NVALT-4 study. J Clin Oncol. 2011;29:4320–6.
37. Gubin MM, Zhang X, Schuster H, Caron E, Ward JP, Noguchi T, Ivanova Y, Hundal J, Arthur CD, Krebber WJ, et al. Checkpoint blockade cancer immunotherapy targets tumour-specific mutant antigens. Nature. 2014;515:577–81.
38. Guo X, Zhang Y, Zheng L, Zheng C, Song J, Zhang Q, Kang B, Liu Z, Jin L, Xing R, et al. Global characterization of T cells in non-small-cell lung cancer by single-cell sequencing. Nat Med. 2018a;24:978–85.
39. Guo Y, Lei K, Tang L. Neoantigen vaccine delivery for personalized anticancer immunotherapy. Front Immunol. 2018b;9:1499.
40. Hanahan D, Weinberg RA. Hallmarks of cancer: the next generation. Cell. 2011;144:646–74.
41. Hensley CT, Faubert B, Yuan Q, Lev-Cohain N, Jin E, Kim J, Jiang L, Ko B, Skelton R, Loudat L, et al. Metabolic heterogeneity in human lung tumors. Cell. 2016;164:681–94.

42. Herber DL, Cao W, Nefedova Y, Novitskiy SV, Nagaraj S, Tyurin VA, Corzo A, Cho HI, Celis E, Lennox B, et al. Lipid accumulation and dendritic cell dysfunction in cancer. Nat Med. 2010;16:880–6.
43. Hiraoka K, Miyamoto M, Cho Y, Suzuoki M, Oshikiri T, Nakakubo Y, Itoh T, Ohbuchi T, Kondo S, Katoh H. Concurrent infiltration by CD8+ T cells and CD4+ T cells is a favourable prognostic factor in non-small-cell lung carcinoma. Br J Cancer. 2006;94:275–80.
44. Hsu YL, Hung JY, Chiang SY, Jian SF, Wu CY, Lin YS, Tsai YM, Chou SH, Tsai MJ, Kuo PL. Lung cancer-derived galectin-1 contributes to cancer associated fibroblast-mediated cancer progression and immune suppression through TDO2/kynurenine axis. Oncotarget. 2016;7:27584–98.
45. Iyengar P, Gerber DE. Locally advanced lung cancer: an optimal setting for vaccines and other immunotherapies. Cancer J. 2013;19:247–62.
46. Jin S, Deng Y, Hao JW, Li Y, Liu B, Yu Y, Shi FD, Zhou QH. NK cell phenotypic modulation in lung cancer environment. PLoS One. 2014;9:e109976.
47. Joyce JA, Fearon DT. T cell exclusion, immune privilege, and the tumor microenvironment. Science. 2015;348:74–80.
48. Kawai O, Ishii G, Kubota K, Murata Y, Naito Y, Mizuno T, Aokage K, Saijo N, Nishiwaki Y, Gemma A, et al. Predominant infiltration of macrophages and CD8(+) T Cells in cancer nests is a significant predictor of survival in stage IV nonsmall cell lung cancer. Cancer. 2008;113:1387–95.
49. Kikuchi E, Yamazaki K, Torigoe T, Cho Y, Miyamoto M, Oizumi S, Hommura F, Dosaka-Akita H, Nishimura M. HLA class I antigen expression is associated with a favorable prognosis in early stage non-small cell lung cancer. Cancer Sci. 2007;98:1424–30.
50. Kinoshita T, Ishii G, Hiraoka N, Hirayama S, Yamauchi C, Aokage K, Hishida T, Yoshida J, Nagai K, Ochiai A. Forkhead box P3 regulatory T cells coexisting with cancer associated fibroblasts are correlated with a poor outcome in lung adenocarcinoma. Cancer Sci. 2013;104:409–15.
51. Koebel CM, Vermi W, Swann JB, Zerafa N, Rodig SJ, Old LJ, Smyth MJ, Schreiber RD. Adaptive immunity maintains occult cancer in an equilibrium state. Nature. 2007;450:903–7.
52. Lambrechts D, Wauters E, Boeckx B, Aibar S, Nittner D, Burton O, Bassez A, Decaluwe H, Pircher A, Van den Eynde K, et al. Phenotype molding of stromal cells in the lung tumor microenvironment. Nat Med. 2018;24:1277–89.
53. Li B, Huang X, Fu L. Impact of smoking on efficacy of PD-1/PD-L1 inhibitors in non-small cell lung cancer patients: a meta-analysis. OncoTargets Ther. 2018a;11:3691–6.
54. Li X, Li J, Wu P, Zhou L, Lu B, Ying K, Chen E, Lu Y, Liu P. Smoker and non-smoker lung adenocarcinoma is characterized by distinct tumor immune microenvironments. Oncoimmunology. 2018b;7:e1494677.
55. Liu Y, Luo F, Xu Y, Wang B, Zhao Y, Xu W, Shi L, Lu X, Liu Q. Epithelial-mesenchymal transition and cancer stem cells, mediated by a long non-coding RNA, HOTAIR, are involved in cell malignant transformation induced by cigarette smoke extract. Toxicol Appl Pharmacol. 2015;282:9–19.
56. Loyher PL, Hamon P, Laviron M, Meghraoui-Kheddar A, Goncalves E, Deng Z, Torstensson S, Bercovici N, Baudesson de Chanville C, Combadiere B, et al. Macrophages of distinct origins contribute to tumor development in the lung. J Exp Med. 2018;215:2536–53.
57. Mantovani A, Sozzani S, Locati M, Allavena P, Sica A. Macrophage polarization: tumor-associated macrophages as a paradigm for polarized M2 mononuclear phagocytes. Trends Immunol. 2002;23:549–55.
58. Mariathasan S, Turley SJ, Nickles D, Castiglioni A, Yuen K, Wang Y, Kadel EE III, Koeppen H, Astarita JL, Cubas R, et al. TGFbeta attenuates tumour response to PD-L1 blockade by contributing to exclusion of T cells. Nature. 2018;554:544–8.
59. Masopust D, Vezys V, Marzo AL, Lefrancois L. Preferential localization of effector memory cells in nonlymphoid tissue. Science. 2001;291:2413–7.

60. McGranahan N, Furness AJ, Rosenthal R, Ramskov S, Lyngaa R, Saini SK, Jamal-Hanjani M, Wilson GA, Birkbak NJ, Hiley CT, et al. Clonal neoantigens elicit T cell immunoreactivity and sensitivity to immune checkpoint blockade. Science. 2016;351:1463–9.
61. Michalek RD, Gerriets VA, Jacobs SR, Macintyre AN, MacIver NJ, Mason EF, Sullivan SA, Nichols AG, Rathmell JC. Cutting edge: distinct glycolytic and lipid oxidative metabolic programs are essential for effector and regulatory CD4+ T cell subsets. J Immunol. 2011;186:3299–303.
62. Nizard M, Roussel H, Diniz MO, Karaki S, Tran T, Voron T, Dransart E, Sandoval F, Riquet M, Rance B, et al. Induction of resident memory T cells enhances the efficacy of cancer vaccine. Nat Commun. 2017;8:15221.
63. Noman MZ, Desantis G, Janji B, Hasmim M, Karray S, Dessen P, Bronte V, Chouaib S. PD-L1 is a novel direct target of HIF-1alpha, and its blockade under hypoxia enhanced MDSC-mediated T cell activation. J Exp Med. 2014;211:781–90.
64. Nyunoya T, Monick MM, Klingelhutz A, Yarovinsky TO, Cagley JR, Hunninghake GW. Cigarette smoke induces cellular senescence. Am J Respir Cell Mol Biol. 2006;35:681–8.
65. O'Callaghan DS, O'Donnell D, O'Connell F, O'Byrne KJ. The role of inflammation in the pathogenesis of non-small cell lung cancer. J Thorac Oncol. 2010;5:2024–36.
66. Ostrand-Rosenberg S. Immune surveillance: a balance between protumor and antitumor immunity. Curr Opin Genet Dev. 2008;18:11–8.
67. Ott PA, Hu Z, Keskin DB, Shukla SA, Sun J, Bozym DJ, Zhang W, Luoma A, Giobbie-Hurder A, Peter L, et al. An immunogenic personal neoantigen vaccine for patients with melanoma. Nature. 2017;547:217–21.
68. Peranzoni E, Lemoine J, Vimeux L, Feuillet V, Barrin S, Kantari-Mimoun C, Bercovici N, Guerin M, Biton J, Ouakrim H, et al. Macrophages impede CD8 T cells from reaching tumor cells and limit the efficacy of anti-PD-1 treatment. Proc Natl Acad Sci U S A. 2018;115:E4041–50.
69. Perrot I, Blanchard D, Freymond N, Isaac S, Guibert B, Pacheco Y, Lebecque S. Dendritic cells infiltrating human non-small cell lung cancer are blocked at immature stage. J Immunol. 2007;178:2763–9.
70. Ratto GB, Zino P, Mirabelli S, Minuti P, Aquilina R, Fantino G, Spessa E, Ponte M, Bruzzi P, Melioli G. A randomized trial of adoptive immunotherapy with tumor-infiltrating lymphocytes and interleukin-2 versus standard therapy in the postoperative treatment of resected nonsmall cell lung carcinoma. Cancer. 1996;78:244–51.
71. Ridker PM, MacFadyen JG, Thuren T, Everett BM, Libby P, Glynn RJ, Group CT. Effect of interleukin-1beta inhibition with canakinumab on incident lung cancer in patients with atherosclerosis: exploratory results from a randomised, double-blind, placebo-controlled trial. Lancet. 2017;390:1833–42.
72. Rizvi NA, Hellmann MD, Snyder A, Kvistborg P, Makarov V, Havel JJ, Lee W, Yuan J, Wong P, Ho TS, et al. Cancer immunology. Mutational landscape determines sensitivity to PD-1 blockade in non-small cell lung cancer. Science. 2015;348:124–8.
73. Rodriguez PC, Hernandez CP, Quiceno D, Dubinett SM, Zabaleta J, Ochoa JB, Gilbert J, Ochoa AC. Arginase I in myeloid suppressor cells is induced by COX-2 in lung carcinoma. J Exp Med. 2005;202:931–9.
74. Rodriguez PC, Popa X, Martinez O, Mendoza S, Santiesteban E, Crespo T, Amador RM, Fleytas R, Acosta SC, Otero Y, et al. A phase III clinical trial of the epidermal growth factor vaccine CIMAvax-EGF as switch maintenance therapy in advanced non-small cell lung cancer patients. Clin Cancer Res. 2016;22:3782–90.
75. Salmon H, Franciszkiewicz K, Damotte D, Dieu-Nosjean MC, Validire P, Trautmann A, Mami-Chouaib F, Donnadieu E. Matrix architecture defines the preferential localization and migration of T cells into the stroma of human lung tumors. J Clin Invest. 2012;122:899–910.
76. Schumacher TN, Scheper W, Kvistborg P. Cancer neoantigens. Annu Rev Immunol. 2018. https://www.ncbi.nlm.nih.gov/pubmed/29226910.

77. Shankaran V, Ikeda H, Bruce AT, White JM, Swanson PE, Old LJ, Schreiber RD. IFNgamma and lymphocytes prevent primary tumour development and shape tumour immunogenicity. Nature. 2001;410:1107–11.
78. Sharma S, Yang SC, Zhu L, Reckamp K, Gardner B, Baratelli F, Huang M, Batra RK, Dubinett SM. Tumor cyclooxygenase-2/prostaglandin E2-dependent promotion of FOXP3 expression and CD4+ CD25+ T regulatory cell activities in lung cancer. Cancer Res. 2005;65:5211–20.
79. Sharma SK, Chintala NK, Vadrevu SK, Patel J, Karbowniczek M, Markiewski MM. Pulmonary alveolar macrophages contribute to the premetastatic niche by suppressing antitumor T cell responses in the lungs. J Immunol. 2015;194:5529–38.
80. Shintani Y, Fujiwara A, Kimura T, Kawamura T, Funaki S, Minami M, Okumura M. IL-6 secreted from cancer-associated fibroblasts mediates chemoresistance in NSCLC by increasing epithelial-mesenchymal transition signaling. J Thorac Oncol. 2016;11:1482–92.
81. Skillrud DM, Offord KP, Miller RD. Higher risk of lung cancer in chronic obstructive pulmonary disease. A prospective, matched, controlled study. Ann Intern Med. 1986;105:503–7.
82. Smith C, Chang MY, Parker KH, Beury DW, DuHadaway JB, Flick HE, Boulden J, Sutanto-Ward E, Soler AP, Laury-Kleintop LD, et al. IDO is a nodal pathogenic driver of lung cancer and metastasis development. Cancer Discov. 2012;2:722–35.
83. So T, Takenoyama M, Mizukami M, Ichiki Y, Sugaya M, Hanagiri T, Sugio K, Yasumoto K. Haplotype loss of HLA class I antigen as an escape mechanism from immune attack in lung cancer. Cancer Res. 2005;65:5945–52.
84. Spranger S, Dai D, Horton B, Gajewski TF. Tumor-residing Batf3 dendritic cells are required for effector T cell trafficking and adoptive T cell therapy. Cancer Cell. 2017;31:711–723 e714.
85. Stoyanov E, Uddin M, Mankuta D, Dubinett SM, Levi-Schaffer F. Mast cells and histamine enhance the proliferation of non-small cell lung cancer cells. Lung Cancer. 2012;75:38–44.
86. Suzuki K, Kadota K, Sima CS, Nitadori J, Rusch VW, Travis WD, Sadelain M, Adusumilli PS. Clinical impact of immune microenvironment in stage I lung adenocarcinoma: tumor interleukin-12 receptor beta2 (IL-12Rbeta2), IL-7R, and stromal FoxP3/CD3 ratio are independent predictors of recurrence. J Clin Oncol. 2013;31:490–8.
87. Takahashi Y, Ishii G, Taira T, Fujii S, Yanagi S, Hishida T, Yoshida J, Nishimura M, Nomori H, Nagai K, et al. Fibrous stroma is associated with poorer prognosis in lung squamous cell carcinoma patients. J Thorac Oncol. 2011;6:1460–7.
88. Thommen DS, Koelzer VH, Herzig P, Roller A, Trefny M, Dimeloe S, Kiialainen A, Hanhart J, Schill C, Hess C, et al. A transcriptionally and functionally distinct PD-1(+) CD8(+) T cell pool with predictive potential in non-small-cell lung cancer treated with PD-1 blockade. Nat Med. 2018;24:994–1004.
89. Thommen DS, Schreiner J, Muller P, Herzig P, Roller A, Belousov A, Umana P, Pisa P, Klein C, Bacac M, et al. Progression of lung cancer is associated with increased dysfunction of T cells defined by coexpression of multiple inhibitory receptors. Cancer Immunol Res. 2015;3:1344–55.
90. Thommen DS, Schumacher TN. T cell dysfunction in cancer. Cancer Cell. 2018;33:547–62.
91. Tomita M, Matsuzaki Y, Onitsuka T. Effect of mast cells on tumor angiogenesis in lung cancer. Ann Thorac Surg. 2000;69:1686–90.
92. Vansteenkiste JF, Cho BC, Vanakesa T, De Pas T, Zielinski M, Kim MS, Jassem J, Yoshimura M, Dahabreh J, Nakayama H, et al. Efficacy of the MAGE-A3 cancer immunotherapeutic as adjuvant therapy in patients with resected MAGE-A3-positive non-small-cell lung cancer (MAGRIT): a randomised, double-blind, placebo-controlled, phase 3 trial. Lancet Oncol. 2016;17:822–35.
93. Wang L, Cao L, Wang H, Liu B, Zhang Q, Meng Z, Wu X, Zhou Q, Xu K. Cancer-associated fibroblasts enhance metastatic potential of lung cancer cells through IL-6/STAT3 signaling pathway. Oncotarget. 2017;8:76116–28.
94. Weynants P, Thonnard J, Marchand M, Delos M, Boon T, Coulie PG. Derivation of tumor-specific cytolytic T-cell clones from two lung cancer patients with long survival. Am J Respir Crit Care Med. 1999;159:55–62.

95. Wherry EJ. T cell exhaustion. Nat Immunol. 2011;12:492–9.
96. Xi KX, Wen YS, Zhu CM, Yu XY, Qin RQ, Zhang XW, Lin YB, Rong TH, Wang WD, Chen YQ, et al. Tumor-stroma ratio (TSR) in non-small cell lung cancer (NSCLC) patients after lung resection is a prognostic factor for survival. J Thorac Dis. 2017;9:4017–26.
97. Zeisberg EM, Potenta S, Xie L, Zeisberg M, Kalluri R. Discovery of endothelial to mesenchymal transition as a source for carcinoma-associated fibroblasts. Cancer Res. 2007;67:10123–8.
98. Ziani L, Chouaib S, Thiery J. Alteration of the antitumor immune response by cancer-associated fibroblasts. Front Immunol. 2018;9:414.

KRAS-Mutated Lung Cancer

Arnab Basu and Jorge Nieva

Abstract A mutation in the Kirsten rat sarcoma virus transforming protein (KRAS) is the most common genomic driver identified in patients with lung adenocarcinoma. It is a key component of the PI3K and MAPK pathways and is an important regulator of cell proliferation and survival. Tobacco use and mutations in KRAS are strongly correlated and co-mutation of p53 or STK11 is common. KRAS is affected by upstream signaling from a variety of tyrosine kinase inhibitors including the epidermal growth factor receptor (EGFR) and ERBB2. Affected patients have a higher risk of death than with other driver mutations and, despite dozens of clinical trials attempting to find a specific inhibitor that is effective in this population, it has been a difficult drug target. There is substantial experience attempting to treat KRAS-mutated lung adenocarcinoma with the use of RAS/RAF multikinase inhibitors as well as inhibitors of both upstream and downstream proteins important in RAS signaling. We review the disappointing results from these clinical trials in lung cancer. However, more recently, there appears to be some improvement in outcome with immune checkpoint inhibitors in these patients.

Keywords KRAS · Lung cancer · EGFR · RAS signaling · Lung adenocarcinoma

Introduction

KRAS alterations (Fig. 1a, b) are among the most common identifiable driver mutations in lung cancer, affecting up to one-third of patients with non-small cell lung cancer (NSCLC). Unlike many other driver mutations, KRAS alterations are commonly seen with tobacco use and rarely occur in younger patients. KRAS-mutated lung cancer has been quite difficult to target directly, and attempts to inactivate

A. Basu · J. Nieva (✉)
Department of Medicine, Norris Comprehensive Cancer Center, University of Southern California, Los Angeles, CA, USA
e-mail: jorge.nieva@med.usc.edu

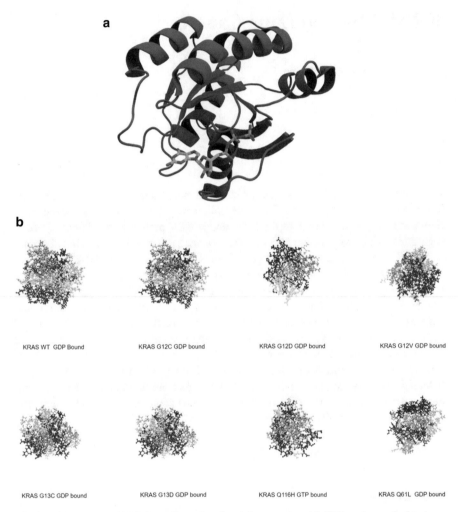

Fig. 1 (**a**) Wild-type KRAS three-dimensional protein structure with GTP analogue depicted attached, (**b**) Common KRAS mutants 3D conformal structures

either upstream and downstream proteins involved in RAS signaling have met with limited success to date. KRAS alterations are unlike the targetable tyrosine kinases epidermal growth factor receptor (EGFR), ERBB2, and MET and rearrangements of the anaplastic lymphoma kinase (ALK), RET, and ROS1 genes. These oncogenic drivers of lung cancer are highly druggable, with successful tyrosine kinase inhibitors, and targeted therapy has supplanted chemotherapy in the first-line treatment. However, to date, there has been no similar success with KRAS.

KRAS Biology

RAS genes were originally discovered in the 1960s through the study of oncogenic viruses in humans, a mouse leukemia virus found to induce sarcoma in rats by Kirsten and Harvey. Eventually, the Kirsten rat sarcoma virus transforming protein (KRAS) was first sequenced by Tsuchida and colleagues and other groups in 1982 [1]. Essentially, KRAS is a replication-defective transforming virus that encodes a protein originally described as p21. It is a component of the PI3K and MAPK pathways and hence is involved in cellular signaling related to proliferation and survival. KRAS is a proto-oncogene, in that in its mutated form, it transforms cells to a malignant phenotype. Abnormalities in KRAS have been associated with lung adenocarcinoma, colorectal carcinoma, and pancreatic carcinoma. In the Cancer Genome Atlas study (TCGA), 33% of lung adenocarcinomas were found to have mutations in KRAS. This is second in frequency only to mutations in p53. While KRAS amplification is associated with colorectal cancers, it is infrequently amplified in lung cancer [2]. The KRAS gene in humans is located on the short arm of chromosome 12 (12p12.1). KRAS undergoes alternative splicing, resulting in two proteins (KRAS4A/B) differing at their carboxyl terminals which are 188 and 189 amino acids in length. There are only minor differences in their biochemistry, KRAS4A undergoes palmitoylation, while KRAS4B does not [3].

The initial 165 codons are conserved across the RAS superfamily and the carboxyl terminal is associated with posttranslational modifications. Posttranslational modifications are important in the transport of the proteins to the correct locations in the cell to be active. All RAS proteins undergo farnesylation to their functional forms. While all newly translated RAS proteins are cytosolic, they are modified by the enzyme farnesyltransferase (FTase). The enzyme moves a moiety of FPP (farnesyl pyrophosphate) to the carboxyl terminal of the RAS protein, such as KRAS. This enables the KRAS protein to associate with the intracellular membrane, which is where it can respond to signals from upstream receptors as described below. Farnesylation provides a therapeutic target against KRAS and will be discussed in later sections. However, given the importance of the transport of KRAS to the plasma membrane, there are redundant systems such as geranylgeranylation by GGTase (geranylgeranyltransferase) which can rescue the protein. Figure 2 illustrates the simplified posttranslational processing of KRAS.

KRAS Signaling

KRAS is allosterically activated and binds to GTP in its active state, converting it to GDP. It is activated by several upstream tyrosine kinase receptors which include EGFR and integrins. The first step to activation is through the binding of such a ligand such as EGFR leading to its dimerization and phosphorylation [4]. RAS phosphorylation is determined by a balance of pro-phosphorylating

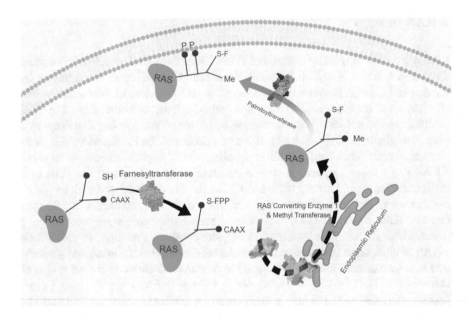

Fig. 2 Posttranslational modifications of RAS

guanine nucleotide exchange factors (GEFs) and negatively regulating GTPase-activating proteins (GAPs). Activated RAS can activate downstream effector rapidly accelerated fibrosarcoma (RAF) kinases which comprise ARAF, BRAF, and c-RAF or RAF1. The acronym RAF stands for rapidly accelerated fibrosarcoma [5]. Activated RAF in turn phosphorylates and activates the mitogen activated protein kinases MEK1 and MEK2 and in sequence the extracellular signal regulated kinases ERK1 and ERK2. These kinases are transported into the nucleus. ERK phosphorylates nuclear transcription factors like the ETS and c-JUN which ultimately lead to expression of cyclin-D and other cell cycle-promoting kinases [6]. RAS phosphorylation is determined by a balance of pro-phosphorylating guanine nucleotide exchange factors (GEFs) and negatively regulating GTPase-activating proteins (GAPs). Important RAS GEFs include son of sevenless 1 and 2 (SOS1 and SOS2) [7].

Apart from its action on the MAPK pathway, RAS can also directly activate the type 1 phosphatidylinositol-3-kinases (PI3K) which bind to membrane-bound PIP-2 converting it to PIP-3 and resulting in cascade activation of AKT. AKT is a serine threonine kinase and is a potent oncoprotein with several downstream targets including mTOR and BAX [8]. BAX is a negative regulator of apoptosis, while mTOR positively impacts protein synthesis in ribosomes through intermediary factors such as S6K. AKT also ubiquitinates FOXO, forkhead transcription factor of the class O, which leads to its destruction. Forkhead proteins are important in cell cycle progression regulation [9]. Figure 3 illustrates the major signaling effects of RAS in the cell.

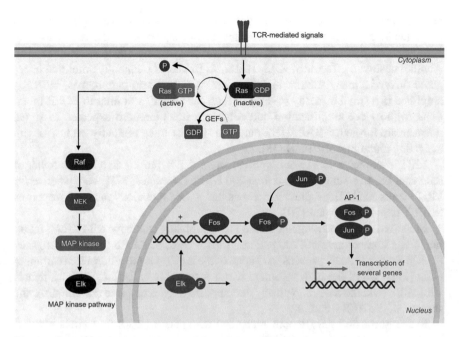

Fig. 3 KRAS-mediated intracellular signaling process: simplified representation

Table 1 Tyrosine kinase receptors that interact with KRAS in NSCLC

TKRs interacting with RAS	Expression/alteration (NSCLC)	References
EGFR	~25% (mutation)	[10]
ALK	~3% (rearrangement)	[22]
FGFR1	~3–5% (overexpression)	[14]
ErBB2	~4–6% (amplification/mutation)	[17]
MET	~30% (amplification/mutation)	[20]
Ddr1	~50% (expression)	[82]

KRAS Upstream Effectors

Upstream effectors of KRAS are primarily the tyrosine kinase receptors (TKRs) (Table 1). The most important upstream TKR effector of KRAS is the epidermal growth factor receptor or EGFR. Activation of the EGFR receptor leads to the dimerization and consequent phosphorylation of adaptor protein Grb-2 which in turns leads to SOS-mediated KRAS activation [10]. Mutations in KRAS are associated with decreased efficacy of EGFR blockade in lung cancer [11, 12]. Similar resistance also occurs in colorectal cancers, and EGFR inhibitors are hence not indicated in KRAS-mutated colorectal tumors [13]. However, other abnormal tyrosine kinase signaling also is affected by the KRAS status. For example, the fibroblast growth factor receptor (FGFR) is a TKR that signals through the RAS-RAF pathway [14]. It also activates the PI3K and JAK-STAT pathways [15]. FGFR is amplified in 20% and mutated in about 5% of lung squamous cell carcinomas [16]. Amplification of FGFR occurs in only about 5% of lung adenocarcinomas [14]. Another upstream effector of RAS, HER2, or ErBB2 is frequently amplified oncogenic driver in many tumors including breast and gastric carcinomas. HER2 is amplified in a small minority (4–6%) of lung cancers [17]. Similar to EGFR mutations, while Her2 amplification and activating mutations are expected to signal downstream through KRAS, Her2 mutations appear to be mutually exclusive with activating mutations of KRAS [18].

MET is another mutated or amplified target that is present in a large number of lung cancers. In a study of more than 200 NSCLC samples, 37% were positive for MET expression [19]. Studies have shown that KRAS mutations can mute responses to MET targeted therapies [20].

Mutations, ALK rearrangements tend to be mutually exclusive with KRAS mutations; in a study of almost 1700 patients, only 4 cases of KRAS mutants were seen to have abnormal ALK patterns, and none of these did met the criteria for rearrangement [21]. One of the rearrangement partners for ALK is EML4. EML4 interacts with KRAS via the MAPK pathway and appears to be a required condition for the survival of the ALK+ cell [22].

Recently, the discoidin domain receptor 1 (Ddr1) was a TKR found to be upregulated in the early phases of KRAS-mutated lung adenocarcinoma [23]. Ddr1 binds collagen and is involved in remodeling of the extracellular matrix and in cell migration. It acts via the MAPK as well as PI3K and notch pathways. In vivo murine models show potential therapeutic utility for DDR1 targeting in KRAS mutant tumor cell lines.

Mutant KRAS and Molecular Epidemiology

RAS proteins cycle between "on" and "off" conformations that are conferred by the binding of GTP and GDP. The most common types of KRAS mutation are G12C, G12 V, and G12D. These point mutations occurring in tumors result in the loss of intrinsic GTPase activity and consequently in the deregulation of cell proliferation signals. These oncogenic substitutions in residues G12 and G13 prevent the formation of van der Waals bonds between RAS and the GTPase-activating proteins through steric hindrance and so perturb the proper orientation of the catalytic glutamine (Q61) in RAS, which results in the pronounced attenuation of GTP hydrolysis [24]. The outcome of these substitutions is the persistence of the GTP-bound state of RAS and, consequently, the incessant activation of a multitude of RAS-dependent downstream effector pathways.

TCGA project recently comprehensively profiled 230 resected lung adenocarcinomas. TP53 mutations were the most common mutations found (46%) followed only by KRAS mutations (33%) [25]. A recent analysis of the Lung Cancer Mutation Consortium (LCMC), the largest multi-institutional database of patients with metastatic KRAS mutant lung adenocarcinomas, found an overall rate of 23% [26]. Mutations in KRAS occur predominantly in codons 12 and 13 and, in rarer cases, codon 61 [27]. The estimates for KRAS mutations vary across studies, ranging up to 30% depending on ethnicity, smoking status, and mutant variants analyzed. Mutations appear most commonly in adenocarcinomas, with almost no pathologic KRAS mutants seen in squamous cell carcinoma of the lung. Ethnicity and smoking status are other important determinants. East Asians appear to have lower incidence of KRAS mutations, likely due to a corresponding higher incidence of EGFR mutations, with which they are largely mutually exclusive. Smoking increases the risk of having KRAS mutant lung cancer. An analysis of lung adenocarcinomas from non-smokers in East Asia had a very low estimate of KRAS mutants of 2% (1 of 52 samples) [28], although this ranged up to 15% in a larger study on 482 Chinese patients [29]. A large Dutch cohort study found a KRAS mutation prevalence of 33% in unselected lung cancer cases and 39% in lung adenocarcinomas, marking an upper estimate across several published studies [30]. In another large cohort of 3026 patients with adenocarcinoma of the lung, 26% harbored pathogenic mutations in KRAS [31]. While an increase in KRAS mutations is associated with smoking, the pattern of KRAS mutations in smokers and nonsmokers are distinctive. Exposure to aromatic polycyclic hydrocarbons found in tobacco smoke predisposes to transversion events, which is the characteristic subtype of KRAS mutation in smokers. This data is corroborated by the previously mentioned study of 3026 patients. KRAS mutations were found in 34% of smokers and 6% of never smokers when tested for only codon 12 and 13 abnormalities. G12C was the commonest mutation in smokers (former/current) (258/670), followed by G12 V (131/670) and G12D (114/670), while among nonsmokers, G12D was by far the most common (24/43). G12C mutants were also more common in women and occurred at a younger age in these patients, suggesting that these KRAS mutation signatures may signal different tumor biology in these patients [31]. Table 2 below provides an overview of some studies across different populations with associated estimates for KRAS incidence and their relationship with smoking status. The list is not comprehensive and only representative. It should be noted that secular trends in estimates may reflect improvement in molecular detection techniques and expanded testing.

Prognostic Implication of KRAS Mutations

Prognostic analysis of KRAS mutant lung cancer continues to produce ambiguous results through several decades. A meta-analysis of as many as 28 studies, combining 5200 patients, arrived at a combined hazard ratio for death of 1.35 (95% CI, 1.16–1.56), showing a worse survival for NSCLC with KRAS mutations or overexpression. Specifically, adenocarcinomas with KRAS mutations had a hazard ratio of 1.59 (95% CI 1.26–2.02). The analysis suggested that the method of assessment of KRAS status via IHC versus PCR was important, with detection via PCR a more robust estimator of poor prognosis [32]. However, several large and robust

Table 2 Lung KRAS mutations, estimates of prevalence, and distribution by smoking status

Author-date	Subtype(s) studied	N	Population studied	KRAS mutant frequency	Smokers	Nonsmokers	References
Fong et al. 1998	All NSCLC	108	Australian	11/108 (10%)	NR	NR	[83]
Tam et al. 2006	Adenocarcinomas	215	Hong Kong (China)	21/215 (10%)	11/58 (12%)	10/167 (5.9%)	[84]
Dogan et al. 2012	Adenocarcinomas	3026	North America	670/2529[a] (26%)	627/1860 (34%)	43/669 (6%)	[31]
Smits et al. 2012	All NSCLC	832	Europe	277/832(33%) unselected 244/625 (39%) adenocarcinomas	93/244 (38%)	3/12 (12%)	[30]
Zheng et al. 2016	Adenocarcinomas	1368	East Asia	113/1368 (8.3%)	79/369 (21%)	34/920 (4%)	[85]
Boch et al. 2013	All NSCLC	552	Europe	85/552 (15%) unselected 67/254 (26%) adenocarcinomas	NR	NR	[86]
Brose et al. 2002	Lung adenocarcinomas and melanomas[b]	147*	North America	14/147* (10%)	NR	NR	[87]
Rodenhuis et al. 1988	Adenocarcinomas	77	Europe	14/77 (18%)	13/67 (19%)	1/10 (10%)	[88]
Sun et al. 2008	Adenocarcinomas	52	East Asia	1/52 (2%)	Nonsmoking population	NA	[28]
Riely et al. 2008	Adenocarcinomas	482	North America	102/482 (21%)	90/405 (22%)	12/81 (15%)	[29]

[a]2529 evaluated for KRAS
[b]Melanomas not included
NR - Not Reported
*signifies lung cancer cases only

individual studies have provided contradictory results. For example, in the E4592 study of 182 patients receiving adjuvant chemotherapy, KRAS mutations or TP53 mutations were not associated with any differences either with progression-free survival or overall survival [33]. The JBR.10 study was a randomized controlled trial where patients with early stage lung cancer were given adjuvant doublet chemotherapy based on nodal status; again KRAS mutations were not prognostic of survival with a HR for OS of 1.23 (95% CI, 0.76–1.97) [34]. Similar results were obtained from the International Adjuvant Lung Cancer Trial as well as the European Early Lung Cancer Project, although in this latter study of 762 lung cancer specimens, the presence of concurrent mutations in TP53 and KRAS appeared to be significantly associated with a worse prognosis (HR 3.26 [1.07–9.90]) [35].

While there remains a lack of definitive evidence for KRAS mutations as a poor prognostic factor when analyzed as a solitary group, some experts hypothesize that the heterogeneity in the molecular makeup of KRAS mutant lung cancer may drive some of the discordance. There is emerging evidence for several distinct phenotypic clusters for KRAS mutant lung adenocarcinoma, such as one with concurrent alterations in STK11/LKB1, a tumor suppressor gene, another with mutations in TP53, and thirdly with inactivation of the cyclin dependent kinases CDKN2A/B combined with a low expression of the transcription factor TTF-1 [36]. KRAS mutants with low TTF-1 expression also appear to have significantly higher expression of HNF4A and PDX1. In these tumors, markers of mucinous differentiation such as CK20, MUC5B, and AGR2 are also upregulated and have been hypothesized to lead to a GI-like differentiation program [37, 38]. Tumors with STK11 mutations are characterized by mutations in KEAP1 and an associated upregulation of a NRF2-driven protective program against oxidative stress, suggesting these tumors may be susceptible to targeting of this axis. These tumors show an increased sensitivity to HSP90 inhibition as well [36]. STK-11 co-mutations appear to be associated with poorer prognosis within the KRAS mutant groups [26]. Relapsed/treatment-refractory lung adenocarcinoma has a larger number of TP53 mutations and concurrent mutations with LKB1, suggesting that these genomic changes may reflect tumor evolution during metastasis or platinum resistance. Specific mutations may also be an important determinant of prognosis and tumor behavior. In some studies, tumors with either mutant KRAS G12C or G12 V appear to have worse outcomes compared with patients whose tumors had other mutant KRAS proteins or wild-type KRAS, with these studies showing almost double progression-free survival (FPS) in non-G12C patients [39, 40]. Analysis of the large LCMC cohort showed patients with KRAS mutations may have a trend toward shorter survival (median (overall survival) OS 1.96 vs. 2.22 years; $p = 0.08$) [26]. Pooled analysis of the prognostic roles of specific mutations continue to remain ambiguous; when four adjuvant lung cancer trials were combined in a meta-analysis, there was no significant prognostic effect on survival for codon 12 (HR 1.04; [0.77–1.40]) or codon 13 mutations (HR 1.01; [0.47–2.17]) [41].

Clinical Trials in KRAS-Mutated NSCLC

Several strategies have been used to target the KRAS mutation in lung cancers, including upstream mediators, downstream effectors, as well as mutant KRAS protein itself. The following section summarizes some of these clinical trial findings.

RAS/RAF Inhibitors

Direct inhibition of RAS and RAF is intuitively the most likely efficacious therapy for KRAS mutant tumors with the lowest expected rate of off-target toxicity. However, it has proven to be challenging to develop direct inhibitors of mutant KRAS. Heterogeneity in mutation profiles and the resistance of KRAS to inhibition due to high GTP affinity are challenges to the development of inhibitors. Previous strategies have focused on attempting to disrupt regions on the protein for GEF interaction, blocking effector binding or nucleotide binding sites and targeting shallow surface pockets for binding areas for these drugs. A drug development challenge appears to be that there appear to be no large pockets on the KRAS protein that can accommodate small molecule inhibitors. An approach at directly blocking the translation of KRAS through RNA interference using antisense oligonucleotides has also been attempted as a strategy but has been limited by the availability of effective vectors as well as acquired resistance to RNAi-based therapies [42]. Recently, newer molecules are being developed that are able to bind and trap oncogenic KRAS (KRASG12C) in an inactive state with potent preclinical activity and are expected in clinical trials soon [43, 44].

Some multikinase inhibitors with RAS/RAF inhibition have been explored in this space. Sorafenib is a multikinase inhibitor with action primarily on C-RAF and B-RAF in both mutant and wild states resulting in downstream inhibition of KRAS. The MISSION trial was a phase III design to evaluate sorafenib versus placebo in advanced relapsed NSCLC patients, there was no overall survival benefit with a minimal improvement in PFS in the unselected population (2.8 vs. 1.4 months 95% CI, 0.51–0.72) unfortunately; in the retrospective analysis of the KRAS-positive subset, differences in overall survival (6.4 vs. 5.1 months) and PFS (2.6 vs. 1.7 months) were nonsignificant. Prospectively, in a study of KRAS mutant NSCLC only, 9 patients with codon 12 mutations and 1 with a codon 13 alteration were treated with sorafenib up to 400 mg BID. Three partial responses and three minimal responses were observed as the best response with a median PFS of 3 months (95% CI, 2.2–3.8 months) [45]. An analysis looking at KRAS status of patients on randomized phase II clinical trials of erlotinib in combination with sorafenib or pazopanib, another similar RAF/RAS inhibitor, showed that in KRAS mutant tumors, the addition of RAS/RAF inhibition improved both progression-free survival minimally at 2.6 months (95% CI 2.2, 3.6) vs. 1.6 months (95% CI 0.92, 1.68) and OS at 5.3 months (95% CI 3.15, 11.33) vs. 3.6 months (95% CI 1.25, 5.85) [46].

More RAS/RAF specific molecules are being developed. LY3009120, a RAF inhibitor with effects on BRAF, NRAS, and KRAS, has been evaluated in a phase I clinical trial in 34 patients with multiple solid tumors, including 18 with N/KRAS mutations; the drug was well tolerated with stable disease (SD) in 5 patients at the dose-escalation phase. Published data from dose-escalation phase is awaited and may provide information on activity in KRAS mutant lung cancer [47]. An inhibitor of CRAF and BRAF, LXH254, has been recently investigated in multiple solid tumor patients with MAPK pathway alterations. This included NSCLC with KRAS mutations. In the first human trial, there was only one partial response noted in a KRAS mutant tumor [48]. A recent phase II trial examined a direct RAS inhibitor salirasib in stage IIIB/IV NSCLC; two cohorts were recruited—including treatment-refractory KRAS mutant cancer and those with previous >15 pack year smoking history. Thirty-three patients were enrolled, and primary end point was PFS at 10 weeks. Thirty percent of previously treated and 40% of treatment-naïve patients had disease stabilization; there were no partial responses (PRs) noted on the trial. Mean OS was 15 months for patients with prior therapy. Further development was abandoned in this space [49]. As evident, the current landscape for direct RAS/RAF targeted therapies in lung cancer is bland with limited to no success with the current generation of inhibitors.

MEK Inhibitors

MEK and ERK signaling are biologically the closest downstream point from RAS and RAF activation; as a result, there is considerable interest in the use of MEK inhibitors in the KRAS mutant population. The evidence of significant synergism and activity of these molecules in combination with RAF inhibition in other sub-types has led to the development of several MEK inhibitors; some as noted below have been explored in KRAS mutant NSCLC.

Selumetinib (AZD6244; ARRY-142886) is an oral MEK inhibitor. In a random-ized trial, NSCLC patients with wild-type KRAS were randomized to erlotinib alone or combination therapy with selumetinib, while mutant KRAS patients were randomized to selumetinib alone or combination therapy. The primary end points were PFS for the KRAS wild-type cohort and objective response rate (ORR) for the KRAS mutant cohort. Results were not impressive, with no PFS difference in the KRAS wild-type arm (2.4 vs. 2.1 months) and no ORR difference in the KRAS-mutated subgroup (0% vs. 10%) [50]. A planned trial of selumetinib in combination with the anti-PD-L1 antibody durvalumab has since been suspended (NCT03004105).

Trametinib (GSK1120212) is an oral MEK inhibitor which has demonstrated excellent results in combination therapy for BRAF-mutated melanoma and is FDA approved in combination with BRAF inhibitors for that indication. Trametinib was evaluated initially as a single agent in KRAS mutant NSCLC in comparison with docetaxel and pemetrexed. Results as a single agent were not impressive, with an ORR of only 12% in these patients [51]. A follow-up trial of trametinib in combination with pemetrexed or docetaxel in a phase Ib design produced more encouraging results. In 25 patients with mutant KRAS given trametinib with docetaxel, there were 6 partial responses for an overall response rate of 24% with a comparison rate of 18% in the KRAS wild-type arm. In 23 KRAS mutant patients who received trametinibin combination with pemetrexed, the ORR was 17% in comparison to 11% in KRAS wild-type tumors. This study presented an encouraging signal for the use of trametinib as combination therapy as these rates were higher than expected with docetaxel or pemetrexed alone [52]. Given these results, there are several clinical trials currently recruiting combining trametinib in several strategies, such as with Her2-directed therapy with lapatinib (NCT02230553), anti-PD-1 therapy with pembrolizumab (NCT03299088), novel ERK inhibitors (NCT02974725), and also patients with locally advanced inoperable lung cancer in combination with chemoradiation (NCT01912625).

Among investigational molecules, RO5126766 is an oral MEK inhibitor with functional RAF inhibition that has demonstrated some activity in KRAS mutant NSCLC. In a phase Ib basket trial for KRAS-, NRAS-, or BRAF-mutated tumors, 20 patients were evaluated including 10 with KRAS mutant lung cancer. Six of these patients had tumor regression with a 30% PR rate with a manageable toxicity profile. This is very exciting data in this population, and further follow-up studies are awaited [53].

MET Inhibitors

MET is a tyrosine kinase that leads to downstream activation of several pathways including RAS and MAPK. As a result, it is quite possible that MET inhibition can be active in RAS mutant tumors and maybe associated with EGFR resistance in NSCLC. Two MET inhibitors, tivantinib and onartuzumab, have been examined in KRAS mutant NSCLC with others in clinical trials at this time. A phase II study of erlotinib in combination with tivantinib in comparison to erlotinib alone did not have impressive results with similar ORR (10% combination vs. 7% erlotinib), and PFS (3.8 vs. 2.3 months [HR], 0.81; 95% CI, 0.57–1.16) but was significant for several responses in the KRAS mutant subset of patients [54]. This led to the combination being examined in only a KRAS mutant population, where 96 patients were enrolled and randomized to erlotinib with tivantinib versus dealer's choice of second-line chemotherapy. The results were discouraging, with no benefit in progression-free survival (4.3 months with chemotherapy vs. 1.7 months with erlotinib and tivantinib) and no difference in overall survival [55]. It is appreciated that tivantinib may not be a specific MET inhibitor.

Onartuzumab, another orally available MET inhibitor, initially was evaluated in a phase II trial in an unselected NSCLC population either as single agent or in combination with erlotinib. There was no improvement in overall survival or progression-free survival in the unselected cohort. However, 66 patients were MET positive and showed improvement in both PFS and OS [56].

PI3K Inhibitors

The PI3Kinases are important downstream effectors of KRAS signaling. In pre-clinical studies, buparlisib (BKM120), a PI3K inhibitor, when combined with MEK inhibitor (PD1056309) led to significant synergistic activity in KRAS mutant NSCLC cell lines [57]. In a phase II trial of BKM-120 in NSCLC, one patient out of three with KRAS mutations had a PR. Further studies of BKM120 are ongoing in combination with traditional chemotherapy (e.g. NCT01723800) should lead to more data in this molecular subset [58].

mTOR Inhibitors

Some mTOR inhibitors have been evaluated in KRAS mutant NSCLC due to its location downstream of activated KRAS on the signaling cascade. Preclinical models suggested improved responses to everolimus, a PI3K inhibitor in patients with KRAS mutations. In its initial trials, everolimus showed some activity in patients with NSCLC [59]. Testing was expanded in phase II studies; however, these were not powered or enriched with KRAS mutants to assess for benefit, but KRAS mutant tumors showed responses [60]. A combination trial of gefitinib and everolimus in advanced NSCLC was notable for only minor response rates of 13%, but the two patients with KRAS G12F mutations had partial responses on the therapy [61]. The SORAVE trial evaluated the combination of sorafenib with everolimus with the scientific rationale for dual blockade on the MAPK and PI3K axes related to RAS activation; an extension phase of only KRAS mutant NSCLC was being recruited as of last report with moderate activity reported at short interval follow-up [62].

Another example of combining inhibitors of the MAPK and PI3K pathways for these tumors was the combination of a MEK inhibitor, pimasertib (MSC1936369B), and a PI3K/mTOR inhibitor, SAR245409, in patients with advanced solid tumors. While there were responses in the phase I trial in patients with KRAS mutant colorectal and ovarian tumors, none were reported for NSCLC [63]. A similar combination of SAR245409 in combination with erlotinib also did not impress, with no partial or complete responses in its early trial [64]. Ridaforolimus is a mTOR inhibitor that has been examined exclusively in the KRAS mutant NSCLC population in a phase II trial. In this trial stage IIIB/IV chemotherapy-refractory patients with KRAS mutations were randomized 1:1 to ridaforolimus versus placebo, at 8 weeks; those who had a >30% decrease in tumor volume remained on therapy, those with stable disease were again randomized 1:1 to placebo, and those without a response discontinued therapy. This trial tested the hypothesis that mTOR inhibitors may be associated with prolonged stable disease in those who respond to therapy. By investigator assessment, PFS was 4 months in the treatment arm and 2 months in the placebo arm, and median OS was 18 months in treatment arm versus 5 months in the placebo arm [65].

Single Agent Immunotherapy Trials

Immunotherapy has had a major impact on the treatment of multiple solid tumors and particularly NSCLC. Immunotherapy with checkpoint blockade is standard of care in several tumor types in the first line. Cancers with a driver mutation such as EGFR tend to not benefit from checkpoint blockade to the extent that genetically diverse tumors with a high tumor mutational burden (TMB) or PD-L1 expression do. In the BIRCH trial, a phase II trial of atezolizumab, an anti-PD-L1 antibody, which evaluated 659 patients with PD-L1 positive NSCLC progressive on chemotherapy, patients with KRAS mutations ($n = 185$) had overall good responses to therapy with the reported median OS of 20.1 months, 15.1 months, and 13.8 months in the IC1/2and 3 populations, respectively [66]. A recent meta-analysis combined data from two other studies of atezolizumab (POPLAR, OAK) and Checkmate057 which examined nivolumab in NSCLC for data on KRAS mutant tumors. From these studies, a total of 138 patients with KRAS mutant and 371 KRAS wild-type patients were analyzed. Overall survival was improved significantly in KRAS mutant patients when compared with those who received chemotherapy (HR 0.64 95% CI = 0.43–0.96], $p = 0.03$), while it did not improve outcomes significantly in wild-type patients (HR = 0.88 [95% CI = 0.68–1.13], $p = 0.30$) [67]. Given the limited toxicity profile of these therapies and the possibility that immunotherapy may be more effective in KRAS mutant NSCLC, further studies are now evaluating immune-oncology combinations in this subset.

Immune-Oncology Combination Trials

While several combination immune-oncology trials have been completed in NSCLC to date, a KRAS subset analysis is frequently not reported. Some trials are however being conducted in specific KRAS mutant subsets. Some preclinical studies have shown that immune checkpoint therapy in combination with MEK inhibition may be effective in RAS mutated NSCLC by multiple mechanisms including the targeting of myeloid derived stem cells. A single institution clinical trial (NCT03299088) is examining a combination of pembrolizumab with MEK inhibitor trametinib in patients with KRAS mutant NSCLC. There was also a trial of durvalumab in combination with selumetinib which has since been withdrawn. Finally, a trial combining atezolizumab with MEK inhibitor cobimetinib (NCT0300701) is currently recruiting, and results should be expected in upcoming months.

Novel Therapeutic Targets in KRAS Mutant NSCLC

CDK Inhibition

Cyclin-dependent kinase (CDK) inhibition provides an attractive strategy of inhibition of the cell division checkpoint and should potentially work equally well in KRAS mutant versus wild-type tumors. CDK inhibitors have been extremely successful in breast cancer therapy, becoming front-line agents for the therapy of these cancers. The recently reported JUNIPER trial examined the CDK4/6 inhibitor abemaciclib in comparison to single erlotinib in patients with KRAS mutant NSCLC. Although there was no improvement in overall survival (7.4 months with abemaciclib versus 7.8 months with erlotinib), there appeared to be some improvement in PFS (3.6 months vs. 1.9 months) and disease control rate (54.4% vs. 31.7%) [68].

HSP90 Inhibition

We have discussed previously about HSP90 targeting as a potential targeting strategy in some populations of KRAS mutant tumors [36]. The GALAXY-1 trial was a large phase II randomized trial of ganetespib in combination with docetaxel versus docetaxel alone in patients with either an elevated LDH or KRAS-mutated tumors. Three hundred and eighty-one patients were treated, there was a statistically nonsignificant trend toward improved PFS ($N = 253$, adjusted HR = 0.82, $p = 0.0784$) and overall survival (OS) (adjusted HR = 0.84, $p = 0.1139$) in adenocarcinoma patients only [69]. Another HSP90 inhibitor, IPI-504 was examined in a small phase Ib trial ($n = 23$) of NSCLC patients. The study was interesting due to the high rates of response in squamous cell subtypes with three of seven patients with squamous cell carcinoma of the lung having partial responses; however, responses in KRAS mutant tumors were lower than in wild type [70].

FAK Inhibition

Focal adhesion kinase or FAK is a tyrosine kinase concentrated in focal adhesions that cells make with the extracellular matrix; it is thought to be involved in helping cell migration and metastases. FAK is a critical downstream mediator of oncogenic RAS signaling [71]. Defactinib(VS-6063) is a cancer stemness inhibitor that is now in trials for KRAS mutant NSCLC. In the first phase II trial, several patients were recruited based on having a KRAS mutation, and then subclassified into additional cohorts based on concurrent p16 and or p53 mutation status. As of last report at IASLC 2018, 36% of 44 patients were progression-free at 12 weeks with a median PFS of 11.7 weeks indicating moderate activity. Treatment was tolerated well with limited constitutional symptoms, p53 or p16 were not associated with differences in outcomes. Further combination studies were being planned [72].

HDAC Inhibition

The MAPK pathway contributes to tumorigenesis by affecting FOXO proteins. Histone deacetylase (HDAC) inhibitors can negatively impact the expression of these proteins and have been studied in pre-clinical models of RAS mutant NSCLC with encouraging results [73]. Romidepsin is a HDAC inhibitor that is approved for the treatment of cutaneous T-cell lymphomas but also investigated in several tumor types. A recent phase I study established safety of the drug when used in combination with erlotinib. Among 10 evaluable patients, 7 patients had SD as the best response, with a 3.3 month median progression-free survival. Patients with KRAS mutation and an SCC patient had stable disease >6 months on trial, indicating signs of drug activity. Dose-limiting toxicity (DLT) on the trial was nausea and vomiting [74].

FASN Inhibition

Fatty acid synthase (FASN) is an enzyme that is essential in neoplastic cell proliferation due to its essential role in generation of necessary lipogenesis through palmitate biosynthesis and has been examined as a therapeutic target. Highly potent FASN inhibitors are being developed, the first in class molecule TVB-2640 was examined in multiple solid tumors, include KRAS mutant NSCLC as either as single agent versus in combination with IV paclitaxel. The medication was associated with some uncommon side effects such as hand foot syndrome in 36% and ocular side effects such as dry eyes (13%), excessive lacrimation (11%), and corneal edema in 3% of a total of 100 patients. However, there were also encouraging responses: 16 NSCLC patients were part of the trial and of 6 with KRAS mutations, half were able to achieve prolonged stable disease [75].

Proteasome Inhibitors

Bortezomib is a proteasome inhibitor with marked activity in multiple myeloma—it has a down regulatory effect on the NF-kB pathway and hence has scientific rationale for activity in KRAS mutant tumors. A phase II trial of patients with NSCLC patients with KRAS G12D mutations was recently conducted, and 16 patients were recruited. 40% patients had stable disease as best response, which was prolonged >5 months in 12%. Median PFS however was only 1 month, with median OS of 13 months in the cohort. Therapy was well tolerated with fatigue, diarrhea, nausea, and rash the reported side effects of any grade. No further studies of bortezomib were pursued [76].

Farnesyltransferase Inhibition

Farnesylation of KRAS is an important step leading to preparation of the protein for transport to the intracellular membrane where it can be effective. Hence, it made strong biological sense to use FTase inhibitors for KRAS mutant tumors. These molecules were tried initially for another indication, progeria, a rare genetic disease characterized by production of a protein called progerin. Farnesylation inhibition had led to impressive results preclinically. Lonafarnib (SCH66336) was initially examined in a phase I study in 20 patients with mixed solid tumors; a patient with NSCLC had a partial response lasting 14 months and the drug was relatively well tolerated [77]. Further, in a phase I study of lonafarnib in combination with paclitaxel in 21 patients, the drug was well tolerated and also led to durable partial responses in 6 of 15 treatment-refractory patients and 2 patients with taxane-refractory NSCLC had partial responses [78]. This further led an expansion cohort in NSCLC with 33 patients enrolled, 29 of whom were evaluable for response. Ten percent had PR and 38% SD as best responses median OS was 39 weeks and the median PFS was 16 weeks. The combination of lonafarnib and paclitaxel was well tolerated with minimal toxicity. Grade 3 toxicities included fatigue (9%), diarrhea (6%), and dyspnea (6%). Grade 3 neutropenia occurred in only 1 patient (3%) [79]. A phase III trial was launched as first-line NSCLC using lonafarnib in combination with carboplatin and paclitaxel; however, the trial failed to produce a survival benefit [80]. In contrast, tipifarnib (R115777), another farnesyltransferase inhibitor, was examined in 44 patients with NSCLC with no objective responses and only 15% patients with stable disease as best response [81]. Importantly, none of these trials have published information on KRAS-specific responses of these tumors.

Conclusion

KRAS mutant tumors represent a large fraction of NSCLC, particularly the adenocarcinomas. Increasingly, we are recognizing that these tumors have variations in molecular pathology and underlying biology, with the most common smoking-associated subtypes differing from rarer KRAS mutants in younger nonsmokers and with several categories of co-occurring mutations. While controversial, KRAS mutations likely represent more aggressive disease and are particularly problematic to manage since these tumors tend to be mutually exclusive from other driver mutations like EGFR and ALK. KRAS has been an extremely difficult molecular target driven by its high GTP affinity and difficult chemical structure to target. Upstream and downstream inhibition has led to only moderate success. KRAS mutant NSCLC remains an area of unmet high need for therapeutic targeting.

References

1. Tsuchida N, Ryder T, Ohtsubo E. Nucleotide sequence of the oncogene encoding the p21 transforming protein of Kirsten murine sarcoma virus. Science. 1982;217(4563):937–9.
2. Chen Y, McGee J, Chen X, et al. Identification of druggable cancer driver genes amplified across TCGA datasets. PLoS One. 2014;9(5):e98293.

3. Westcott PM, To MD. The genetics and biology of KRAS in lung cancer. Chin J Cancer. 2013;32(2):63–70.
4. Reuter CW, Morgan MA, Bergmann L. Targeting the Ras signaling pathway: a rational, mechanism-based treatment for hematologic malignancies? Blood. 2000;96(5):1655–69.
5. Zebisch A, Troppmair J. Back to the roots: the remarkable RAF oncogene story. Cell Mol Life Sci. 2006;63(11):1314–30.
6. Jirmanova L, Afanassieff M, Gobert-Gosse S, Markossian S, Savatier P. Differential contributions of ERK and PI3-kinase to the regulation of cyclin D1 expression and to the control of the G1/S transition in mouse embryonic stem cells. Oncogene. 2002;21(36):5515–28.
7. Pierre S, Bats AS, Coumoul X. Understanding SOS (Son of Sevenless). Biochem Pharmacol. 2011;82(9):1049–56.
8. Sadidi M, Lentz SI, Feldman EL. Hydrogen peroxide-induced Akt phosphorylation regulates Bax activation. Biochimie. 2009;91(5):577–85.
9. Zhang X, Tang N, Hadden TJ, Rishi AK. Akt, FoxO and regulation of apoptosis. Biochim Biophys Acta. 2011;1813(11):1978–86.
10. Lowenstein EJ, Daly RJ, Batzer AG, et al. The SH2 and SH3 domain-containing protein GRB2 links receptor tyrosine kinases to ras signaling. Cell. 1992;70(3):431–42.
11. Giaccone G, Gallegos Ruiz M, Le Chevalier T, et al. Erlotinib for frontline treatment of advanced non-small cell lung cancer: a phase II study. Clin Cancer Res. 2006;12(20 Pt 1):6049–55.
12. Pao W, Wang TY, Riely GJ, et al. KRAS mutations and primary resistance of lung adenocarcinomas to gefitinib or erlotinib. PLoS Med. 2005;2(1):e17.
13. Siddiqui AD, Piperdi B. KRAS mutation in colon cancer: a marker of resistance to EGFR-I therapy. Ann Surg Oncol. 2010;17(4):1168–76.
14. Bockorny B, Rusan M, Chen W, et al. RAS-MAPK reactivation facilitates acquired resistance in FGFR1-amplified lung cancer and underlies a rationale for upfront FGFR-MEK blockade. Mol Cancer Ther. 2018.
15. Desai A, Adjei AA. FGFR signaling as a target for lung cancer therapy. J Thorac Oncol. 2016;11(1):9–20.
16. Hashemi-Sadraei N, Hanna N. Targeting FGFR in squamous cell carcinoma of the lung. Target Oncol. 2017;12(6):741–55.
17. Ugocsai K, Mandoky L, Tiszlavicz L, Molnar J. Investigation of HER2 overexpression in non-small cell lung cancer. Anticancer Res. 2005;25(4):3061–6.
18. Shigematsu H, Takahashi T, Nomura M, et al. Somatic mutations of the HER2 kinase domain in lung adenocarcinomas. Cancer Res. 2005;65(5):1642–6.
19. Salgia R. MET in lung cancer: biomarker selection based on scientific rationale. Mol Cancer Ther. 2017;16(4):555–65.
20. Leiser D, Medova M, Mikami K, et al. KRAS and HRAS mutations confer resistance to MET targeting in preclinical models of MET-expressing tumor cells. Mol Oncol. 2015;9(7):1434–46.
21. Gainor JF, Varghese AM, Ou SH, et al. ALK rearrangements are mutually exclusive with mutations in EGFR or KRAS: an analysis of 1683 patients with non-small cell lung cancer. Clin Cancer Res. 2013;19(15):4273–81.
22. Hrustanovic G, Bivona TG. RAS signaling in ALK fusion lung cancer. Small GTPases. 2016;7(1):32–3.
23. Ambrogio C, Nadal E, Villanueva A, et al. KRAS-driven lung adenocarcinoma: combined DDR1/Notch inhibition as an effective therapy. ESMO Open. 2016;1(5):e000076.
24. Scheffzek K, Ahmadian MR, Kabsch W, et al. The Ras-RasGAP complex: structural basis for GTPase activation and its loss in oncogenic Ras mutants. Science. 1997;277(5324):333–8.
25. Cancer Genome Atlas Research N. Comprehensive molecular profiling of lung adenocarcinoma. Nature. 2014;511(7511):543–50.
26. El-Osta B, Behera M, Kim S, et al. Characteristics and outcomes of patients (pts) with metastatic KRAS mutant lung adenocarcinomas: lung cancer mutation consortium (LCMC) database. ASCO Annual Meet. 2017; 2017; Chicago: JCO; 2017.

27. Quinlan MP, Settleman J. Isoform-specific ras functions in development and cancer. Future Oncol. 2009;5(1):105–16.
28. Sun Y, Ren Y, Fang Z, et al. Lung adenocarcinoma from East Asian never-smokers is a disease largely defined by targetable oncogenic mutant kinases. J Clin Oncol. 2010;28(30):4616–20.
29. Riely GJ, Kris MG, Rosenbaum D, et al. Frequency and distinctive spectrum of KRAS mutations in never smokers with lung adenocarcinoma. Clinical Cancer Res. 2008;14(18):5731–4.
30. Smits AJ, Kummer JA, Hinrichs JW, et al. EGFR and KRAS mutations in lung carcinomas in the Dutch population: increased EGFR mutation frequency in malignant pleural effusion of lung adenocarcinoma. Cell Oncol (Dordr). 2012;35(3):189–96.
31. Dogan S, Shen R, Ang DC, et al. Molecular epidemiology of EGFR and KRAS mutations in 3026 lung adenocarcinomas: higher susceptibility of women to smoking-related KRAS-mutant cancers. Clinical Cancer Res. 2012;18(22):6169–77.
32. Mascaux C, Iannino N, Martin B, et al. The role of RAS oncogene in survival of patients with lung cancer: a systematic review of the literature with meta-analysis. Br J Cancer. 2005;92(1):131–9.
33. Schiller JH, Adak S, Feins RH, et al. Lack of prognostic significance of p53 and K-ras mutations in primary resected non-small-cell lung cancer on E4592: a laboratory ancillary study on an eastern cooperative oncology group prospective randomized trial of postoperative adjuvant therapy. J Clin Oncol. 2001;19(2):448–57.
34. Winton T, Livingston R, Johnson D, et al. Vinorelbine plus cisplatin vs. observation in resected non-small-cell lung cancer. New England J Med. 2005;352(25):2589–97.
35. Scoccianti C, Vesin A, Martel G, et al. Prognostic value of TP53, KRAS and EGFR mutations in nonsmall cell lung cancer: the EUELC cohort. Eur Respir J. 2012;40(1):177–84.
36. Skoulidis F, Byers LA, Diao L, et al. Co-occurring genomic alterations define major subsets of KRAS-mutant lung adenocarcinoma with distinct biology, immune profiles, and therapeutic vulnerabilities. Cancer Discov. 2015;5(8):860–77.
37. Maeda Y, Tsuchiya T, Hao H, et al. Kras(G12D) and Nkx2–1 haploinsufficiency induce mucinous adenocarcinoma of the lung. J Clin Invest. 2012;122(12):4388–400.
38. Snyder EL, Watanabe H, Magendantz M, et al. Nkx2–1 represses a latent gastric differentiation program in lung adenocarcinoma. Mol Cell. 2013;50(2):185–99.
39. Ihle NT, Byers LA, Kim ES, et al. Effect of KRAS oncogene substitutions on protein behavior: implications for signaling and clinical outcome. J Natl Cancer Inst. 2012;104(3):228–39.
40. Park S, Kim JY, Lee SH, et al. KRAS G12C mutation as a poor prognostic marker of pemetrexed treatment in non-small cell lung cancer. Korean J Intern Med. 2017;32(3):514–22.
41. Shepherd FA, Lacas B, Le Teuff G, et al. Pooled analysis of the prognostic and predictive effects of TP53 comutation status combined with KRAS or EGFR mutation in early-stage resected non-small-cell lung cancer in four trials of adjuvant chemotherapy. J Clin Oncol. 2017;35(18):2018–27.
42. Tomasini P, Walia P, Labbe C, Jao K, Leighl NB. Targeting the KRAS pathway in non-small cell lung cancer. Oncologist. 2016;21(12):1450–60.
43. Janes MR, Zhang J, Li LS, et al. Targeting KRAS mutant cancers with a covalent G12C-specific inhibitor. Cell. 2018;172(3):578–89.e17.
44. Statsyuk AV. Let K-Ras activate its own inhibitor. Nat Struct Mol Biol. 2018.
45. Smit EF, Dingemans AM, Thunnissen FB, Hochstenbach MM, van Suylen RJ, Postmus PE. Sorafenib in patients with advanced non-small cell lung cancer that harbor K-ras mutations: a brief report. J Thorac Oncol. 2010;5(5):719–20.
46. David Michael Waterhouse DMS, Davey B. Daniel, Paula L. Griner, F Anthony Greco, Howard A. Burris, John D. Hainsworth, David R. Spigel KRAS subset analysis from randomized phase II trials of erlotinib versus erlotinib plus sorafenib or pazopanib in refractory non-small cell lung cancer (NSCLC). JCO. 2013;31.
47. David S, Hong AH, Gordon MS, Flaherty KT, Shapiro G, Rodon J, Millward M, Ramdas N, Zhang W, Gao L, Sykes A, Willard MD, Yu D, Schade A, Flynn DL, Kaufman M, Peng S-B, Conti I, Tiu RV, Sullivan RJ. A first-in-human dose phase 1 study of LY3009120 in advanced cancer patients. JCO. Chicago 2017.

48. Janku F, Iyer G, Spreafico A, et al. A phase I study of LXH254 in patients (pts) with advanced solid tumors harboring MAPK pathway alterations. J Clin Oncol. 2018;36(15_suppl):2586.
49. Riely GJ, Johnson ML, Medina C, et al. A phase II trial of Salirasib in patients with lung adenocarcinomas with KRAS mutations. J Thorac Oncol. 2011;6(8):1435–7.
50. Carter CA, Rajan A, Keen C, et al. Selumetinib with and without erlotinib in KRAS mutant and KRAS wild-type advanced nonsmall-cell lung cancer. Ann Oncol. 2016;27(4):693–9.
51. Blumenschein GR, Smit EF, Planchard D, et al. MEK114653: a randomized, multicenter, phase II study to assess efficacy and safety of trametinib (T) compared with docetaxel (D) in KRAS-mutant advanced non–small cell lung cancer (NSCLC). J Clin Oncol. 2013;31(15_suppl):8029.
52. Gandara DR, Leighl N, Delord JP, et al. A phase 1/1b study evaluating trametinib plus docetaxel or pemetrexed in patients with advanced non-small cell lung cancer. J Thorac Oncol. 2017;12(3):556–66.
53. Chenard-Poirier M, Kaiser M, Boyd K, et al. Results from the biomarker-driven basket trial of RO5126766 (CH5127566), a potent RAF/MEK inhibitor, in RAS- or RAF-mutated malignancies including multiple myeloma. J Clin Oncol. 2017;35(15_suppl):2506.
54. Sequist LV, Jv P, Garmey EG, et al. Randomized phase II study of erlotinib plus tivantinib versus erlotinib plus placebo in previously treated non–small-cell lung cancer. J Clin Oncol. 2011;29(24):3307–15.
55. Gerber DE, Socinski MA, Neal JW, et al. Randomized phase 2 study of tivantinib plus erlotinib versus single-agent chemotherapy in previously treated KRAS mutant advanced non-small cell lung cancer. Lung Cancer. 2018;117:44–9.
56. Spigel DR, Ervin TJ, Ramlau RA, et al. Randomized phase II trial of Onartuzumab in combination with erlotinib in patients with advanced non-small-cell lung cancer. J Clin Oncol. 2013;31(32):4105–14.
57. Jiang ZB, Huang J, Xie C, et al. Combined use of PI3K and MEK inhibitors synergistically inhibits lung cancer with EGFR and KRAS mutations. Oncol Rep. 2016;36(1):365–75.
58. Vansteenkiste JF, Canon JL, De Braud F, et al. Safety and efficacy of Buparlisib (BKM120) in patients with PI3K pathway-activated non-small cell lung cancer: results from the phase II BASALT-1 study. J Thorac Oncol. 2015;10(9):1319–27.
59. O'Donnell A, Faivre S, Judson I, et al. A phase I study of the oral mTOR inhibitor RAD001 as monotherapy to identify the optimal biologically effective dose using toxicity, pharmacokinetic (PK) and pharmacodynamic (PD) endpoints in patients with solid tumors. Proc Am Soc Clin Oncol. 2003;2003:200.
60. Owonikoko TK, Ramalingam SS, Miller DL, et al. A translational, pharmacodynamic, and pharmacokinetic phase IB clinical study of everolimus in resectable non-small cell lung cancer. Clin Cancer Res. 2015;21(8):1859–68.
61. Price KA, Azzoli CG, Krug LM, et al. Phase II trial of gefitinib and everolimus in advanced non-small cell lung cancer. J Thorac Oncol. 2010;5(10):1623–9.
62. Nogova L, Mattonet C, Gardizi M, et al. SORAVE: Sorafenib and everolimus for treatment of patients with relapsed solid tumors and with KRAS mutated NSCLC—a phase I study. J Clin Oncol. 2013;31(15_suppl):8112.
63. Heist RS, Gandhi L, Shapiro G, et al. Combination of a MEK inhibitor, pimasertib (MSC1936369B), and a PI3K/mTOR inhibitor, SAR245409, in patients with advanced solid tumors: Results of a phase Ib dose-escalation trial. Am Soc Clin Oncol. 2013.
64. Janne PA, Cohen RB, Laird AD, et al. Phase I safety and pharmacokinetic study of the PI3K/mTOR inhibitor SAR245409 (XL765) in combination with erlotinib in patients with advanced solid tumors. J Thorac Oncol. 2014;9(3):316–23.
65. Riely GJ, Brahmer JR, Planchard D, et al. A randomized discontinuation phase II trial of ridaforolimus in non-small cell lung cancer (NSCLC) patients with KRAS mutations. J Clin Oncol. 2012;30(15_suppl):7531.
66. Peters S, Gettinger S, Johnson ML, et al. Phase II trial of atezolizumab as first-line or subsequent therapy for patients with programmed death-ligand 1-selected advanced non-small-cell lung cancer (BIRCH). J Clin Oncol. 2017;35(24):2781–9.

67. Kim JH, Kim HS, Kim BJ. Prognostic value of KRAS mutation in advanced non-small-cell lung cancer treated with immune checkpoint inhibitors: a meta-analysis and review. Oncotarget. 2017;8(29):48248–52.
68. Goldman JW, Mazieres J, Barlesi F, et al. A randomized phase 3 study of abemaciclib versus erlotinib in previously treated patients with stage IV NSCLC with KRAS mutation: JUNIPER. J Clin Oncol. 2018;36(15_suppl):9025.
69. Ramalingam S, Goss G, Rosell R, et al. A randomized phase II study of ganetespib, a heat shock protein 90 inhibitor, in combination with docetaxel in second-line therapy of advanced non-small cell lung cancer (GALAXY-1). Ann Oncol. 2015;26(8):1741–8.
70. Riely GJ, Gettinger SN, Stoller RG, et al. Safety and activity of IPI-504 (retaspimycin hydrochloride) and docetaxel in pretreated patients (pts) with metastatic non-small cell lung cancer (NSCLC). J Clin Oncol. 2011;29(15_suppl):7516.
71. Schlaepfer DD, Hunter T. Focal adhesion kinase overexpression enhances ras-dependent integrin signaling to ERK2/mitogen-activated protein kinase through interactions with and activation of c-Src. J Biol Chem. 1997;272(20):13189–95.
72. Gerber DE, Ramalingam SS, Morgensztern D, et al. A phase 2 study of defactinib (VS-6063), a cancer stem cell inhibitor that acts through inhibition of focal adhesion kinase (FAK), in patients with KRAS-mutant non-small cell lung cancer. J Clin Oncol. 2014;32(15_suppl):TPS8126–TPS.
73. Yamada T, Amann JM, Tanimoto A, et al. Histone deacetylase inhibition enhances the antitumor activity of a MEK inhibitor in lung cancer cells harboring RAS mutations. Mol Cancer Ther. 2018;17(1):17–25.
74. Gerber DE, Boothman DA, Fattah FJ, et al. Phase 1 study of romidepsin plus erlotinib in advanced non-small cell lung cancer. Lung Cancer. 2015;90(3):534–41.
75. Dean EJ, Falchook GS, Patel MR, et al. Preliminary activity in the first in human study of the first-in-class fatty acid synthase (FASN) inhibitor, TVB-2640. J Clin Oncol. 2016;34(15_suppl):2512.
76. Litvak AM, Drilon AE, Rekhtman N, et al. Phase II trial of bortezomib in KRAS G12D mutant lung cancers. J Clin Oncol. 2015;33(15_suppl):e19002–e.
77. Adjei AA, Erlichman C, Davis JN, et al. A Phase I trial of the farnesyl transferase inhibitor SCH66336: evidence for biological and clinical activity. Cancer Res. 2000;60(7):1871–7.
78. Khuri FR, Glisson BS, Kim ES, et al. Phase I study of the farnesyltransferase inhibitor lonafarnib with paclitaxel in solid tumors. Clin Cancer Res. 2004;10(9):2968–76.
79. Kim ES, Kies MS, Fossella FV, et al. Phase II study of the farnesyltransferase inhibitor lonafarnib with paclitaxel in patients with taxane-refractory/resistant nonsmall cell lung carcinoma. Cancer. 2005;104(3):561–9.
80. Blumenschein GR, Khuri F, Gatzemeier U, et al. A randomized phase III trial comparing bexarotene/carboplatin/paclitaxel versus carboplatin/paclitaxel in chemotherapy-naive patients with advanced or metastatic non-small cell lung cancer (NSCLC). J Clin Oncol. 2005;23(16_suppl):LBA7001–LBA.
81. Adjei AA, Mauer A, Bruzek L, et al. Phase II study of the farnesyl transferase inhibitor R115777 in patients with advanced non-small-cell lung cancer. J Clin Oncol. 2003;21(9):1760–6.
82. Yang SH, Baek HA, Lee HJ, et al. Discoidin domain receptor 1 is associated with poor prognosis of non-small cell lung carcinomas. Oncol Rep. 2010;24(2):311–9.
83. Fong KM, Zimmerman PV, Smith PJ. KRAS codon 12 mutations in Australian non-small cell lung cancer. Aust N Z J Med. 1998;28(2):184–9.
84. Tam IY, Chung LP, Suen WS, et al. Distinct epidermal growth factor receptor and KRAS mutation patterns in non-small cell lung cancer patients with different tobacco exposure and clinicopathologic features. Clin Cancer Res. 2006;12(5):1647–53.
85. Zheng D, Wang R, Zhang Y, et al. The prevalence and prognostic significance of KRAS mutation subtypes in lung adenocarcinomas from Chinese populations. Onco Targets Ther. 2016;9:833–43.

86. Boch C, Kollmeier J, Roth A, et al. The frequency of EGFR and KRAS mutations in non-small cell lung cancer (NSCLC): routine screening data for central Europe from a cohort study. BMJ Open. 2013;3(4).
87. Brose MS, Volpe P, Feldman M, et al. BRAF and RAS mutations in human lung cancer and melanoma. Cancer Res. 2002;62(23):6997–7000.
88. Rodenhuis S, Slebos RJ, Boot AJ, et al. Incidence and possible clinical significance of K-ras oncogene activation in adenocarcinoma of the human lung. Cancer Res. 1988;48(20):5738–41.

Targeting Epigenetic Regulators in Cancer to Overcome Targeted Therapy Resistance

Dan J. Raz

Abstract Therapies targeting epigenetic changes hold promise to prevent drug resistance and improve durability of therapy responses in lung and other cancers. Epigenetic control of gene expression occurs through a variety of dynamic mechanisms, including DNA methylation and histone modifications. Currently, the only epigenetic therapies approved for use in humans are DNA methyltransferase (DNMT) inhibitors and histone deacetylase (HDAC) inhibitors. Clinical trials in lung cancer have shown some promise for combination therapy of DNMT and HDAC inhibitors and for combination of epigenetic inhibitors with targeted therapies. In this review, we describe the rationale for use of epigenetic inhibitors to overcome therapy resistance in cancer, with a focus on the role of epigenetics in resistance to targeted therapies. We also summarize completed and ongoing clinical trials utilizing epigenetic inhibitors in combination with chemotherapy, immunotherapy, and targeted therapies.

Keywords Epigenetics · DNA methylation · Histone modification · Immunotherapy · Targeted therapy · Lung cancer

Introduction

Although there have been significant advances in lung cancer therapy, including targeted therapies and immunotherapies, survival after a diagnosis of advanced stage lung cancer remains poor for the vast majority of patients. While many patients respond to systemic chemotherapy and targeted therapies, resistance to these therapies is inevitable. Understanding the mechanisms of resistance to specific therapies can lead to the identification of new treatments that can be used to overcome this resistance and prolong survival.

D. J. Raz (✉)
Department of Surgery, City of Hope National Medical Center, Duarte, CA, USA
e-mail: draz@coh.org

© Springer Nature Switzerland AG 2019   217
R. Salgia (ed.), *Targeted Therapies for Lung Cancer*, Current Cancer Research,
https://doi.org/10.1007/978-3-030-17832-1_11

There are a number of mechanisms involved in acquired drug resistance. These include selection for specific mutations that confer resistance to specific therapies, expression of transporter proteins that confer drug resistance, and epigenetic changes that lead to drug resistance. Epigenetic changes refer to changes in chromatin modifications that result in gene expression without mutations in the DNA. Epigenetic regulation of gene expression is responsible for differentiation of pluripotent stem cells into various tissue-specific cell types during embryologic development [1]. Epigenetic modifications lead to stark phenotypic differences between various cells in the body or within organs, even though these cells all originated from similar parent cells and have the same DNA sequence. Similarly, cancer is thought to originate from a population of tumorigenic cells, which have been called cancer stem cells (CSC) or tumor initiating cells. This small population of cancer cells has a different pattern of gene expression, mostly explained by differences in epigenetic modifications, than the remaining population of cancer cells [3]. CSCs are more drug resistant, including cytotoxic chemotherapy and certain targeted therapies. CSCs are thought to be responsible in part for tumor cell heterogeneity through differentiation into cells with different epigenetically controlled gene expression. CSCs have been challenging to define, as there are no cell surface markers that are specific for CSCs. A number of cell surface markers, including CD133 and CD 24, have been described, but it is the phenotype of highly tumorigenic and therapy-resistant cells that are the hallmark of this cancer cell population [49].

There has been interest using epigenetic therapies as an adjunct to other therapies, most commonly cytotoxic chemotherapy in lung and other cancers. "Reprogramming" resistant populations of cancer cells to drug-sensitive phenotypes is the goal of epigenetic therapies.

Epigenetic Dysregulation in Lung Cancer

DNA Methylation

DNA methylation is the most well-studied epigenetic modification in lung cancer. DNA affects gene expression via CpG island methylation in the promoter region of a gene. CpG island methylation is a dynamic process that most commonly leads to repression of gene transcription. A large number of oncogenes are regulated in lung cancer through promoter-region methylation. Three different DNA methyltransferases (DNMTs) exist that transfer a methyl group to the 5′-cytosine carbon on a CpG island. DNMT1 is primarily involved in maintenance of methylation after DNA replication, whereas DNMT3a and 3b are primarily involved in de novo methylation [8, 24].

Clinical Trials of DNMT-Inhibitors in NSCLC

There are two FDA-approved DNMT inhibitors, 5-azacitidine and decitabine (Table 1). Both received their initial approval for myelodysplastic syndrome, but are used in other hematologic malignancies, most commonly certain types of AML. 5-azacytidine is incorporated into both DNA and RNA, leading to covalent binding with DNMTs and proteasomal degradation. Decitabine is incorporated into DNA and not RNA [8, 51]. The hypomethylating effects of these agents in vitro are achieved with lower dosages and prolonged administration. Although effective in preclinical models of lung cancer, single agent treatment with decitabine has led to unacceptable toxicity. In one phase I/II trial, heavily pretreated patients with NSCLC were treated with high dose decitabine (Table 2). Although there were no objective responses, four patients had stable disease for 6 months, with only one patient completing more than one cycle due to toxicity [47]. Trials utilizing lower doses of decitabine did not report any significant objective responses to therapy, although there were several patients who achieved stable disease [58]. A novel oral formulation of azacitidine, CC-486, was tested in combination with pembrolizumab, but there was no difference in objective response compared to pembrolizumab alone [39]. That drug was also tested in combination with nab-paclitaxel as a second-line therapy in NSCLC in a randomized phase II trial comparing the combination with nab-paclitaxel alone, but there was no difference in objective response in that trial either [48].

Histone Modifications

Histones are proteins that make up the nucleosome, around which DNA is wrapped. Histones can be modified by methylation, acetylation, phosphorylation, sumoylation, and ubiquitylation. These various modifications affect gene expression through a variety of mechanisms, including DNA relaxation for RNA expression and by affecting DNA methylation [31]. Histone modifications have been

Table 1 FDA-approved epigenetic therapies

Drug	Mechanism	Approved disease treatment	Year approved
5-Azacytidine (Vidaza)	DNMT inhibitor	MDS, AML	2004
Decitabine (Dacogen)	DNMT inhibitor	MDS, AML	2006
Vorinostat (Zolinza)	HDAC inhibitor	CTCL	2006
Romidepsin (Istodax)	HDAC inhibitor	CTCL, PTCL	2009
Belinostat (Beleodaq)	HDAC inhibitor	PTCL	2014
Panobinostat (Farydak)	HDAC inhibitor	Multiple myeloma	2015

Abbreviations: *DNMT* DNA methyltransferase, *HDAC* histone deacetylase, *MDS* myelodysplastic syndromes, *AML* acute myelogenous leukemia, *CTCL* cutaneous T-cell lymphoma, *PTCL* peripheral T-cell lymphoma

Table 2 Clinical trials using epigenetic combination therapies in NSCLC (ongoing or completed)

DNMT-inhibitor combination trials		
Drug	*Patients*	*Study population and notes*
Decitabine+cisplatin	35	Phase 1/2; no objective responses [59]
Azacitidine+erlotinib	30	Two patients with NSCLC, benefit unclear [2]
CC486 + pembrolizumab	90	Randomized controlled trial IIIb/IV NSCLC, no benefit [39]
CC486 + nab-paclitaxel	161	Randomized controlled trial IIIb/IV NSCLC, no benefit [48]
FdCyd+tetrahydrouridine	~185	Ongoing multi-histology phase 2 study
HDAC-inhibitor combination trials		
Drug	*Patients*	*Study population and notes*
Vorinostat+carboplatin+paclitaxel	253	Phase II randomized, improved response rate [55]
Panobinostat+erlotinib	33	Phase I, well tolerated, efficacy unclear [29]
Entinostat+erlotinib	132	Phase I/II, elevated E-cadherin associated with improved survival [56]
Entinostat+pembrolizumab	158	Phase I/II, second line, improved responses with PDL1 < 1% [36]
Vorinostat+sorafenib	35	Phase I, 15 NSCLC patients, 1 partial response [12]
Belinostat, carboplatin, paclitaxel, bevacizumab		Phase I/II, ongoing
Belinostat+erlotinib		Phase I/Ib, ongoing
Vorinostat+gemcitabine+platinum		Phase I, ongoing
Combination DNMT/HDAC inhibitor trials		
Drug	*Patients*	*Study population and notes*
Azacitidine+entinostat	34	One partial response, one complete response, 10 stable disease [37]
Azacitidine+entinostat		Phase 2, ongoing
Azacitidine+entinostat+chemotherapy		Phase 2, ongoing
Azacitidine+entinostat+nivolumab		Phase 2, ongoing

found to have important roles in lung cancer development, cancer progression, metastasis, and response to therapy. Inhibition of histone acetylation, methylation, and ubiquitylation is associated with cell death and response to chemotherapy in a variety of lung cancer cell lines in vitro [46, 70, 75, 77]. In addition, expression patterns of histone deacetylases (HDACs) and histone acetyltransferases (HATs) are correlated with lung cancer prognosis [50, 60]. Currently, the only inhibitors of histone modification that are approved for treatment are HDAC inhibitors. Vorinostat, romidepsin, belinostat, and panobinostat have been approved by the Food and Drug Administration (FDA) for treatment of cutaneous T-cell lymphoma, peripheral T-cell lymphoma, and multiple myeloma (Table 1). There are at least 18 HDACs identified in humans. HDAC inhibitors result in cancer cell death by inducing apoptosis, cell cycle arrest, suppressing tumor angiogenesis, and immune modulation [31].

Currently approved HDACS are non-specific and affect the expression of a number of cancer-related genes. Most importantly, they upregulate proapoptotic genes, including TRAIL, DR5, Bax, Bak, and APAF1, and downregulate BCL-2 [31, 46, 57]. As mentioned, HDAC inhibitors have immune-modulating features, possibly related to cytokine secretion modulation and upregulation of costimulatory molecules such as CD80 and CD86 [14, 57]. Although HDAC inhibitors have a variety of possible mechanisms leading to alteration of gene expression, it is thought that HDAC inhibitors lead to a more open chromatin configuration, which results in transcription of tumor suppressor genes.

Clinical Trials of HDAC-Inhibitors in NSCLC

Vorinostat given in combination with carboplatin and paclitaxel in a phase II study of advanced NSCLC was found to significantly improve response rate compared to carboplatin and paclitaxel alone, and there was trend toward improved survival [55]. The Wisconsin Oncology Network phase II study by Traynor et al. showed that monotherapy with vorinostat in patients with relapsed NSCLC provided significant benefit regarding time to progression; however, no objective antitumor activity was observed [69]. Panobinostat is a novel HDAC inhibitor that was recently demonstrated to sensitize *EGFR*-mutated and wild-type NSCLC cells to the antiproliferative activity of erlotinib in vitro. Furthermore, this combination enhanced the induced acetylation of histone H3 [30]. As will be described later in this review, a small phase I trial of combination therapy with panobinostat and erlotinib in patients with advanced NSCLC and head-and-neck cancer was well-tolerated but had limited clinical efficacy [29], and additional combinations of epigenetic therapies and erlotinib have also been studied with limited success. However, larger randomized controlled studies are needed to elucidate its clear benefits in erlotinib-resistant NSCLC [11].

Combination Epigenetic Therapy

Although so far targeting DNA methylation and histone acetylation alone has yielded disappointing clinical results in lung cancer patients, there is rationale for combination therapy of epigenetic drugs. While hypomethylating agents cause CpG island demethylation leading to enhanced expression of tumor suppressor genes, HDAC inhibitors lead to chromatin relaxation, which promote the expression of tumor suppressor genes [18, 37]. Targeting both processes simultaneously may result in synergism. Synergism of decitabine with the HDAC inhibitor trichostatin A (TSA) has been observed in colorectal cancer [6], while the combination of decitabine and the HDAC inhibitor phenylbutyrate resulted in synergistic therapeutic effect in lung cancer cell lines [4]. These and other studies have led to small clinical trials evaluating the combination of demethylating with HDAC therapy. Although initial trials including one with decitabine and vorinostat did not show any clinical benefit [7, 9, 40, 64], a more recent clinical trial reported by Juergens and colleagues combining azacitidine and entinostat showed several striking responses in a heavily pretreated population of patients with NSCLC. In that phase II study, 10 of 34 participants had stable disease, 1 patient had a partial response for 8 months, and another patient had a complete response [37]. This finding has demonstrated that some patients do in fact derive great clinical benefit from epigenetic therapy, but toxicity and identification of appropriate patients who benefit from therapy remains a challenge.

Epigenetic Reprogramming

Lung and other cancers are typically comprised of genomically heterogeneous populations of cells that vary in their ability to grow and respond to therapy. The phenomena of drug resistance, including resistance to certain targeted therapies, appear to be linked to tumor heterogeneity and populations of self-renewing CSCs [15]. There is accumulating evidence that epigenetic mechanisms play a critical role in mediating drug resistance in these highly tumorigenic cell populations. The concept of "epigenetic reprogramming" refers to modulating epigenetic modifications to switch drug-resistant cell populations to drug-sensitive cell populations [65]. In the study by Juergens and colleagues, four of the patients who went on to receive additional cancer therapies exhibited a major objective response, including two who survived more than 3 years after failing epigenetic therapy [37]. A phase II trial randomized patients to two different regimens of 5-AZA and entinostat with second-line chemotherapy for patients who had stable or progressive disease or second-line chemotherapy. Unfortunately, this trial was terminated early due to poor enrollment, and few patients who did enroll completed therapy for unclear reasons. As lung cancer therapy has incorporated immunotherapy and targeted therapies into a great number of patients, the effects of epigenetic reprogramming on a variety of therapies or in select groups of patients who are undergoing specific therapies needs to be examined. Moreover, identification of more selective epigenetic therapies that may result in similar improvements in treatment sensitivity without the toxicity, particularly hematologic toxicity, that is seen with DNA demethylating agents, which can limit its use alongside cytotoxic chemotherapy.

Immunotherapy and Epigenetics

Immunotherapy with monoclonal antibodies that block the PD-1/PD-L1 interactions has become an important therapy in the treatment of NSCLC and is used as first-line therapy alone or in combination with chemotherapy for most patients with metastatic or unresectable lung cancer who do not have actionable mutations [16]. PD-1 inhibits T-cell receptor signaling and is often expressed on activated CD4 and CD8+ T-cells and other immune cells. PD-1 is activated by PD-L1 and PD-L2 which are variably expressed in cancers. Lung cancer cells often express PD-L1 as an adaptive response to T-cell recognition resulting in activation of the inhibitory PD-1 receptor on T cells that have infiltrated the tumor microenvironment [62]. Although PDL-1 is the most widely used biomarker to help select responders to checkpoint inhibitors in lung cancer, other markers including tumor mutational burden (TMB) and T lymphocyte infiltration (TIL) also have a role in predicting response to immunotherapy [44].

Combination Immunotherapy and Epigenetic Therapy

Recently, the role of epigenetics in immune evasion has uncovered a role for epigenetic drugs in modulating immune cell pathways to decrease tumor evasion from the immune system. Analogous to epigenetic reprogramming, epigenetic therapies may prime the host immune response for subsequent immunotherapy [32, 63, 68]. Several preclinical studies have demonstrated the efficacy of combined epigenetic therapy and immunotherapy in a variety of cancers including hematologic malignancies, breast cancer, and melanoma [42, 45, 66, 67]. Immune priming with epigenetic therapies has been described in combination with immunotherapies other than checkpoint inhibition including adoptive cellular immunotherapy [33, 67], cytokine-based therapy [27, 42], and tumor vaccines [38]. A phase Ib/II trial of entinostat and pembrolizumab demonstrated a clinical benefit for this therapy combination. The ENCORE-601 study evaluated the combination of entinostat and pembrolizumab in patients with recurrent or metastatic NSCLC who progressed on anti-PD-1/PD-L1 therapy. Five of 57 participants enrolled had an objective partial response. Moreover, of the responders, four (80%) had PDL1 expression of less than 1%. Investigators reported that elevated baseline levels of monocytes had a significantly higher response rate than those with low levels of monocytes. It is unclear if patients with low PDL1 expression have improved response to anti-PD-1/PD-L1 up front with the addition of entinostat or other epigenetic therapy [36]. Together, these discoveries establish a highly promising basis for combination studies using epigenetic and immunotherapeutic agents in cancer patients.

Targeted Therapies and Epigenetics

Targeted therapies have markedly improved survival and reduced toxicities for patients with lung cancers that carry specific actionable genetic changes, including EGFR, EML-ALK, and ROS1 rearrangements, and less common actionable changes such as BRAF and MET mutation and RET amplification [5].

While receptor tyrosine kinases (RTK) on the cell surface are activated by ligand binding in normal cells, lung cancer cells with the mentioned genetic changes have deregulated kinase activity, amplifying the signaling produced downstream of the tyrosine kinase and creating a new physiologic state where the cells become "oncogene-addicted." Targeting the responsible oncogenic kinase drivers has proved highly successful in leading to cancer cell death. Currently, tyrosine kinase inhibitors (TKIs) are the mainstay of targeted therapies. Commonly used inhibitors include EGFR-TKIs (including osimertinib, erlotinib, afatinib, and gefitinib) and ALK-TKIs (including alectinib, ceritinib, brigatinib, and crizotinib) [5].

Unfortunately, all patients eventually develop resistance to TKIs. The mechanisms of acquired resistance to TKI therapy are still to be understood, and there are several mechanisms that are thought to be responsible. Gatekeeper mutations, including the T790 M mutation in EGFR mutant lung cancers, arise in multiple tumor types with driver mutations. Clonal populations arise most commonly during the course of treatment in which the TKI is no longer effective, but cancer cells continue to strongly depend on the kinase signaling but not with a gatekeeper mutation that has rendered the cells resistant to the TKI [72, 73]. This has led to development of next-generation TKIs that are still able to effectively block kinase activity, for example, with osimertinib and the T790 M mutation [78]. Another mechanism of resistance to TKIs is gene amplification, either changes in copy numbers of driver mutations (as seen in BRAF mutation), or amplification of alternative RTKs [10]. For example, MET amplification is observed in some patients with resistance to EGFR TKIs [17]. A variety of mechanisms of pathway reactivation have been described in BRAF, MEK, and MAPK pathways in other cancers [22, 35, 53].

It is unclear to what extent preexisting clonal populations of cells harboring changes that lead to resistance to TKIs are responsible for acquired resistance as opposed to adaptive resistance mechanisms whereby certain cell populations develop genetic changes necessary for resistance. Sharma et al. described the expansion of a reversibly gefitinib-resistant population in lung adenocarcinoma cells characterized by an altered chromatin state that requires the histone demethylase RBP2/KDM5A/Jarid1A. The drug-resistant population could be eliminated with treatment of a histone deacetylase inhibitor [61]. This finding was one of the early descriptions of the role of epigenetics in adaptive resistance to TKIs. It is becoming clear that epigenetic events may be driving TKI resistance rather than being passenger events. Moreover, the complexity of epigenetic changes and chromatin modifications that occur with drug resistance is mounting.

Chromatin writers (e.g., histone methyltransferases) and erasers (e.g., histone lysine methylases, histone deacetylases), responsible for laying down marks of modification including histone and DNA modifications, as well as chromatin readers (e.g., proteins containing chromo or bromodomains such as Brg1), responsible for recognizing marks, each are capable of contributing to adaptive resistance. While there is emerging evidence on the importance of these dynamic chromatin modifications and their effect on therapy resistance or expression of key resistance genes in other cancers, there is scant data specifically in lung cancers. Yun and colleagues recently reported that the histone 2B deubiquitinase USP22 is an important chromatin eraser whose expression is associated with therapy resistance and expression of stem cell markers in lung adenocarcinomas [75]. In breast cancer cells, the H3K36 histone methyltransferase NSD2 regulates transcription of genes downstream of the estrogen receptor and recruited by the bromodomain chromatin readers BRD3 and 4, which enhance chromatin openness and elongation via control of the P-TEFb complex through binding to acetylated histones and other chromatin-related proteins [19, 34, 41]. Along these lines, the bromodomain inhibitor JQ1 inhibited growth of tamoxifen-resistant breast cancer cells compared with sensitive cells. These effects were reported to be related to suppression of ER and MYC pathway transcription by displacement of the NSD2/BRD4 promoter complex by JQ1 in vitro [20]. This is an example of resistance to targeted therapy (in this case estrogen receptor targeted) mediated at the level of chromatin reader/writer complex.

In acute myelogenous leukemia (AML), resistance to chemotherapy is regulated in part by EZH2, a H3K27 methyltransferase and a component of the polycomb repressive complex 2. Gollner and colleagues found that in chemotherapy-resistant AML cells, EZH2 levels were lower which occurs via phosphorylation of EZH2 at T487, which leads to enhanced proteasomal degradation of EZH2 [26]. This results in expression of several genes associated with chemotherapy resistance including the drug transporter ABCC1. In addition, proteasomal inhibition with bortezomib restores EZH2 expression and resensitizes AML cells to chemotherapy. Meanwhile, lung cancer cell lines have been reported to have high EZH2 expression, and inhibition of EZH2 has been reported to sensitize lung cancer cell lines to etoposide treatment [21]. Moreover, in lung cancer cell lines, expression of SMARCA4, a critical component of chromatin-modifying complexes involved in DNA/histone interactions, is increased. This suggests that proteins involved in chromatin remodeling may be involved in the adaptive response, potentially through intrinsic helicase activity (the helicase TOP2A is targeted by etoposide) and their importance in scaffolding between HDACs and histone lysine acetyltransferases [13].

Another potential epigenetic mechanism of resistance to targeted therapies is through enhancer-mediated control of transcriptional adaptive resistance. Enhancers are DNA elements that control gene transcription at a distance. Enhancers contain transcription factor binding sites and are associated with nearby specific histone modifications. They control transcription through direct interaction or looping to interact with the promoter region of target genes. Super-enhancers are a class of regulatory regions with strong enrichment for binding of transcriptional activators, specifically Med1 and the presence of H3K27ac marks [52]. Zawistowski and colleagues reported that in triple negative breast cancer patients treated with the MEK inhibitor trametinib, BRD4-rich enhancers and super-enhancers were formed in response to drug treatment at multiple loci, including at RTK, which is known to drive resistance to trametinib in breast cancer [76]. BET bromodomain inhibition treatment in conjunction with trametinib markedly reduced enhancer formation in vitro and resulted in improved suppression of tumor growth [54]. BET inhibition with JQ1 and BRD4 knockdown have been reported to decrease lung cancer cell proliferation; however, its effects on therapy resistance, including TKI resistance, have not yet been reported in lung cancer [25].

The relationship between enhancer control and adaptive transcriptional response to drug therapy is undoubtedly complex and involves chromatin conformational changes that are just starting to be elucidated. For example, chromosome conformational changes are observed in melanoma cells with BRAF-targeted therapy as a result of looping between an enhancer region and the transcriptional start site of MET, and this is associated with therapy resistance [71]. Topologically associating domains (TADs) are chromatin regions which form megabase-scale DNA loops. TADs are bordered by CCCTC-binding factor (CTCF) and cohesin and typically span several genes [28, 43]. Other smaller regions which have similar interactions with enhancers have been identified. One example of the emerging importance of TADs in cancer therapy is the finding that IDH1 mutant gliomas exhibit enhanced methylation of CpG islands at CTCF binding sites, which may inhibit the transcriptional effects of TAD-related conformational changes. PDGFRA, a critical oncogene in glioma, is aberrantly controlled by CTCF methylation, and this was partially rescued by demethylation therapy with 5-azacytidine [23]. The role of and manipulation of these topological domains in response to therapy warrant further study to more fully comprehend the impact of epigenetic changes on adaptive transcription in response to targeted therapy.

Clinical Trials of Combination Epigenetic and Targeted Therapies

The clinical benefit of combining epigenetic therapy with targeted therapies is unknown. It is unclear which epigenetic therapies may help prevent resistance to targeted therapies and how best to select patients who may benefit. A limited number of early phase clinical trials have been conducted in lung cancer combining epigenetic therapies with targeted therapies. In a phase I trial which included 2 patients with NSCLC, Bauman et al. showed that azacitidine plus erlotinib was well tolerated. Both patients had prolonged stable disease, but it is not clear what their EGFR mutational status was (although one patient was noted to be EGFR wild type) and what prior therapies the patients received. Moreover, it is unclear whether the patients would have derived similar benefit from azacitidine alone [2].

In another phase 1 trial, the HDAC inhibitor panobinostat was combined with erlotinib in 33 patients with NSCLC and head and neck cancer. The combination was overall well tolerated and resulted in an OS of 41 in EGFR-mutated patients compared with 5.2 months in patients in EGFR wild-type patients. The responding patients were all EGFR-TKI naive. These results make it difficult to determine whether the addition of the HDAC inhibitor contributed to the degree of the response or not, but the prolonged response time warrants further study of this combination [29].

Another phase I/II study which included 33 EGFR-mutated NSCLC patients who had progressed on erlotinib treated participants with vorinostat combined with erlotinib. Although the combination was well tolerated, there was little clinical activity identified [56]. A randomized phase II trial of erlotinib in combination with entinostat versus erlotinib alone in 132 stage III and IV NSCLC patients who had failed 1 or 2 other therapies did not show a significant clinical benefit to the addition of HDAC therapy. Interestingly though, patients with high E-cadherin levels on pretreatment biopsies had longer OS with the combination treatment compared to erlotinib alone [74].

Another phase I study that included 3 NSCLC patients and a dose expansion cohort of 12 additional NSCLC studied the combination of vorinostat and sorafenib. Although there was one partial response seen, the drugs were not well tolerated due to toxicities. Moreover, participants were not selected based on specific molecular profiles and were heavily pretreated [12].

Conclusions

Epigenetic therapies hold promise to improve treatment response in a variety of cancers including lung cancer. The complex role of epigenetics in chemotherapy resistance and adaptive resistance to targeted therapies is just starting to be understood. Further study of the mechanisms by which epigenetics can be modulated to improve treatment sensitivity in lung cancer is critical to developing more specific epigenetic therapies that improve sensitivity to platinum chemotherapy and targeted therapies. In addition, identification of biomarkers that predict response is critical to developing novel epigenetic therapies.

References

1. Allis CD, Caparros M-L, Jenuwein T, Reinberg D. *Epigenetics*. Cold Spring Harbor, New York: CSH Press, Cold Spring Harbor Laboratory Press; 2015.
2. Bauman J, Verschraegen C, Belinsky S, Muller C, Rutledge T, Fekrazad M, Ravindranathan M, Lee SJ, Jones D. A phase I study of 5-azacytidine and erlotinib in advanced solid tumor malignancies. Cancer Chemother Pharmacol. 2012;69:547–54.
3. Beck B, Blanpain C. Unravelling cancer stem cell potential. Nat Rev Cancer. 2013;13:727–38.
4. Boivin AJ, Momparler LF, Hurtubise A, Momparler RL. Antineoplastic action of 5-aza-2′-deoxycytidine and phenylbutyrate on human lung carcinoma cells. Anti-Cancer Drugs. 2002;13:869–74.
5. Buffery D. Innovation tops current trends in the 2016 oncology drug pipeline. Am Health Drug Benefits. 2016;9:233–8.
6. Cameron EE, Bachman KE, Myohanen S, Herman JG, Baylin SB. Synergy of demethylation and histone deacetylase inhibition in the re-expression of genes silenced in cancer. Nat Genet. 1999;21:103–7.
7. Candelaria M, Gallardo-Rincon D, Arce C, Cetina L, Aguilar-Ponce JL, Arrieta O, Gonzalez-Fierro A, Chavez-Blanco A, de La Cruz-Hernandez E, Camargo MF, Trejo-Becerril C, Perez-Cardenas E, Perez-Plasencia C, Taja-Chayeb L, Wegman-Ostrosky T, Revilla-Vazquez A, Duenas-Gonzalez A. A phase II study of epigenetic therapy with hydralazine and magnesium valproate to overcome chemotherapy resistance in refractory solid tumors. Ann Oncol. 2007;18:1529–38.

8. Christman JK. 5-Azacytidine and 5-aza-2'-deoxycytidine as inhibitors of DNA methylation: mechanistic studies and their implications for cancer therapy. Oncogene. 2002;21:5483–95.

9. Chu BF, Karpenko MJ, Liu Z, Aimiuwu J, Villalona-Calero MA, Chan KK, Grever MR, Otterson GA. Phase I study of 5-aza-2'-deoxycytidine in combination with valproic acid in non-small-cell lung cancer. Cancer Chemother Pharmacol. 2013;71:115–21.

10. Corcoran RB, Dias-Santagata D, bergethon K, Iafrate AJ, Settleman J, Engelman JA. BRAF gene amplification can promote acquired resistance to MEK inhibitors in cancer cells harboring the BRAF V600E mutation. Sci Signal. 2010;3:ra84.

11. Damaskos C, Tomos I, Garmpis N, Karakatsani A, Dimitroulis D, Garmpi A, Spartalis E, Kampolis CF, Tsagkari E, Loukeri AA, Margonis GA, Spartalis M, Andreatos N, Schizas D, Kokkineli S, Antoniou EA, Nonni A, Tsourouflis G, Markatos K, Kontzoglou K, Kostakis A, Tomos P. Histone deacetylase inhibitors as a novel targeted therapy against non-small cell lung cancer: where are we now and what should we expect? Anticancer Res. 2018;38:37–43.

12. Dasari A, Gore L, Messersmith WA, Diab S, Jimeno A, Weekes CD, Lewis KD, Drabkin HA, Flaig TW, Camidge DR. A phase I study of sorafenib and vorinostat in patients with advanced solid tumors with expanded cohorts in renal cell carcinoma and non-small cell lung cancer. Investig New Drugs. 2013;31:115–25.

13. Direnzo J, Shang Y, Phelan M, Sif S, Myers M, Kingston R, Brown M. BRG-1 is recruited to estrogen-responsive promoters and cooperates with factors involved in histone acetylation. Mol Cell Biol. 2000;20:7541–9.

14. Dunn J, Rao S. Epigenetics and immunotherapy: the current state of play. Mol Immunol. 2017;87:227–39.

15. Easwaran H, Tsai HC, Baylin SB. Cancer epigenetics: tumor heterogeneity, plasticity of stem-like states, and drug resistance. Mol Cell. 2014;54:716–27.

16. Ellis PM, Vella ET, Ung YC. Immune checkpoint inhibitors for patients with advanced non-small-cell lung cancer: a systematic review. Clin Lung Cancer. 2017;18(444–459):e1.

17. Engelman JA, Zejnullahu K, Mitsudomi T, Song Y, Hyland C, Park JO, Lindeman N, Gale CM, Zhao X, Christensen J, Kosaka T, Holmes AJ, Rogers AM, Cappuzzo F, Mok T, Lee C, Johnson BE, Cantley LC, Janne PA. MET amplification leads to gefitinib resistance in lung cancer by activating ERBB3 signaling. Science. 2007;316:1039–43.

18. Esteller M. Cancer epigenetics for the 21st century: what's next? Genes Cancer. 2011;2:604–6.

19. Feng Q, Zhang Z, Shea MJ, Creighton CJ, Coarfa C, Hilsenbeck SG, Lanz R, He B, Wang L, Fu X, Nardone A, Song Y, Bradner J, Mitsiades N, Mitsiades CS, Osborne CK, Schiff R, O'Malley BW. An epigenomic approach to therapy for tamoxifen-resistant breast cancer. Cell Res. 2014;24:809–19.

20. Filippakopoulos P, Qi J, Picaud S, Shen Y, Smith WB, Fedorov O, Morse EM, Keates T, Hickman TT, Felletar I, Philpott M, Munro S, Mckeown MR, Wang Y, Christie AL, West N, Cameron MJ, Schwartz B, Heightman TD, La Thangue N, French CA, Wiest O, Kung AL, Knapp S, Bradner JE. Selective inhibition of BET bromodomains. Nature. 2010;468:1067–73.

21. Fillmore CM, Xu C, Desai PT, Berry JM, Rowbotham SP, Lin YJ, Zhang H, Marquez VE, Hammerman PS, Wong KK, Kim CF. EZH2 inhibition sensitizes BRG1 and EGFR mutant lung tumours to TopoII inhibitors. Nature. 2015;520:239–42.

22. Flaherty KT, Infante JR, Daud A, Gonzalez R, Kefford RF, Sosman J, Hamid O, Schuchter L, Cebon J, Ibrahim N, Kudchadkar R, Burris HA 3rd, Falchook G, Algazi A, Lewis K, Long GV, Puzanov I, Lebowitz P, Singh A, Little S, Sun P, Allred A, Ouellet D, Kim KB, Patel K, Weber J. Combined BRAF and MEK inhibition in melanoma with BRAF V600 mutations. N Engl J Med. 2012;367:1694–703.

23. Flavahan WA, Drier Y, Liau BB, Gillespie SM, Venteicher AS, Stemmer-Rachamimov AO, Suva ML, Bernstein BE. Insulator dysfunction and oncogene activation in IDH mutant gliomas. Nature. 2016;529:110–4.

24. Forde PM, Brahmer JR, Kelly RJ. New strategies in lung cancer: epigenetic therapy for non-small cell lung cancer. Clin Cancer Res. 2014;20:2244–8.

25. Gao Z, Yuan T, Zhou X, Ni P, Sun G, Li P, Cheng Z, Wang X. Targeting BRD4 proteins suppresses the growth of NSCLC through downregulation of eIF4E expression. Cancer Biol Ther. 2018;19:407–15.
26. Gollner S, Oellerich T, Agrawal-Singh S, Schenk T, Klein HU, Rohde C, Pabst C, Sauer T, Lerdrup M, Tavor S, Stolzel F, Herold S, Ehninger G, Kohler G, Pan KT, Urlaub H, Serve H, Dugas M, Spiekermann K, Vick B, Jeremias I, Berdel WE, Hansen K, Zelent A, Wickenhauser C, Muller LP, Thiede C, Muller-Tidow C. Loss of the histone methyltransferase EZH2 induces resistance to multiple drugs in acute myeloid leukemia. Nat Med. 2017;23:69–78.
27. Gollob JA, Sciambi CJ. Decitabine up-regulates S100A2 expression and synergizes with IFN-gamma to kill uveal melanoma cells. Clin Cancer Res. 2007;13:5219–25.
28. Gomez-Marin C, Tena JJ, Acemel RD, Lopez-Mayorga M, Naranjo S, de La Calle-Mustienes E, Maeso I, Beccari L, Aneas I, Vielmas E, Bovolenta P, Nobrega MA, Carvajal J, Gomez-Skarmeta JL. Evolutionary comparison reveals that diverging CTCF sites are signatures of ancestral topological associating domains borders. Proc Natl Acad Sci U S A. 2015;112:7542–7.
29. Gray JE, Haura E, Chiappori A, Tanvetyanon T, Williams CC, Pinder-Schenck M, Kish JA, Kreahling J, Lush R, Neuger A, Tetteh L, Akar A, Zhao X, Schell MJ, Bepler G, Altiok S. A phase I, pharmacokinetic, and pharmacodynamic study of panobinostat, an HDAC inhibitor, combined with erlotinib in patients with advanced aerodigestive tract tumors. Clin Cancer Res. 2014;20:1644–55.
30. Greve G, Schiffmann I, Pfeifer D, Pantic M, Schuler J, Lubbert M. The pan-HDAC inhibitor panobinostat acts as a sensitizer for erlotinib activity in EGFR-mutated and -wildtype non-small cell lung cancer cells. BMC Cancer. 2015;15:947.
31. Grunstein M. Histone acetylation in chromatin structure and transcription. Nature. 1997;389:349–52.
32. Heninger E, Krueger TE, Lang JM. Augmenting antitumor immune responses with epigenetic modifying agents. Front Immunol. 2015;6:29.
33. Ishibashi K, Kumai T, Ohkuri T, Kosaka A, Nagato T, Hirata Y, Ohara K, Oikawa K, Aoki N, Akiyama N, Sado M, Kitada M, Harabuchi Y, Celis E, Kobayashi H. Epigenetic modification augments the immunogenicity of human leukocyte antigen G serving as a tumor antigen for T cell-based immunotherapy. Oncoimmunology. 2016;5:e1169356.
34. Jang MK, Mochizuki K, Zhou M, Jeong HS, Brady JN, Ozato K. The bromodomain protein Brd4 is a positive regulatory component of P-TEFb and stimulates RNA polymerase II-dependent transcription. Mol Cell. 2005;19:523–34.
35. Johannessen CM, Boehm JS, Kim SY, Thomas SR, Wardwell L, Johnson LA, Emery CM, Stransky N, Cogdill AP, Barretina J, Caponigro G, Hieronymus H, Murray RR, Salehi-Ashtiani K, Hill DE, Vidal M, Zhao JJ, Yang X, Alkan O, Kim S, Harris JL, Wilson CJ, Myer VE, Finan PM, Root DE, Roberts TM, Golub T, Flaherty KT, Dummer R, Weber BL, Sellers WR, Schlegel R, Wargo JA, Hahn WC, Garraway LA. COT drives resistance to RAF inhibition through MAP kinase pathway reactivation. Nature. 2010;468:968–72.
36. Johnson ML, Gonzalez R, Opyrchal M, Gabrilovich D, Ordentlich P, Brouwer S, Sankoh S, Schmidt EV, Meyers ML, Agarwala SS. ENCORE 601: a phase II study of entinostat (ENT) in combination with pembrolizumab (PEMBRO) in patients with melanoma. J Clin Oncol. 2017;35:9529.
37. Juergens RA, Wrangle J, Vendetti FP, Murphy SC, Zhao M, Coleman B, Sebree R, Rodgers K, Hooker CM, Franco N, Lee B, Tsai S, Delgado IE, Rudek MA, Belinsky SA, Herman JG, Baylin SB, Brock MV, Rudin CM. Combination epigenetic therapy has efficacy in patients with refractory advanced non-small cell lung cancer. Cancer Discov. 2011;1:598–607.
38. Krishnadas DK, Shusterman S, Bai F, Diller L, Sullivan JE, Cheerva AC, George RE, Lucas KG. A phase I trial combining decitabine/dendritic cell vaccine targeting MAGE-A1, MAGE-A3 and NY-ESO-1 for children with relapsed or therapy-refractory neuroblastoma and sarcoma. Cancer Immunol Immunother. 2015;64:1251–60.

39. Levy BP, Giaccone G, Besse B, Felip E, Garassino MC, Domine GM, Garrido P, Piperdi B, Ponce-Aix S, Menezes D, Macbeth KJ, Risueno A, Slepetis R, Wu X, Fandi A, Paz-Ares L. Randomised phase 2 study of pembrolizumab plus CC-486 versus pembrolizumab plus placebo in patients with previously treated advanced non-small cell lung cancer. Eur J Cancer. 2019;108:120–8.

40. Lin J, Gilbert J, Rudek MA, Zwiebel JA, Gore S, Jiemjit A, Zhao M, Baker SD, Ambinder RF, Herman JG, Donehower RC, Carducci MA. A phase I dose-finding study of 5-azacytidine in combination with sodium phenylbutyrate in patients with refractory solid tumors. Clin Cancer Res. 2009;15:6241–9.

41. Liu W, Ma Q, Wong K, Li W, Ohgi K, Zhang J, Aggarwal A, Rosenfeld MG. Brd4 and Jmjd6-associated anti-pause enhancers in regulation of transcriptional pause release. Cell. 2013;155:1581–95.

42. Lucarini V, Buccione C, Ziccheddu G, Peschiaroli F, Sestili P, Puglisi R, Mattia G, Zanetti C, Parolini I, Bracci L, Macchia I, Rossi A, D'urso MT, Macchia D, Spada M, De Ninno A, Gerardino A, Mozetic P, Trombetta M, Rainer A, Businaro L, Schiavoni G, Mattei F. Combining Type I Interferons and 5-Aza-2′-Deoxycitidine to improve anti-tumor response against melanoma. J Invest Dermatol. 2017;137:159–69.

43. Lupianez DG, Kraft K, Heinrich V, Krawitz P, Brancati F, Klopocki E, Horn D, Kayserili H, Opitz JM, Laxova R, Santos-Simarro F, Gilbert-Dussardier B, Wittler L, Borschiwer M, Haas SA, Osterwalder M, Franke M, Timmermann B, Hecht J, Spielmann M, Visel A, Mundlos S. Disruptions of topological chromatin domains cause pathogenic rewiring of gene-enhancer interactions. Cell. 2015;161:1012–25.

44. Maleki Vareki S, Garrigos C, Duran I. Biomarkers of response to PD-1/PD-L1 inhibition. Crit Rev Oncol Hematol. 2017;116:116–24.

45. Mikyskova R, Indrova M, Vlkova V, Bieblova J, Simova J, Parackova Z, Pajtasz-Piasecka E, Rossowska J, Reinis M. DNA demethylating agent 5-azacytidine inhibits myeloid-derived suppressor cells induced by tumor growth and cyclophosphamide treatment. J Leukoc Biol. 2014;95:743–53.

46. Miyanaga A, Gemma A, Noro R, Kataoka K, Matsuda K, Nara M, Okano T, Seike M, Yoshimura A, Kawakami A, Uesaka H, Nakae H, Kudoh S. Antitumor activity of histone deacetylase inhibitors in non-small cell lung cancer cells: development of a molecular predictive model. Mol Cancer Ther. 2008;7:1923–30.

47. Momparler RL, Bouffard DY, Momparler LF, Dionne J, Belanger K, Ayoub J. Pilot phase I-II study on 5-aza-2′-deoxycytidine (Decitabine) in patients with metastatic lung cancer. Anti-Cancer Drugs. 1997;8:358–68.

48. Morgensztern D, Cobo M, Ponce Aix S, Postmus PE, Lewanski CR, Bennouna J, Fischer JR, Juan-Vidal O, Stewart DJ, Fasola G, Ardizzoni A, Bhore R, Wolfsteiner M, Talbot DC, Jin Ong T, Govindan R, On Behalf Of The Abound, L Investigators. ABOUND.2L+: a randomized phase 2 study of nanoparticle albumin-bound paclitaxel with or without CC-486 as second-line treatment for advanced nonsquamous non-small cell lung cancer (NSCLC). Cancer. 2018;124:4667–75.

49. Nguyen LV, Vanner R, Dirks P, Eaves CJ. Cancer stem cells: an evolving concept. Nat Rev Cancer. 2012;12:133–43.

50. Ozdag H, Teschendorff AE, Ahmed AA, Hyland SJ, Blenkiron C, Bobrow L, Veerakumarasivam A, Burtt G, Subkhankulova T, Arends MJ, Collins VP, Bowtell D, Kouzarides T, Brenton JD, Caldas C. Differential expression of selected histone modifier genes in human solid cancers. BMC Genomics. 2006;7:90.

51. Patel K, Dickson J, Din S, Macleod K, Jodrell D, Ramsahoye B. Targeting of 5-aza-2′-deoxycytidine residues by chromatin-associated DNMT1 induces proteasomal degradation of the free enzyme. Nucleic Acids Res. 2010;38:4313–24.

52. Pott S, Lieb JD. What are super-enhancers? Nat Genet. 2015;47:8–12.

53. Poulikakos PI, Persaud Y, Janakiraman M, Kong X, Ng C, Moriceau G, Shi H, Atefi M, Titz B, Gabay MT, Salton M, Dahlman KB, Tadi M, Wargo JA, Flaherty KT, Kelley MC, Misteli T, Chapman PB, Sosman JA, Graeber TG, Ribas A, Lo RS, Rosen N, Solit DB. RAF inhibitor resistance is mediated by dimerization of aberrantly spliced BRAF(V600E). Nature. 2011;480:387–90.

54. Prat A, Parker JS, Karginova O, Fan C, Livasy C, Herschkowitz JI, He X, Perou CM. Phenotypic and molecular characterization of the claudin-low intrinsic subtype of breast cancer. Breast Cancer Res. 2010;12:R68.

55. Ramalingam SS, Maitland ML, Frankel P, Argiris AE, Koczywas M, Gitlitz B, Thomas S, Espinoza-Delgado I, Vokes EE, Gandara DR, Belani CP. Carboplatin and paclitaxel in combination with either vorinostat or placebo for first-line therapy of advanced non-small-cell lung cancer. J Clin Oncol. 2010;28:56–62.

56. Reguart N, Rosell R, Cardenal F, Cardona AF, Isla D, Palmero R, Moran T, Rolfo C, Pallares MC, Insa A, Carcereny E, Majem M, De Castro J, Queralt C, Molina MA, Taron M. Phase I/II trial of vorinostat (SAHA) and erlotinib for non-small cell lung cancer (NSCLC) patients with epidermal growth factor receptor (EGFR) mutations after erlotinib progression. Lung Cancer. 2014;84:161–7.

57. Riggs MG, Whittaker RG, Neumann JR, Ingram VM. n-Butyrate causes histone modification in HeLa and Friend erythroleukaemia cells. Nature. 1977;268:462–4.

58. Schrump DS, Fischette MR, Nguyen DM, Zhao M, Li X, Kunst TF, Hancox A, Hong JA, Chen GA, Pishchik V, Figg WD, Murgo AJ, Steinberg SM. Phase I study of decitabine-mediated gene expression in patients with cancers involving the lungs, esophagus, or pleura. Clin Cancer Res. 2006;12:5777–85.

59. Schwartsmann G, Schunemann H, Gorini CN, Filho AF, Garbino C, Sabini G, Muse I, Dileone L, Mans DR. A phase I trial of cisplatin plus decitabine, a new DNA-hypomethylating agent, in patients with advanced solid tumors and a follow-up early phase II evaluation in patients with inoperable non-small cell lung cancer. Investig New Drugs. 2000;18:83–91.

60. Seligson DB, Horvath S, Mcbrian MA, Mah V, Yu H, Tze S, Wang Q, Chia D, Goodglick L, Kurdistani SK. Global levels of histone modifications predict prognosis in different cancers. Am J Pathol. 2009;174:1619–28.

61. Sharma SV, Lee DY, Li B, Quinlan MP, Takahashi F, Maheswaran S, Mcdermott U, Azizian N, Zou L, Fischbach MA, Wong KK, Brandstetter K, Wittner B, Ramaswamy S, Classon M, Settleman J. A chromatin-mediated reversible drug-tolerant state in cancer cell subpopulations. Cell. 2010;141:69–80.

62. Sharpe AH, Pauken KE. The diverse functions of the PD1 inhibitory pathway. Nat Rev Immunol. 2018;18:153–67.

63. Sigalotti L, Fratta E, Coral S, Maio M. Epigenetic drugs as immunomodulators for combination therapies in solid tumors. Pharmacol Ther. 2014;142:339–50.

64. Stathis A, Hotte SJ, Chen EX, Hirte HW, Oza AM, Moretto P, Webster S, Laughlin A, Stayner LA, Mcgill S, Wang L, Zhang WJ, Espinoza-Delgado I, Holleran JL, Egorin MJ, Siu LL. Phase I study of decitabine in combination with vorinostat in patients with advanced solid tumors and non-Hodgkin's lymphomas. Clin Cancer Res. 2011;17:1582–90.

65. Suva ML, Riggi N, Bernstein BE. Epigenetic reprogramming in cancer. Science. 2013;339:1567–70.

66. Tellez CS, Grimes MJ, Picchi MA, Liu Y, March TH, Reed MD, Oganesian A, Taverna P, Belinsky SA. SGI-110 and entinostat therapy reduces lung tumor burden and reprograms the epigenome. Int J Cancer. 2014;135:2223–31.

67. Terracina KP, Graham LJ, Payne KK, Manjili MH, Baek A, Damle SR, Bear HD. DNA methyltransferase inhibition increases efficacy of adoptive cellular immunotherapy of murine breast cancer. Cancer Immunol Immunother. 2016;65:1061–73.

68. Terranova-Barberio M, Thomas S, Munster PN. Epigenetic modifiers in immunotherapy: a focus on checkpoint inhibitors. Immunotherapy. 2016;8:705–19.

69. Traynor AM, Dubey S, Eickhoff JC, Kolesar JM, Schell K, Huie MS, Groteluschen DL, Marcotte SM, Hallahan CM, Weeks HR, Wilding G, Espinoza-Delgado I, Schiller JH. Vorinostat (NSC# 701852) in patients with relapsed non-small cell lung cancer: a Wisconsin Oncology Network phase II study. J Thorac Oncol. 2009;4:522–6.
70. Van Den Broeck A, Brambilla E, Moro-Sibilot D, Lantuejoul S, Brambilla C, Eymin B, Khochbin S, Gazzeri S. Loss of histone H4K20 trimethylation occurs in preneoplasia and influences prognosis of non-small cell lung cancer. Clin Cancer Res. 2008;14:7237–45.
71. Webster DE, Barajas B, Bussat RT, Yan KJ, Neela PH, Flockhart RJ, Kovalski J, Zehnder A, Khavari PA. Enhancer-targeted genome editing selectively blocks innate resistance to oncokinase inhibition. Genome Res. 2014;24:751–60.
72. Weisberg E, Manley PW, Cowan-Jacob SW, Hochhaus A, Griffin JD. Second generation inhibitors of BCR-ABL for the treatment of imatinib-resistant chronic myeloid leukaemia. Nat Rev Cancer. 2007;7:345–56.
73. Whittaker S, Kirk R, Hayward R, Zambon A, Viros A, Cantarino N, Affolter A, Nourry A, Niculescu-Duvaz D, Springer C, Marais R. Gatekeeper mutations mediate resistance to BRAF-targeted therapies. Sci Transl Med. 2010;2:35ra41.
74. Witta SE, Jotte RM, Konduri K, Neubauer MA, Spira AI, Ruxer RL, Varella-Garcia M, Bunn PA Jr, Hirsch FR. Randomized phase II trial of erlotinib with and without entinostat in patients with advanced non-small-cell lung cancer who progressed on prior chemotherapy. J Clin Oncol. 2012;30:2248–55.
75. Yun X, Zhang K, Wang J, Pangeni RP, Yang L, Bonner M, Wu J, Wang J, Nardi IK, Gao M, Raz DJ. Targeting USP22 suppresses tumorigenicity and enhances cisplatin sensitivity through ALDH1A3 downregulation in cancer-initiating cells from lung adenocarcinoma. Mol Cancer Res. 2018;16:1161–71.
76. Zawistowski JS, Bevill SM, Goulet DR, Stuhlmiller TJ, Beltran AS, Olivares-Quintero JF, Singh D, Sciaky N, Parker JS, Rashid NU, Chen X, Duncan JS, Whittle MC, Angus SP, Velarde SH, Golitz BT, He X, Santos C, Darr DB, Gallagher K, Graves LM, Perou CM, Carey LA, Earp HS, Johnson GL. Enhancer remodeling during adaptive bypass to MEK inhibition is attenuated by pharmacologic targeting of the P-TEFb complex. Cancer Discov. 2017;7:302–21.
77. Zhang K, Wang J, Tong TR, Wu X, Nelson R, Yuan YC, Reno T, Liu Z, Yun X, Kim JY, Salgia R, Raz DJ. Loss of H2B monoubiquitination is associated with poor-differentiation and enhanced malignancy of lung adenocarcinoma. Int J Cancer. 2017;141:766–77.
78. Zhou W, Ercan D, Chen L, Yun CH, Li D, Capelletti M, Cortot AB, Chirieac L, Iacob RE, Padera R, Engen JR, Wong KK, Eck MJ, Gray NS, Janne PA. Novel mutant-selective EGFR kinase inhibitors against EGFR T790M. Nature. 2009;462:1070–4.

Index

R. Salgia (ed.), *Targeted Therapies for Lung Cancer*, Current Cancer Research,
https://doi.org/10.1007/978-3-030-17832-1

Printed in the United States
By Bookmasters